FOREWORD BY ROBERT

EVERY KNOCK IS A BOOST

BOOK TWO
THE REPRODUCTIVE, PRODUCTIVE, AND REFLECTIVE YEARS

MEMOIRS OF A 20TH CENTURY PSYCHOANALYST

Melvin S. Heller, MD
WITH FONDNESS
AND BEST WISHES

Melvin S. Heller, M.D.

Every Knock Is a Boost: Book Two, The Reproductive, Productive, and Reflective Years
Memoirs of a 20th Century Psychoanalyst
All Rights Reserved.
Copyright © 2016 Melvin S. Heller, M.D.
v3.0 r1.0

Cover Image by Melvin S. Heller, M.D.
Irmgard's Azalea Gardens at our Elk River home in Maryland.

Outskirts Press, Inc.
http://www.outskirtspress.com

Paperback ISBN: 978-1-4787-6186-0
Hardback ISBN: 978-1-4787-6418-2

Outskirts Press and the "OP" logo are trademarks belonging to Outskirts Press, Inc.

PRINTED IN THE UNITED STATES OF AMERICA

Contents

Part Two: Some Things I Ponder and Believe

Acknowledgements

I MUST THANK again the same helpful persons acknowledged in Book One. They still include my two attentive sons, David and Paul Heller, their sister, Joan Heller Miller, and her husband, Ken, who have all kept me well and working hard at age ninety-three to finish these memoirs before the job finishes me. Joan and Ken's adult daughters, Cara and Julie, have previewed both oral and written parts of my story, along with their very bright brother, Jeremy, who has served as my "point man" in moving this manuscript through the publication process at Outskirts Press. I want also to thank the members of our very adept and talented Writers' Group here at our fine Quadrangle retirement facility, where they have each read sections of these memoirs and provided their feedback, suggestions, and encouragement as experienced peers and fellow writers.

The things I have written about my academic career in these memoirs are simply my own reflections of those days, and not an official history of Temple University's Unit in Law and Psychiatry. Although detailed, these recollections make no effort to record the dates, amounts, and specifics of our pioneering service contracts between Temple University and our courts and correctional facilities before the current days of "outsourcing." There is no place or room here to record our programs' staffing patterns, caseloads, payrolls, and other expenditures, including university overhead fees, all of which may still reside somewhere in Temple University's accounting and budget records for its law and medical schools from the late 1950s to the early 1990s.

What I wish to record here is that neither Professor Sam Polsky nor I (nor Professor William Traylor and I subsequently) worked alone in our efforts to provide clinical services in the public sector of forensic psychiatry. We were particularly grateful for the personal support of Deans Benjamin Boyer and Robert Bucher of Temple's Law and Medical Schools, respectively, as well as the ongoing help of Dr. O. Spurgeon English, chairman of the Department of Psychiatry. It would take many additional pages, however, to describe the individual contributions of the many faculty members, friends, lawyers, judges, psychiatric residents and forensic fellowship recipients, as well as officials of the Pennsylvania Office of Mental Health, and others who participated and helped enormously in our interdisciplinary forensic psychiatry efforts. I know that a number are now be deceased, but let me take a very deep breath at age ninety-three to acknowledge at least some of them alphabetically, but most fondly and sincerely, as follows:

Judge Edward Blake, Dr. Arthur Boxer, Judge Edward Bradley, Warden Joseph Brierley, Judge Berel Caesar, Dr. Edward Camiel, Dr. William Camp, MD, Judge Vincent Carroll, James Crawford, Alan Cristal, MD, Alan J. Davis, Sandra H. Ehrlich, MSW, Miriam Gafni, Dr. Martin Gay, Dr. Gino Grosso, Dr. Edward B. Guy, Robert Haigh, Dr. Claude B. Harms, Dr. Fred Herring III, Dr. Francis Hoffman, Dr. Janet Hoopes, Dr. Norman Jablon, Judge D. Donald Jamieson, Dr. Kenneth Kool, Dr. Lidia Kopernic, Dr. George Lasota, Dr. Elizabeth A. Lawder, Dr. David Lester, Judge Herbert Levin, Dr. Ned Levine, Dr. Al Levitt, Commissioner Ronald Marks, Dr. Paul E. McQuaid, Prof. Earl Finbar Murphy, Dr. J. Martin Myers, Ralph Phelleps, Dr. Jonas Rappeport, Judge Lisa Aversa Richette, Dr. Philip Quentin Roche, Dr. Larry Rotenberg, Dr. Robert L. Sadoff, Dr. David Sall, Dr. Sheila Scott, Dr. Alex Von Schlichten, Dr. Richard Schwartzman, Dr. Brij Sethi, and Judge Joseph Sloane.

Last, but most important of all, let me whisper a fond word of thanks to my many patients, who shall remain unnamed whether I helped them or not. For those I helped, my deepest gratitude for the professional privilege of sharing the intimate feelings, thoughts, and very personal history of a fellow human being, who taught me that my patients and I differed mainly quantitatively, and often not by that much, as we bonded slowly, successfully and dynamically in our psychotherapeutic efforts. To those that I did not help much, if at all, my deepest apologies and sincerest hopes that I did you no harm in referring you, or not referring you, to another therapist, clinic, or hospital. Having already lived for almost a full century, I have a collection of long neglected regrets that need to be processed and digested, if possible, before I depart from this life. We practice a very privileged profession in which we have much to learn.

Finally, in view of my recent need for brighter, sharper, and younger eyes pending cataract surgery and other postponed events, I have been benefited by the excellent typing and copyediting help of Katelynn Luczkow, along with the ongoing editorial suggestions of my very loyal and knowledgeable niece, Dr. Karen Heller.

Dedication

TO MY UNBORN great-grandchildren, wondering if they will ever read these pages.

Foreword
by Robert L. Sadoff, MD

I AM HONORED that my mentor and teacher has asked me to write the Foreword to his memoirs, especially the productive years in which he has made such significant contributions to medicine, psychiatry and forensic psychiatry.

The first questions I asked are: Why write one's memoirs? Who will read them? Of what value are they? Who is interested? Who is the audience for such details of one's life? Dr. Heller asked similar questions and responded that memory is important to our species and the ability to communicate history is essential for survival. His children and grandchildren have asked him to "tell his story." Fortunately, Mel Heller has a prodigious memory for details even at his advanced age and has the ability to effectively express his ideas and to impart his wisdom in his writing.

Many people would like to write their memoirs for a number of reasons but have little of interest to say except perhaps for their children and grandchildren. Most memoirs are best for family only, but I have found Dr. Heller's insights and general knowledge and wisdom to be exceptional and of value to most of us. He is not only a physician with a background in surgery, but a psychiatrist, child psychiatrist, and psychoanalyst with experience in legal matters and prison work.

After reading the history of his professional, personal, and family life, one is treated to his beliefs and thoughts based on almost a century of living, observing, teaching, and pondering. I was most impressed with the depth and breadth of his knowledge, the astuteness of his observations, and the extent of his wisdom. The final brief Chapters 25 through 31 are exceptional and reflect the genius of Mel Heller.

As his student, I was privy to his teaching skills and the significant contributions he has made to the many institutions in Pennsylvania that continue to this day. He brought psychiatry to our prison system, forensic psychiatry to our criminal justice system, and psychoanalysis to our dynamic understanding of criminal and violent behavior. I have been privileged to receive his teachings and have imparted them to my students, many of whom have taught a third generation of forensic psychiatrists who will impart Mel's teaching to the next generation, and on and on. "L'Dor Va'Dor." From generation to generation, as we say.

That is the value of Mel's memoirs that are passed on not only to his progeny, but also through his students and "grand-students". Examples of his beliefs are expressed in brief Chapters 25 through 31, the final pages that include his concepts of Truth, Justice, War, and most importantly, Mortality. He believes that mortality is what drives people to accomplish. Even Death is a Boost. Man may not be immortal, but through such memoirs as Mel has written, he achieves a legacy that will live for many generations. He has given a "Boost" to us all.

Robert L. Sadoff, M.D.
Clinical Professor of Forensic Psychiatry,
Perelman School of Medicine
University of Pennsylvania

Introduction
The Human Importance of Our Memories and Memoirs

WHY WRITE MEMOIRS? Why recollect and try to remember? It was only after I began writing and examining my own recollections that I fully grasped the importance of memory in my own development as an individual. More important, in the larger perspective of our human development as our solar system's apparently sole species with the powerful ability to record our extensive experiences and wide-ranging observations of our earthly environment and each other, I submit that it is our unique propensity to recall and record our human experiences that makes us the formidable species we have become.

What renders us so markedly different from all other species is not merely the dexterity and skill of our fingers, but our even more remarkable ability to record and share the events, thoughts, and emotional experiences of our daily lives, as well as our scientific discoveries, national histories, and cultural legacies, both oral and written. Our unique human ability to contemplate our feelings, thoughts, and experiences enables us subsequently to evaluate them, and to develop such complex cosmic speculations and scientific concepts as the relationships between time, space, and distance. As individuals, after we are gone, most of us leave behind our children and the products of our various creative efforts in life, but also, what we and others remember and communicate with each other about the events and experiences of our own and others' lives. Indeed, the importance of memory in shaping one's connections to self and others is starkly apparent in people with advanced Alzheimer's disease, in whom the profound loss of memory gradually erodes their sense of personal identity, their ability to relate to others, and their comprehension of events and experiences in their own or others' lives. Those losses are among the most tragic consequences of memory loss in advanced dementia.

Unless we are being observed and studied by some higher power or advanced species, we are apparently the sole scribes of life on this planet as we struggle to find and ponder our own significance, if any, in this barely glimpsed, endlessly vast, and still expanding universe. What we do not recall, record, and communicate with others dies with us.

That brings me back to my recollections of and reflections on what my life was about while I was here. I will be ninety-three this summer, and may not be around much longer. So, why am I writing this now? Well, arguably I've had one of the best seats in the House of Life, and a long time to look around during the twentieth century and more than a decade of the twenty-first. So, while sitting at the end of my life's long train ride, looking back from the rear windows of the caboose, I want to share what I've seen, and where I've been.

Part One
Some Things I Remember

The Ongoing Story of a Long and Lucky Life

AS INDICATED IN the Introduction to *Every Knock Is a Boost: Book One, The Developmental Years – Memoirs of a 20th Century Psychoanalyst*, my grown children and grandchildren kept asking me to tell them what life and work had been like for me when I was at their various ages during what thus far has been almost a century of very eventful and changing times, as I write these sentences today. Their words were, "Dad, tell us your story. Tell us about yourself, our grandparents and yours. What stories did your parents tell you about themselves and each other? Tell us about how you grew up, your friends, what you remember. What were some of the special things and people that made you the way you are, and that really influenced you?"

I had to find a way to frame them as a chronological narrative. That was easier said than done. After I finished Book One, which described my early development and education, like any number of working persons who might want to look back and write about their occupational lives, I needed to deal with two separate but simultaneously occurring developments: my vocational career and my family life as a husband, father, grandfather, uncle and more. Professional persons sometimes refer to their occupational efforts as their "Body of Work." In that vein, I like to think of my family life as the "Work of my Body" (and soul), a more intimate, basic, and potentially more rewarding and ongoing series of work. My so-called Body of Work has also been interesting, personally rewarding, and frequently gratifying, if not of outstanding significance. So, let me get on with my long working life following the completion of my surgical internship in 1949, where I ended Book One, and continue with my career, family, and personal setbacks and bounce backs, the inevitable knocks and boosts for which these memoirs are named.

Chapter 1
Understanding Surgery's Pyramidal System

AS ONE OF the five surgical interns who began our post-doctoral training in 1948 at Boston's Beth Israel Hospital, we found that our experience was, among other things, a very serious, if gentlemanly competition. That was because further surgical residency training was based on a pyramidal system with room for only one at the top. We were friends and companions, reliably supporting and filling in for each other in our patient care on the surgical wards, but only one of us would get to be chief surgical resident, who would get first crack at performing the most desirable, interesting, skillfully challenging, and complex procedures. Why was that? Unlike internal medicine residencies, where there is room for several stethoscopes to be placed sequentially if not simultaneously on the patient's chest, there is room for only one surgeon to be in charge at the operating table and responsible for performing the surgery.

So that was my situation when I reported in the closing days of my internship to Dr. Jacob Fine, the Beth Israel Hospital's highly regarded Chief of Surgery. He offered me a second year of training as a resident in the general surgical pyramid, where I might further prove myself in their surgical research lab. This involved performing important experimental procedures on dogs and other animals. I had done some early research on electroencephalograms (EEGs) in my senior college year, which involved recording brain waves in lab rats. But that had involved merely the pasting of tiny electrodes onto their scalps, and no surgery whatsoever.

By way of contrast, when I went down to explore the hospital's surgical lab, after one look at the sad and trusting eyes of those unfortunate canines in cages, I found the prospect of doing experimental surgery on dogs to be emotionally unattractive, to put it mildly. Of added importance, I felt I could not financially afford to prolong unduly the time when I could be working as a practicing surgeon. Like most young doctors, I was twenty-six when I graduated from medical school, twenty-seven when I finished my internship, and would be twenty-eight when I finished another year at this Beth Israel animal lab assignment. I would still have three more years to complete my basic residency requirements for the surgical specialty Board.

An Alternative Surgical Residency Appeared

Fortunately, an alternative residency prospect appeared. My cousin, Dr. Ray Yesner, about ten years older than I, was at that time chief pathologist at the Newington Veterans Administration Hospital, which had a close teaching affiliation with the nearby Yale Medical School and its Grace-New Haven Hospital. Ray asked, "Why not come down and interview with the Chief of Surgery at Yale's VA Hospital in Newington?" And so I did, and I was accepted as a surgical resident at Newington with rotations through Yale's Grace-New Haven Hospital. I found the surgical training at Newington and Yale to be comparable and every bit as good as that at Boston's Beth Israel.

Doubts About Surgery: Dropping In On A Psychiatric Case Conference

For many reasons, I began to wonder whether general surgery with all its glamour, macho prestige, and remunerative rewards was for me. I was beginning to see patients as segments of anatomy and recall them as appendices, hernias, and hemorrhoids rather than as people with medical or surgical problems, people whom I might have been privileged to know as human beings. Moreover, thinking back now, general surgery seemed to be too rushed and somehow too transient to engender doctor-patient relationships.

Many surgeons seemed not to want such relationships, and the attitude was contagious. I got the idea that maybe if I trained for a surgical sub-specialty like orthopedics, urology, or neurosurgery, I'd have more time to see and treat my patients as individuals rather than pieces or types of surgery.

Soon thereafter, while still in that somewhat discontented and questioning mood, I wandered into one of Yale's regular weekly case conferences in the Department of Psychiatry on a pleasant spring day. With my staff doctor's uniform, it was easy for me to find a seat near the back to quietly look and listen. A couple of psychiatric residents who I knew recognized me and casually nodded. Soon, a senior resident who I did not know began to present a case to the small assembled group consisting of about two dozen psychiatrists, psychologists, nurses, and social workers in the psychiatry department. Although I was a stranger in the room, several people recognized me from around the hospital. I soon felt welcome, and not at all uncomfortable.

I quickly recognized Dr. Fritz Redlich, the department chairman. Seated next to him was a well-dressed gentleman, who turned out to be Dr. Larry Kubie, a prominent psychoanalyst from New York. Dr. Kubie had been invited to discuss the case of a woman with multiple phobias that Dr. Kubie identified as neurotic fears. Although the patient recognized that her fears of driving more than a short distance from home, and especially over a bridge, were irrational, Dr. Kubie explained that she could not overcome them by any amount of willpower alone. She was a captive of an unconscious emotional conflict, which bound her like a chain or leash close to her home, Dr. Kubie explained. How strange, I thought. I was fascinated enough to talk with one of the psychiatric residents named Jack, whom I had briefly encountered a time before at the home of mutual friends.

Jack explained that Yale's Department of Psychiatry under Dr.

Redlich's recent chairmanship had become psychoanalytically-oriented in the early 1950s, but not exclusively so. He described Dr. Redlich as a very capable administrator, an "empire-builder," who had established teaching connections with some of the foremost analysts in the country. I gave the prospect of a year in psychiatry some further thought, perhaps like a semester abroad, just to explore another country or field. As time wore on, I felt inside that it was an increasingly attractive prospect.

A "Sabbatical" Year in Psychiatry?

Torn between the far more prestigious practice of surgery and the specialty of psychiatry, which was lowly regarded among most of my fellow residents and medical colleagues, I mentioned my changing thoughts and potential plans to my parents. My dear mother was aghast. Usually our Ma was very supportive of me, unless it involved such cardinal sins as gambling, smoking, or taking what she regarded as needless risks of injury by playing football. She had been quietly proud of her "son, the doctor," who had been working so diligently to become a surgeon, no less. To our Ma, the idea of my becoming a psychiatrist and delving into the messy and forbidden mysteries of mental illness and, God forbid, insanity, were causes for alarm. In desperation, she played out in full measure her maternal concerns and perceived duty to warn me from making a big mistake. When she saw that she was not getting very far, she blurted out in despair, "How can you think of working with crazy people? They'll drive you crazy!"

I thought that was both sad and funny, as though a part of my old-country Ma feared that mental illness might somehow be contagious, like working in a leper colony. I felt her love for me far more than her fear of the insane, and I reassured her that it would take a lot more than that to drive me crazy—but that I would give her words further thought. Although she was later very proud of my subsequent success as a professor of psychiatry and forensic consultant, her initial distress and words of warning about working with "crazy people" sometimes returned to mind over the years. Beginning in my late fifties, I began to suffer episodes of hearing loss. I eventually had the misfortune of losing much of my adult hearing too early, and too soon after my dear aging mother had lost some of hers, too. So, in my own subsequent elder years, when I sometimes felt her spirit within me and recalled her long-ago warning that working with "crazy people" might drive me crazy, I would whisper fondly to her, "No Ma, not crazy, but just a bit deaf, it seems."

Yale Was a Top Place to Train in Psychiatry

To be truthful, switching from my surgical training to a psychiatric residency had seemed like a most difficult prospect, but I rationalized that I could thereafter resume my surgical training none the worse for my having sampled another field. I consoled myself that I was still single, free of obligations, not yet thirty, and, therefore still "young." I told myself that a single year in psychiatry might be like an interesting "trip abroad," which would satisfy my curiosity, and perhaps enlarge my overall medical perspective. On that optimistic note, I applied for a year of residency training at Yale's prestigious department of psychiatry under Dr. Fritz Redlich's chairmanship, and I was quickly accepted.

At Yale, I spent what would turn out to be a very interesting and career-changing year with a small but very bright and stimulating group of psychiatric residents. Although both Yale and Menninger's, regarded as top psychiatric residency programs, were receptive to psychoanalytic thinking, not all of the faculty and residents, including myself, were completely sold on psychoanalysis. One of our brightest fellow residents, Daniel X. Friedman, dismissed it as no more than "an interesting theory, but clearly lacking scientific proof and methodology," as I recall his oft-repeated rebuttals some sixty years ago. Danny, a good friend, went on to become the very popular and much respected Chairman of Psychiatry at the University of Chicago.

Another holdout was Aaron T. Beck, who was a year or so ahead of me at Yale. He was well liked, and a great guy. The middle initial "T" was for "Tim", which we called him, and which seemed to match the bow ties he always wore. I eventually caught up with him several years later when I came to Philadelphia. Tim Beck went on to achieve international fame as the founder of cognitive therapy. Nevertheless, between the 1950s and 1970s, psychoanalytic thinking was in the ascendancy in American psychiatry. As my year of psychiatric training drew to a close, something more pressing than theoretical and academic arguments presented itself. The time was approaching when I would need to pay back the US Navy for its V-12 program.

I Owed the Government Two Years of Service

In the early summer of 1951, following my exploratory year of psychiatric residency and two prior years as a surgical intern and resident, I received orders to report to the US Naval Hospital at St. Albans, New York for active duty as a lieutenant, junior grade. I was thrilled at this prospect because it gave me a reprieve from making a choice between psychiatry and surgery and a chance to further contemplate my options while performing my patriotic duty and repaying my legal and moral obligation to our government. To my utter dismay, a week before I was to report in my new naval officer's uniform to St. Albans, I received a letter from the Navy that landed like a bombshell. It informed me that my orders were rescinded, that the Navy no longer would grant me a commission, and that I was free to fulfill my government obligation with another uniformed service.

An Unexpected Encounter With McCarthyism

Having no idea of why or what happened to my orders, I felt so shocked, shamed and dishonored with each passing hour that I became more furious than curious. It did not occur to me to see a lawyer, or write to my congressman. By the next morning, I was so dismayed that I tore the letter to pieces, and flushed them down the toilet, which I felt was exactly where they belonged. Through no fault of my own, I had felt knocked down, but not out, by the virus of McCarthyism that was being widely disseminated in the daily news, but which I had not realized was running so rampant.

What could have caused my problem? My father was not some secret conspirator with socialist leanings. He was a wide-open, confirmed, and full-blooded socialist who strongly believed in democracy by repeatedly voting for, and actively supporting, Norman Thomas's campaigns for the presidency of the United States. What kind of subversive threat to the United States Constitution was Norman Thomas, an ordained Presbyterian minister and a distinguished graduate of both Princeton and the Union Theological Seminary? I felt that it was McCarthyism that was un-American and radical. But in 1951, the Navy didn't know that, not until after Joseph McCarthy and Roy Cohn began accusing the Army itself of harboring secret Communists and their sympathizers in high places.

I had nothing to hide and was no secret anything. I felt how unfair and ironic it was for a patriotic son like me, who had been a proud cadet lieutenant in Captain Kelly's well-drilled Memorial High School Corps that had marched proudly down Boston's Commonwealth Avenue in their annual parade, should be smeared by McCarthyism. That boy had always been unabashedly patriotic, and remained that way thereafter. If the Navy didn't want me, it was their loss, I felt. "I'll join the Coast Guard and do just as well," I told myself.

Prize Drill at Roxbury Memorial High School

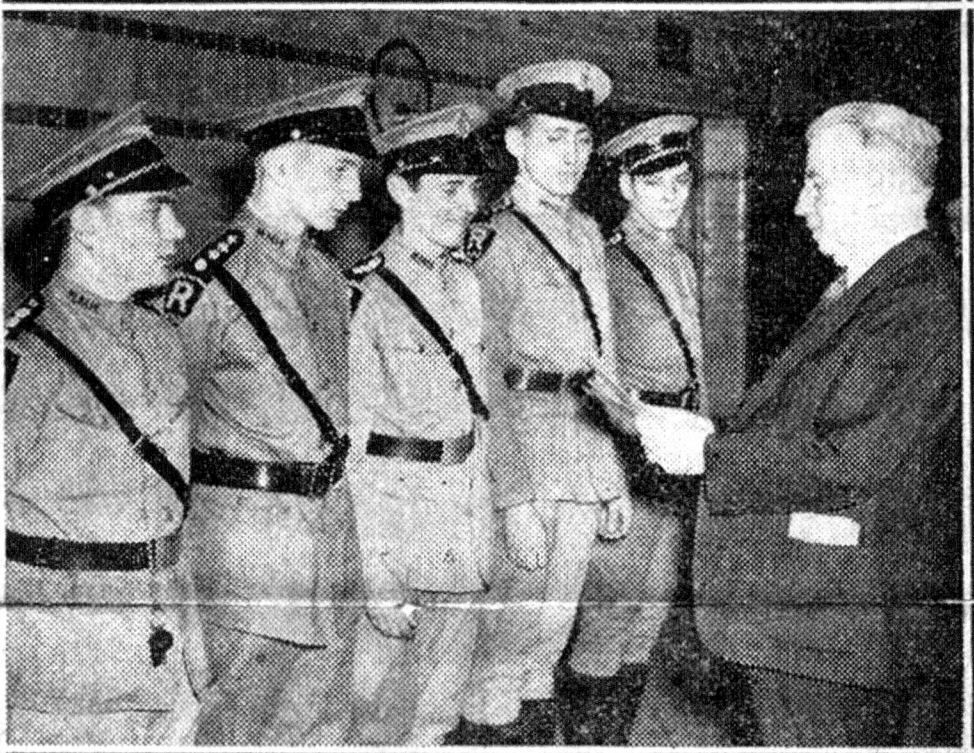

ROXBURY CADETS DRILL.

The Roxbury Memorial High School cadets drilled yesterday and the above were selected as officers of the 21st regiment. Left to right, Cadet Colonel Bernard Leibovitz, Lieutenant-Colonel Francis Kiley, Major Albert Rubin, Major Melvin Heller, Major Robert Harrison and Headmaster Robert B. Masterson.

Author (second from right) as Cadet Major in Roxbury Memorial High School student Drill Team (1939).

If Not the Navy, Why Not the Coast Guard?

So I tried to do just that, and I was told that the Coast Guard's medical services were provided by the U.S. Public Health Service. When I applied for a commission in the U.S. Public Health Service and asked them whether I would be assigned for Coast Guard service, their answer, which I remember clearly to this very day, was, "Oh yes, Doctor Heller, with your academic record, residency training, and letters of recommendation, it is practically guaranteed." Imagine how I felt when I received my commission as a Senior Assistant Surgeon in the U.S. Public Health Service with orders to report in my new uniform for duty at the Federal Penitentiary in Terra Haute, Indiana, on the banks of the Wabash River. That was as close to the water as I ever got, despite my request and deep desire for service to the Coast Guard.

To make matters worse, with two years of surgical training and only one year of psychiatric residency, I had been assigned not as a general medical officer, but to be the chief (and only) psychiatrist for an 1,100 bed, maximum security penitentiary. I must admit that the enthusiastic recruitment officer had mentioned that the U.S. Public Health Service also supplied medical services for our foreign embassies and Indian reservations, but it turned out that the U.S. Penitentiary in Terre Haute was where I landed and would be stationed for two years.

What a setback that seemed. What was it that Mother always said about every knock being a boost? What a knock this setback seemed to be. What about the boost? Little did I know that this unwanted prison assignment would turn out to be more of a boost than I could ever have imagined. It not only enlarged my perspective, but it eventually influenced a substantial part of my subsequent medical and academic career.

Chapter 2
My Early Adventures in Forensic Psychiatry

The Federal Penitentiary at Terre Haute, Indiana: Warden Joseph Overlade

WHERE SHALL I begin? Why not with the Warden? I was age thirty, still single and never suspecting how many very fine, congenial, and genuine people I would meet in Terre Haute, Indiana and rural Illinois. With neither the time nor space to go into the details here, I can list no more than a few of the many interesting staff persons I met in my work at Terre Haute, beginning with the Warden, Joseph Overlade, who was, I was told, a Mormon bishop. I had never known a Mormon before, let alone a bishop, but Warden Overlade turned out to be a very fine, civic-minded person, who, in addition to his supervisory and administrative responsibilities, took an active interest in the relationships between his prison and the surrounding community. Toward that end, he attended regular luncheon meetings of such organizations as the local Chamber of Commerce, Kiwanis, Elks, and similar groups.

Taking an interest in his penitentiary's new young psychiatrist, Warden Overlade invited me in due course to attend some of these luncheons as his guest, where I was invariably asked to say a few words about psychiatrists and prisons. Can you imagine how I felt as a novice with only one year of residency training in psychiatry and, if you would believe, the only psychiatrist in Terre Haute, a town of some 60,000 souls at the time? How quickly one learns not to flounder and sink on such occasions, but to speak up and talk confidently while swimming toward some friendly shore. In addition to such lessons in extemporaneous public speaking, I learned many additional things while working for Warden Overlade and his two associate wardens at Terre Haute.

Associate Warden Paul Madigan

Paul Madigan and Mark Richmond, the Penitentiary's two associate wardens, each added much to my new education as a prison psychiatrist. Paul Madigan was a long-experienced hand. Starting as a guard, he had worked his way up from the bottom to the top tier. Mr. Madigan was from the old school, old enough to be my father. He carried a small notebook and stubby pencil in his breast pocket, and a short, leather, lead-weighted sap or "billy club" in his back pocket, ostensibly to protect himself from unruly prisoners, but no one had ever heard of his actually needing to use it on anyone.

Paul Madigan's official title was Associate Warden, M.T. "M.T." stood for "Mass Treatment," which dealt essentially with security and safety measures. Mass Treatment trumped all other treatment programs and issues. The political strength of his role reflected society's pervasive concerns regarding prison security and the safety of nearby communities. Mentally disturbed inmates were regarded as constituting additional safety risks until proven otherwise. That overriding safety issue frequently brought Mr. Madigan to me regarding inmates whose eccentric behaviors and attitudes moved him to refer them for my psychiatric evaluation and recommendations.

I found Mr. Madigan to be a very polite gentleman, who always respectfully addressed me as "Doctor" when referring numerous mentally ill prisoners whom he had diagnosed as "dingbats," and whom I had been taught at Yale to recognize and diagnose as "schizophrenics." I soon discovered that the very experienced Mr. Madigan was better at diagnosing dingbats than I, with only a single year of psychiatry under my belt, was at recognizing schizophrenics.

Prison Was a Full-Time Job, Learning as I Went Along

There was a lot of work to be done at the Terre Haute Federal Penitentiary. My most demanding medical duty was to examine and write an annual psychiatric evaluation on each of the 1,100 prisoners' parole prospect reports. If you do the simple math, that task, along with my regular weekly "sick-call" duties, would have kept me busy seven days a week. And busy I was, but increasingly fascinated by my new work, and quite happy, too. I suddenly found myself examining, listening to, and talking with—not manifestly ill psychotics or physically impaired persons with hernias, hemorrhoids, or appendicitis—but with murderers, rapists, repeat sex offenders, substance abusers, armed robbers, burglars, and thieves of all types, who knew much more about their different kinds of dangerous and disordered lives than I did.

I soon learned that for many of the prisoners, their behavior and troubles had started far back, even before they knew which end was up, or the way out, if there ever was a way out for them. And so, for far too many of my inmate-patients, I felt that I wasn't going to make many quick cures, if any, no matter how I much I threw myself into the job. I was feeling not very hopeful and confident, but somehow very privileged to open the frequently voluminous case records of violent offenders, and begin to talk with them about their pains, pleasures, efforts, worries, frustrations, and dim prospects in their remaining, still young lives. Most of them were not yet forty, and many were much younger than that. As I was young myself, that sobering glimpse of our unequal personal circumstances and situations might well have been one of the most important single lessons I learned as a psychiatrist in my first year at Terre Haute. What if I were in their shoes and they were in mine? I had a lot more to learn and a lot of work to do.

In that regard, Warden Overlade was quick to come to my rescue. He assigned me not one, but three, inmate secretary-clerks to provide whatever help I needed in the dictation and typing of numerous case reports, filing and fetching records, answering phone calls, scheduling appointments, and so forth. Warden Overlade allowed me to interview and choose my clerks from among the general inmate population. I was able to locate three prisoners who were high school graduates with some college background and good secretarial skills in typing, filing, and record keeping.

My Inmate Clerks and Me

Being a doctor's clerk, orderly, or secretary was a very desirable job for an inmate with basic office skills. There was no shortage of applicants, and the Warden encouraged me to select as many more of those as I could use. So, by way of a further bonus for me, and an educational and vocational boost for them, I found two extra clerks who were excellent readers with good vocabularies and basic typing skills. I put them to work typing key parts of psychiatric texts and psychiatric and medical journal articles that I had brought with me for reference and my own further study. Thus, in 1951, long before continuing medical education (or C.M.E. as it is currently called) became mandatory nationally for re-licensure of doctors and other health professionals, I invented my own C.M.E. for myself in Terre Haute.

One of the books I outlined and studied was Dr. Arthur P. Noyes' textbook on psychiatry. Other books included Dr. Otto Fenichel's *Psychoanalytic Theory of Neurosis*, and several volumes of Freud's work, from which I selected sections. My home study program did me much good, especially when I took a few extra minutes to explain some of the psychoanalytic and psychiatric concepts to my frequently questioning, but increasingly interested and fascinated inmate clerk-typists.

It is repeatedly said that the best way to learn is to teach. So I learned some things about practice-teaching in my very brief, informal, after-work sessions with several eager, but tough-questioning inmate clerks, whose main scholarly qualifications were curiosity, literacy, and a newly nurtured desire to learn from books, preceded by a recurrently failed career in "criminal street smarts."

My inmate clerks and I were about the same age, and we found common masculine ground in our new relationship. I talked about things that I knew, and they talked with increasing candor about things that they knew. What I gained from these mutual learning and teaching exercises stood me in good stead as a model when I returned to complete my residency training at Yale, as well as in my subsequent career when I needed to find common ground in courts and prisons with my forensic patients, as fellow human beings locked in together on planet Earth from which none of us, man or beast, patient or doctor, criminal or cop, will get out alive.

Meet Mark Richmond, Associate Warden

In contrast to Paul Madigan, who had worked himself up from the bottom as a correctional officer to become a warden, Mark Richmond had a college background and a degree in sociology. As Associate Warden I.T., Mark was in charge of individual treatment issues. He and I designed an introductory mental health discussion course for our correctional officers. They showed enough interest for Warden Overlade to bring our in-service training initiative to the attention of the director of the Federal Bureau of Prisons, the much-respected James V. Bennett, Esq.

The Bureau of Prisons, like its more newsworthy and TV-glamorized counterpart, the FBI, reported directly to the U.S. Attorney General as equally situated agencies within the federal justice system. James V. Bennett was one of the most accomplished, brilliant, and politically astute persons I was ever to meet. He was an excellent lawyer and remarkably capable administrator, as well as a respected member of the Bar, who chaired a number of its key committees dealing with crime and corrections.

James V. Bennett's and Dr. Karl Menninger's Shared Prison Interests

On Mr. Bennett's next visit to Terre Haute, Warden Overlade introduced me, purposely I thought, to Mr. Bennett, who very kindly spent a few extra minutes with young, prison-novice-me, chatting about psychiatry and my views about our mentally ill prisoners and their needs. I was surprised to find how much interest Mr. Bennett took in mental illness. He explained that he and Dr. Karl Menninger were longstanding friends with a shared interest in mentally ill prisoners—and would I care to attend a forthcoming meeting on mentally ill prisoners at the Federal Prison Hospital in Lexington, Kentucky? I told him I would be most grateful to be invited. I don't know what else Warden Overlade might have told Mr. Bennett about me, but I soon found myself at the same table with the great Karl Menninger of the famous Menninger Clinic in Topeka, Kansas, as one of the two psychiatrists and several psychologists and penologists who would address the large group.

When it came my turn to speak, painfully knowing how inexperienced I was, especially in comparison to Dr. Menninger, who was sitting right next to me, I simply talked about my work with Terre Haute's prisoners as a newcomer that past year. Despite my understandable fears of failure with these more experienced prison experts, my talk seemed to go well. To top things off, when Dr. Menninger took the podium after me, he graciously complimented me for what he called a sincere and candid presentation, and said, "That's what we need in prison psychiatry—more newcomers. That's what this meeting is about."

Boosted by James V. Bennett, Director of Federal Bureau of Prisons

I don't know if I turned merely pink or bright red, but I was overwhelmed by his kind words. Whether or not they went to my face, I did not let them go to my head. I knew that I had been invited to speak there because of the importance of the position I held as a much needed and newly recruited prison psychiatrist, rather than for my personal importance as an individual. I was fortunate to be doing a good job at filling a position that was desperately needed. I knew that it was not me, but the need for new prison psychiatry that was so great. But how nice it could be to feel needed, and maybe a bit important for a time—how really lovely!

The next day was also unforgettably lovely on my long and leisurely drive back from Lexington to Terre Haute. I mulled over the meeting and how much I had learned there, including what an unexpected boost it actually had been for me to have been assigned to what had seemed initially like such an undesirable and unimportant medical duty as trying to serve as a psychiatrist for a maximum security penitentiary. Had I been working as a junior surgical officer at St. Albans Naval Hospital, what chance would I have had to assist or even meet with a senior surgeon who held as lofty a reputation in surgery as the famous Karl Menninger held in psychiatry? Had I remained at Yale and continued my residency training uninterrupted there, would I have shared a speaker's platform so soon, if ever, with so eminent a psychiatrist as Dr. Menninger? Even so, as I thanked what I had previously thought would be my unlucky stars, I learned that sometimes, if we take what we get and make the most of it, we can reach some very lucky stars indeed. Even on that happy day, I could not have foreseen what further good fortune would await me in the next few years.

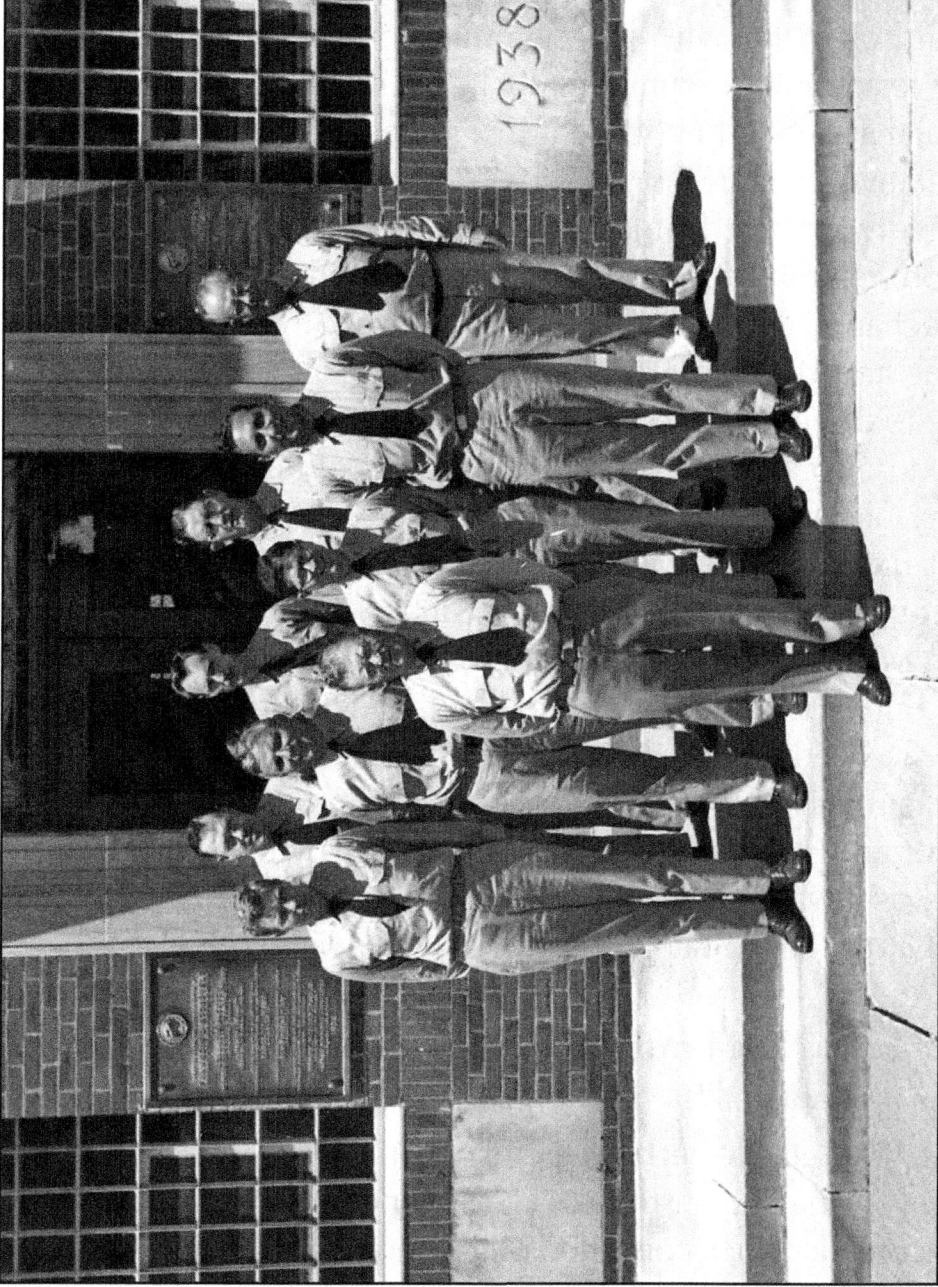

Medical Staff Federal Penitentiary, Terre Haute, Indiana. Dr. Thomas Smith, Medical Director standing in front. Author in first row, far right (1951).

My Speedy Drives to Boston from Terre Haute, Indiana

Before I take leave of Terre Haute, I must tell your how much I grew to enjoy living there as a thirty-year-old single man who, after years of living with below-minimum-wage stipends as an intern or resident in training, finally had a modest, but reasonable living wage as a U.S. Public Health Service Officer. I soon found a better, relatively luxurious, used car—a large, light blue, Olds 98 convertible with nice leather seats and a new top and tires. One of the correctional officers at the penitentiary had a brother who was a mechanic at the Olds agency. He personally checked out the car for me and kept it running fine. With that "as new" machine, I was able to drive all the way across Indiana and Ohio in one day to reach a convenient motel on the outskirts of Pittsburgh without killing myself, or getting a speeding ticket.

Up at dawn the next day, I was able to get back on the road with a couple of freshly made sandwiches, a thermos of coffee, and with one or two pit stops, and reach Boston the next day—a bit tired, but happy to see my Mom, Dad, and older brother and his family, who lived nearby in Brookline. Needless to say, my mother treated me royally, but urged me to take a train or at least a bus the next time, and stop driving so fast and so far by myself. The two-day trip was always worth the effort because it made my folks, and especially our Ma, so happy to see me.

Settling In to Terre Haute and Meeting Midwest Friends

Once I got settled in to Terre Haute, and it didn't take long for me to do that, I was glad to get back there, not only to my work, but to the new life I was making for myself. I had found a very nice apartment on the second floor of a converted private home that must have been a mansion in its day, at least judging from the huge tiled bathroom that had adjoined the master bedroom, which, with a small kitchen, comprised the rest of my apartment. The enormous master bathroom was about fifteen feet by eighteen feet in dimensions, was brightly lit, and had marvelous acoustics. So I unfolded my music stand and practiced my violin etudes there, figuring that a psychiatrist is entitled to a few eccentricities. The neighbors did not seem to object; in fact, they liked me, and one of them knew of a lady who played piano well. She had gone to Radcliffe College, where she met her husband while he was at Harvard Law School. When they married, he brought her home with him to Terre Haute, where he had grown up, and soon built a fine practice. They were about five years older than I, and often invited me as a single man to their large parties, where the wife and I would eventually play a movement or two of a Beethoven or Brahms sonata for violin and piano. They introduced me to their friends, including a few of the faculty members of the Indiana State Teachers College in Terre Haute.

Terre Haute, which had seemed like such a disappointing destination when I was assigned to duty there, turned out to be a very nice, small Midwestern city with a number of vibrant enterprises in addition to the penitentiary. The people were so welcoming and cordial that I soon began to feel much at home there. Terre Haute was also the home of the Champaign Velvet Beer Brewery. The aroma of its fermenting grain seemed often to blow eastward from the Wabash River toward the street where I lived. Terre Haute's most prominent citizen seemed to be Tony Hulman, whom I was told owned not only a controlling interest in the Champaign Velvet Beer Company, but also a major share of the famous Indianapolis Speedway. I was invited to enjoy the annual Indianapolis 500 race in choice seats made available by well-connected friends, who allegedly knew Mr. Hulman and other important Speedway folk.

A Special Friend at the State Teachers College

As a licensed physician, but a very novice psychiatrist, I was rapidly accumulating very real and practical clinical experience in psychiatry at the penitentiary. This brought me to the attention of a very nice psychology professor in the Department of Special Education at Terre Haute's State Teachers College. He asked me to give a few lectures about my work with Terre Haute's federal prisoners. I leaped at the chance to make a new academic friend at the local college, and at the same time, to please Warden Overlade by furthering his efforts at promoting good relations between the penitentiary and its surrounding community.

The psychology professor was only about six or seven years older than I, and finding common interests, it didn't take us long to become friends. He seemed as much interested in my experiences as a resident in Yale's psychiatric training program as he was in learning about my work at the prison. Liking the way I described the behavior and personality disorders, as well as the major mental illnesses I encountered in my prison work, he invited me to serve a few hours in his department, with the impressive title of Visiting Professor. In turn, I was much interested in learning about his perspective as a special education professor, since so many of our prisoners needed remedial education, vocational training, and much more.

We soon became such good friends that he invited me to join him, his wife, and their two young children on what for me was an unforgettable camping trip, with their towed trailer, to the Big Lake State Forest campground in Michigan's Upper Peninsula. There we caught, cleaned, and cooked wall-eye bass over an open campfire. It was all as new to me as my prison work had been, and in its own way, as life-changing. I would one day find a different, but equally captivating outdoor haven on our East Coast's Chesapeake shore.

A Short Love Story and Some Prior Debts

I was beginning to be enthralled by the outdoor beauty of Michigan's Upper Peninsula and Indiana's lovely Brown County, with its fine university in Bloomington. If truth be known, I could have fallen in love with Terre Haute and a number of the people who lived there, including a particularly lovely girl named Mary. Mary was a talented young pianist and a very pretty girl of twenty-two. She had been a student of the well-known composer, conductor, and pianist, Rudolph Ganz, at the Chicago Musical College. We were in love, and the temptation to marry Mary and settle down with her in Terre Haute pulled at my heart for a time. But I had other, older debts to pay—debts to mentors, family, and friends who had invested in me. How does one walk away from such debts? I couldn't.

Chapter 3
Back to Yale: More About How and Why I Chose Psychiatry

Prison Service Had Seemed a Hard Knock But Was an Unexpected Boost

LONG BEFORE I completed my unexpected and unrequested duties as the psychiatrist for Terre Haute's Federal Penitentiary, I more than forgave the Navy for canceling my orders to report for medical officer duty at St. Albans Naval Hospital. I was so grateful for how much I had learned at Terre Haute, and how well things had turned out for me, that I had soon re-developed the warm and loyal feelings I had long felt for our Navy. It had taken two years to fully realize that my severance had not been the Navy's fault. Our Navy had much more important things to do during the Korean Conflict than to take on Senator McCarthy's office on so minor a matter as questioning and blocking my pending commission as a lieutenant, junior grade.

Neither President Eisenhower nor the Navy had seemed to have the inclination or political stomach to challenge Senator McCarthy's increasingly wild and widespread search for Red spies and their sympathizers in high places. It was probably some over-zealous assistant spook in Joseph McCarthy's and Roy Cohn's office that fingered my father for openly supporting Norman Thomas's socialism, and found my name on a prospective list for commissioned officers. No one wanted to take on McCarthy's intimidating record of accusations until attorney Joseph Welch set viewers straight during Senator McCarthy's nationally televised hearings about highly placed Communist spies in the Army.

Under those nasty circumstances, the Navy itself had done

me no unnecessary harm. Instead, they had provided me with an Honorable Discharge, which listed my Naval V-12 service at Tufts College and the Chelsea Naval Hospital, as well as making note of my World War Victory Medal, my American Theater Ribbon, and Good Conduct Medal, to boot. What more could I ask of the Navy thereafter, except for the middle age chance to cheer with a beer for our team in the annual Army-Navy football game? When I got back to Yale, I was momentarily tempted to write to the Navy to thank them for allowing me "to fulfill my V-12 obligation in another uniformed service," as they had put it, but why be a sore winner and rock the boat when the knock had turned into such a boost?

Time Was Marching On

Happily back and busy at Yale, I was now looking forward to completing my third year of residency training requirements for certification by the American Board of Psychiatry and Neurology. Although I had not entirely abandoned the still lingering possibility of a surgical career, after my two years of service at Terre Haute, surgery had become a much diminished option. This was especially so since the American Board of Psychiatry and Neurology had ruled to accept my two years of practice at the penitentiary as the equivalent of a second year of residency training. Thus, when I terminated my tour of duty at Terre Haute, it appeared that I would need only one more year at Yale to complete the residency requirements for Board certification. By comparison, were I to choose to return to surgery, I would need a minimum of three additional years of surgical residencies to become Board-qualified.

I was already thirty-two and ripening on the vine. I knew, however, that ripening on the vine was much better than ripening on the ground. And the vine was academia, where Yale was welcoming me back with open arms to continue my career at what was arguably one of America's top psychiatric training programs at the time. That tipped the scale even further away from any lingering thoughts of returning to surgery.

Completing Residency Training at Yale, 1953-1954

Although the psychiatric residency training at Yale had been essentially eclectic and included clinical considerations of learning theory, operant conditioning, and behavior modification, it was psychoanalytically oriented. Psychoanalytic concepts made sense to me as a system for understanding psychoneurotic symptoms as abnormal, pathological mechanisms of defense against anxieties arising from situational and unconscious emotional conflicts. These unconscious conflicts stemmed largely, it seemed, from unacceptable erotic impulses and aggressive instincts. This new psychodynamic approach appeared both plausible and persuasive to me as a framework for what I regarded as a needed system for understanding the pathological mechanisms of symptom formation.

I was not a PhD candidate embarked on a basic science career. I was a physician in advanced specialty training as a clinician. As a clinical pursuit rather than a demonstrably provable "hard science," psychoanalysis seemed far more promising than psychological studies based on stimulus-response mechanisms. However, as an effective and widely available therapy for even the upper middle classes, not to mention the masses, I felt that "classical analysis" had paved the way, but left much to be desired as an affordable therapy. How could one know, I asked myself, if one had never tried it as a properly trained analyst? At the very least, would there not be much to be learned by studying its theories of psychoneurotic symptom formation? Accordingly, Dr. Fritz Redlich, our department chairman, invited a number of prominent psychoanalysts to provide their interpretations and insights at our clinical case conferences. They included such notables as Drs. Larry Kubie from New York;

Merton Gill, Margaret Brenman, and Robert Knight from the Austin Riggs Foundation in Stockbridge, Massachusetts; and Frieda Fromm-Reichmann from Rockville, Maryland, among others. I was fascinated by their brilliance.

Yale's Unit in Law and Psychiatry

When I returned to Yale as a senior psychiatric resident, Dr. Redlich sensed immediately that my learning experiences at Terre Haute had already made me something of an "expert" in prison work and an emerging sub-specialty, "forensic psychiatry," which dealt with common ground between law and psychiatry and the unavoidable interface between the criminal justice and mental health systems. My thousand or more clinical evaluations in comparing a variety of violent versus non-violent offenders, ranging from murderers to check forgers and confidence men, had placed me somewhat at the head of the short medical line of academically oriented physicians with recent clinical experience in evaluating criminal offenders as parole prospects. Because of my practical experiences with the Federal Bureau of Prisons at Terre Haute, I was invited to join Yale's small new interdisciplinary Unit in Law and Psychiatry, which was led by Professor Harold Lasswell of Yale's Law School and Dr. Larry Z. Friedman of the Medical School's Department of Psychiatry. I was teamed up in their Unit with a very bright, enthusiastic, and capable young Philadelphia lawyer named Lisa Aversa, who had just added a Yale Master's Degree in Law to her credentials. Dr. Redlich also encouraged me as part of my residency experience to serve as psychiatric consultant one day a week at the Connecticut State Penitentiary in nearby Wethersfield. So, life was interesting and good. It would only become even more interesting in terms of my personal life, as I was soon to discover.

My Love Life as a Single Man

I was now thirty-two years old. If these recollections are to be shared as a reasonably comprehensive, meaningful, and candid account of an adult male's life, by this time they ought to have included at least something about adult sex. So first, let me admit that my sex life was active, self-indulgent, and shall we say "illegitimate" for many years prior to my getting married at age thirty-two. It was illegitimate in the sense that one needed to obtain an official license to wed a spouse and then be lawfully entitled to have sex exclusively with that individual person. Before I married, I had tried in vain to live with that impediment to sexual fulfillment. However, as my sexual desires and instincts continued unabated during the many years of my prolonged "singlehood," like many young people before us, our generation strayed not innocently, but furtively.

I say "we" because it took a decent and willing partner to stray. Much of that sexual restraint was to disappear rapidly in the subsequent and successive eras of the contraceptive pill, computer, Internet, social websites, and the currently ubiquitous cell phone. But before all that, what I recall as my suffering singlehood in the early 1940s had extended all the way through college, medical school, my surgical internships, and my subsequent training in psychiatry—adding some twelve additional years during which I was driven to engage surreptitiously in sex without a license.

I use the term "singlehood" instead of independent "bachelorhood," which, to me at least, implies some adequate status, as well as the financial ability and availability to marry. Lacking for years the financial ability, but not the desire to support a wife and children, I was determined to obtain the best training I could find while continuing to frugally support myself during an extended period of post-doctoral study. So how did I feel about all that? Not so good.

My Circumstances and Thoughts of a Family at Age Thirty-Two

I was increasingly trained and productive professionally, but missing out on the loving and reproductive years. I loved children. Having enjoyed my own childhood, I sometimes found my adult self dreaming of a wife and children, perhaps to savor that happy time once more, not as a child but as a parent. I did not abandon my two years of training in surgery to become a run-of-the-mill psychiatrist, however. I wanted the best training I could find to become the best psychiatrist I could be. But "Art is long and Time is fleeting," as Longfellow so succinctly and poetically reminds us.

Now in my thirties, and well beyond the several wild oats that I had sown in my less bridled twenties, I was beginning to wonder if I might be rapidly approaching the first cusp of middle age. There were forebodings when I looked in the mirror. I was no longer in the shape I was in when I played varsity football. I was beginning to feel that my hair, if not my waist, was a bit thinner, and that time was marching on. My friends were marrying, and what was I doing instead of raising a family? I was completing my final year of residency training for certification by the American Board of Psychiatry and Neurology. But I was about to encounter the girl I would soon marry.

Chapter 4
Meeting My Wife and Her Family

Our Fates Unfold

IN MY LAST year of training in adult psychiatry, I passed a very pretty girl pushing an electrocardiograph (EKG) machine through a crowded corridor of Yale's Grace-New Haven Hospital. It was not exactly love at first sight, but she was very good looking, even on second sight. So, on some now forgotten pretext or other, I stopped her and we made a bit of small talk—which soon became larger, and we began dating. Her name was Jane Harris, and she had graduated from Smith College the year before with a degree in child development. Apparently for lack of something more appealing to pursue, she was taking electrocardiograms for her father, Dr. Benedict Harris, a professor of medicine and well-regarded cardiologist, who had been a Yale graduate himself. When he had finished his American training, Dr. Harris had pursued further studies in Europe with a highly regarded cardiologist, Dr. Johann Mönckeberg, famed for describing Mönckeberg's sclerosis (hardening) of the arteries.

Hardening and other blood vessels aside, I soon felt deep in my pulsing heart and adjoining aorta that I had finally found in Jane not only "my true love," but to my added amazement and amusement, that I had finally stumbled upon that proverbially "nice Jewish girl from a good family" that my mother had always hoped that I would marry. My father had no such ethnic specifications. I knew, however, that, if asked, he would have wished only that my fiancé would be sincere, stable, reliable, compassionate, capable, and basically intelligent, in roughly that order. At least unconsciously, I had apparently wanted to please my mother more than my father at the time, and since Jane's mother took to me immediately, it seemed, it did not hurt matters one bit that Jane's father was pleased by the prospect of finally adding a son to their all-female family household.

Courtship or Abandon Ship?

How sincere, cathartic, or candid can memoirs be without some "true confessions"? So let me now confess that during my lengthy bachelorhood, I had been consecutively involved in several intimate, passionate, and ongoing sexual relationships, and broken them off when matters came down to final commitment. I had felt something very akin to the deep guilt and shame of having abandoned ship, so to speak. It was a prolonged, recurrent, and punitive sense of pain. I did not want to go through that again, and would not with Jane. Enamored as I was of her, and feeling inwardly ready to marry, I had little time or cause to pause and dwell upon my father's unspoken, but well-advised checklist of preferred spousal attributes before the wedding itself came quickly to pass. Having known, as I said, a few romantic relationships before, I felt quite sure that a girl with Jane's good background and foreground would do just fine for all my marital needs and desires.

In truth, I had known and dated Jane for only a few months before I proposed and she quickly accepted. She ran upstairs from her father's den, where we had been making out at 1 a.m., to awaken and tell her parents, who came slowly down in their slippers and night robes to grant their approval and share their daughter's happiness and my momentary bewilderment at being so quickly and sincerely embraced by another family. They started almost immediately to make plans for an early June wedding, only a few months away. So, we were officially engaged.

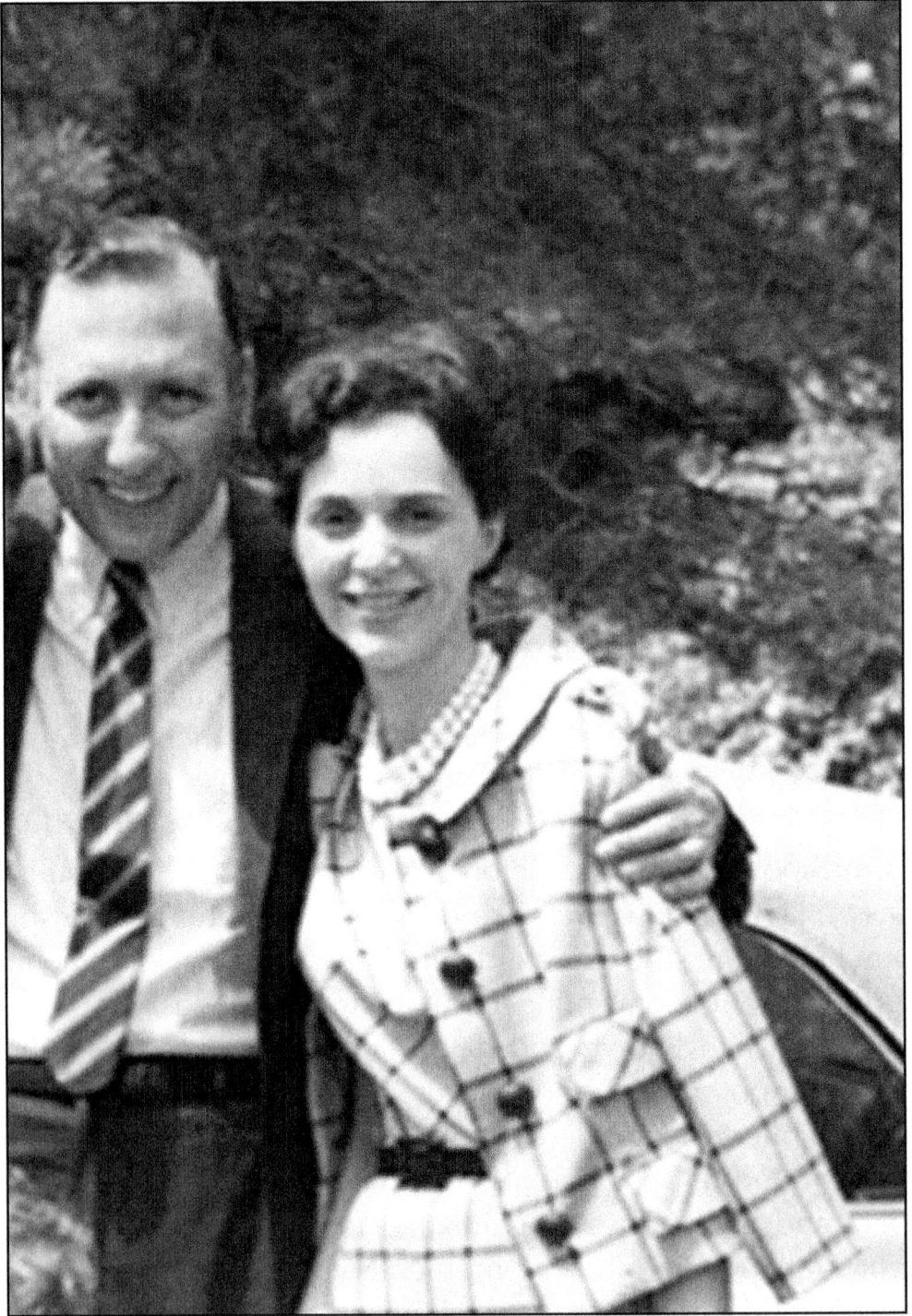

Jane Harris Heller and Author as Happy Newlyweds (1954).

As for our own plans and engagement, Jane and I had engaged only in what people called back then heavy petting or "necking," as old-fashioned and perhaps even ridiculous as that might seem to young people today. Jane had wanted and insisted that we save the grand finale, perhaps as a special late night wedding dessert, if you will, and if I would, and which we did. Not having known any wedding nights of our own before, we got to know each other in a more belated and conservative fashion rather than a prenuptial one. And so, it was only postnuptially that we found ourselves embedded and quickly enfolded in the double helix of marital life, which, in our case, was not punctuated with an initial period, but the unexpected blessing and exclamation point of an unplanned pregnancy. The new pregnancy in our new marriage suddenly confirmed that life was indeed as "real" and "earnest" as Longfellow had contended in his prayerful poem, *A Psalm of Life*.

Lacking the dramatic flair of creative script writers in such television soap operas as *Days of Our Lives*, Jane's and my personal story never made it to network television. But had it been created and cast as a TV "docudrama," its initial storyline would likely have included some of the following.

Jane's Story: A 1950s Docudrama

Jane and her younger sister, Sue, lived with their parents in a lovely suburban home. Their parents belonged to a local country club in Woodbridge, a New Haven suburb, where they provided a large and most impressive wedding party, inviting all their family and many friends, as well. As the wedding celebration went on and on, it became too late to set out from New Haven for our Washington, D.C. honeymoon destination. Almost ten years older than my young bride, I remember getting a bit tired of the tumult, and increasingly anxious to leave with my still peppy bride and get the show on the road. With growing impatience, I stood some paces away from Jane while watching her bestow farewell hugs on each of her suddenly tearful bridesmaids, as well as on seemingly dozens of very jolly, last minute well-wishers on both sides.

Sharing my concern at the hour when Jane would finally change from her wedding gown to her traveling clothes, my brand new father-in-law became my new buddy. He took me aside and said, "Son, you'll never make Washington, D.C. tonight. Let me call the Hotel Barnum in Bridgeport. It's only about a half hour away, and I'll tell them to hold a room for Dr. and Mrs. Heller, and that you'll be there some time tonight, and to charge it to me." What greater male empathy and bonding could I have wanted from my new father-in-law? With a wife and two daughters, it seemed he had waited too long for a son and pal to share his masculine perspective. At any rate and in due course, my bride arrived at the stage of changing from her lovely wedding gown into her going-away street clothes, and then finally to a choice nightgown, in which she sat herself down on the bed to begin our wonderful and unexpectedly fruitful honeymoon.

An Intimate Peek at a Dynamic and Daring Honeymoon Moment

I had assumed that Jane had discussed contraception with her gynecologist or at least with her mother. She had not. If truth be told, I had never felt sexually fulfilled with a condom. Somehow, on the first night of our honeymoon, after Rabbi Goldberg had blessed us and set us off to be fruitful and multiply, and after our guests had thrown handfuls of rice at us, wearing a condom seemed somehow counter-productive, if not sacrilegious. On the other hand, we did not throw contraceptive caution entirely to the wind because Jane had shared with me the key information that she always had regular periods and had completed her most recent period just a few days before the wedding ceremony. And so, as the critical moment arrived, we looked into each other's eyes and silently agreed, as partners in marriage, to try the rhythm method, or Vatican Roulette, at least this one time.

For those unfamiliar with Vatican Roulette, it consists of a mathematical gamble based on the female's proximity to her ovulation time, which is her most fertile phase between two menstrual periods. This method is not highly regarded for its contraceptive reliability. The moral of this brief, sexy story is that not quite nine months later, a fine, healthy, and handsome son was born to us. Let's look in on how that unexpected blessing impacted each of us so early in our marriage.

Suddenly It Was a New Ball Game With A Baby on the Way

Although her pregnancy was most assuredly a biological blessing, and a bit of a miracle as newborn infants seem to be, Jane and I were more than a bit taken aback by its timing. What had seemed initially like post-marital indigestion erroneously attributed to emotional stress was soon correctly diagnosed by an obstetrician as "first-trimester morning sickness." Having so recently returned from our brief honeymoon, and after so short a courtship in which everything had seemed so promising, the diagnosis of our unexpectedly prompt gift of pregnancy was a mixed-feeling event.

As for relatives and other people, their reactions and feelings about Jane's pregnancy depended on who the person was in relation to the bride and groom. For example, to my new mother-in-law, a dear lady named Pearl, the news that her first grandchild was on the way was an unmixed matter of joy. Let me add that Pearl Harris had always made me feel that she loved and approved of me from the time I rang their front doorbell to fetch her Jane for our first date.

My new father-in-law took a more sober view. He knew that his daughter and I would need to work a bit harder in settling down, not only to our new marital life in Philadelphia, but to our first child, due in only a few months. He kept his cool and sense of humor, however, and helped me to keep mine by kidding and calling me "Sure Shot" when we played as a twosome on the golf course. He had been trying in vain to make a decent golfer out of an athletically enthusiastic, six-foot-tall son-in-law who could hit an exuberant 300-yard drive from the tee, only to be followed by an uncontrolled second shot that lay lost somewhere in the woods far from the fairway. He, on the other hand, was a very experienced and controlled golfer, who scored regularly in the low eighties. Concentration and control were what golf and Dr. Benedict Harris were all about.

My Second Family: Good Heads and Hearts From a Different Neighborhood

Ben Harris was not only a respected cardiologist, cool gentleman, and avid golfer who could diagnose the slope of a putting green as though it were an EKG printout. He was a patient instructor in trying to make a least a decent golfer, if not a cardiologist, out of his newly polished psychiatrist son-in-law. We got along, laughed, and felt good about each other, despite his occasionally reminding me that first summer while we were still in New Haven that it was still "not too late to go back into surgery." We had much in common, but we were from different sociological neighborhoods and opposite sides of the track. Although we were both physicians with post-doctoral specialty training, I had not grown up in his circles. For example, I had never been able to get or figure out the inside story of the stock market, in which my substantially different, and quite willing father-figure delved a bit.

By contrast, my own father, who had been a teenage immigrant from Eastern Europe, was a skilled jeweler who regarded himself as a working-class craftsman or skilled "mechanic," as the best ones were called in the trade. Ironically, my father was in actual practice a business man, if only marginally successful in making money. He was, nevertheless, a capitalist in the sense that he created, built, and owned his own profit-seeking business, in which he employed and paid the weekly wages of others. He regarded the stock market as a foolish gambling game for uninformed laymen like himself, who were rounded up by tips and temptation to be regularly fleeced by investment bankers, professional lenders, big-time speculators, and other insiders, who lived lavishly on their interest, dividends, and capital gains in markets that were, in his view, notoriously subject to insider trading and manipulation. "There is no such thing as a free lunch" was the message he gave me whenever I was offered a "hot tip" by a newly encountered, investment-oriented acquaintance. In summary, my first and second father-figures, each of whom I respected and grew to love, were from different walks of life. And I still had much to learn from each of them.

We Encounter Our Newborn Son

Like my earlier prison work, which at first had seemed like such a hard and untimely knock, but had turned out to be such a large and long-term boost, our unexpected child turned out to be an even larger, long-term boost in an initially small package. From the viewpoint of our pre-marital plans and expectations, Jane and I would appear to have lost the "Vatican roulette" bets that we jointly made as we took our honeymoon spins on Mother Nature's biological wheel of fortune. However, along with her happy mother and my own mom, Jane knew deep down what winners we all were with the arrival on January 24th, 1955 of our handsome and healthy first child, whom we promptly and proudly named David Harris Heller.

It was this first child's hasty arrival that stapled us together as a new family of three, rather than other young couples, who perhaps more casually and less firmly were sampling life and each other together for a time to see how things turned out. Like many newly married couples who had not planned on being blessed so soon with a child, Jane and I did what we had to do. We compromised and adapted.

I was very busy with my studies and work, and not focused on the early details of normal infant care while pursuing my additional specialty training and credentials. I prized our infant, but was more of a bystander than an equally active participant at the beginning. Like the labor of childbirth itself, the initial price of our baby had been higher and harder on Jane than me, as she worked diligently at setting up a new home with a new husband in a new city, while heavy with our first child on the way. It was not the most auspicious start for a young bride, who had not planned on getting so very pregnant so very soon.

In marked contrast to the wooded and landscaped suburban home in Woodbridge, Connecticut from which I had plucked my bride, I ensconced us in urban West Philadelphia at 43rd and Osage Avenue. It was the cleanest affordable apartment that we could find close to the Institute of the Pennsylvania Hospital's Child Study Center, where I had previously signed on for a two-year fellowship in child psychiatry. Why had I done that?

Having completed the adult psychiatric residencies at Yale, I still did not feel that I knew anywhere near enough about the underlying causes and psychological mechanisms that make people tick. How one got to be the particular individual one became seemed to be a fundamental mystery locked away in one's genes and child development. We knew next to nothing about our individual genomes back then, and so I felt that more answers might emerge if I obtained additional training in child psychiatry. Were not the first five or six years of our long lives called the formative years? I felt the need to stay close to academia for a bit longer.

Staying Close to Teaching and Academia at The Child Study Center

If truth be told, I was at risk of becoming something of an academic bum when I decided to stay close to "teaching" for two more years at the Institute of the Pennsylvania Hospital. I also had received a fellowship offer from Philadelphia's Child Guidance Clinic, but had been very impressed by Norman Nixon, MD at the Institute of the Pennsylvania Hospital. Dr. Nixon had an interesting and extensive pre-psychiatric background as a prominent pediatrician in California, where, I am told, his pediatric patients included a number of children of film stars and prominent persons in the movie industry. Dr. Nixon became increasingly interested in pediatric psychiatry, and after additional training at the Columbia Psychoanalytic Institute, became the director of the Institute of the Pennsylvania Hospital's Child Study Center.

I liked Dr. Nixon's approach both to children and their families. Although dynamically attuned as a psychoanalyst, he retained his basic pediatric orientation as a clinician. I respected his many years of experience in treating a wide range of children from infancy through adolescence. Young children (and many adults) had little idea of what psychiatry was really about, and what it was that psychiatrists did. To a puzzled three or four year old, Dr. Nixon would explain in understandable terms that he was a "worry doctor" and that everyone had worries—and what were theirs?

Chapter 5
The Further Training of A Child Psychiatrist

Working with Children and Families

I QUICKLY FOUND that working with children was much different than working with adult patients at Yale or with inmates at Terre Haute's federal penitentiary. Psychotherapy and relating to different folks required different strokes, and one size did not fit all. Furthermore, at the Child Study Center, meetings with family members were so routine that it should have been called the Family Study Center. Another difference was that we worked not only as individual therapists, but as interdisciplinary teams assigned to each patient. In that way, the psychiatrist worked directly with the child generally in weekly sessions. A psychiatric social worker worked with the child's parents and family members, while a child psychologist performed a variety of tests and measures that assessed not only the child's cognitive functions and I.Q., but also emotional and perceptive problems elicited through so-called projective tests, using semi-structured stimuli like ink blots which, like clouds in the sky, could resemble different things to different people.

After our initial individual workups, we put our heads together to compare and discuss our findings and recommendations for a treatment plan at a meeting with Dr. Nixon or his next in command, Dr. Bob Prall. Although we sometimes disagreed in our individual assessments of our patients' prospects, as time went on and we learned to listen to each other's notes, our most successful clinical team meetings became more like string trios or quartets rather than individual solos. In listening to each other's tests and instruments instead of hearing only our own, I learned to appreciate more fully the clinical perspectives and methods of our child psychologists and psychiatric social workers as trained and valued mental health professionals. Together, we worked with dozens of individual families for the best interests of their child.

Our small, individually assigned, child psychiatric examination rooms contained our own desk and chair, a smaller chair and a play table for the child, as well as uniform, standard collections of toys and creative play therapy equipment, including an attractive assortment of large and small animal figures, trucks, various dolls, plastic soldiers, hats, bandanas, and other costumes and props, as well as play dough, crayons, clay, and drawing paper.

Play Therapy: Learning by Listening, Observing and Participating

I am not trying to teach you about child psychiatry here. I wish only to share with you some of my clinical experiences and thoughts in learning about it. During my two years of fellowship at the Child Study Center in the mid-1950s, I learned many things, including the diagnostic necessity of reviewing more than some quickly scanned routine check lists. In evaluating children and their circumstances, it was essential to obtain their complete medical records as well as developmental and psychosocial family history. That was only the beginning.

When it came to verbal communication with very young children, we could not expect them to sit and talk for forty-five minutes like grownups in ongoing weekly psychotherapy sessions. Little children related to us through play, in which they often conjured up imaginary playmates to fill assigned roles in episodes they created spontaneously right before our eyes. They did not announce it like the pre-schoolers' game that begins with "Let's play house." They played house, but it was a particular house, their own, that they wanted to play in and depict while revealing thinly disguised renditions of relationships with their parents, siblings, peers and others. A typical performance, for example, might feature a very strict mother punishing her child for such wayward behavior as hitting a little sister, or stealing cookies, or not eating all the vegetables on her plate.

I quickly recognized that it was largely through their spontaneous play that young children expressed themselves and related to each other. It followed that if I wanted them to relate to me, I sometimes needed to get down on the floor with them and participate in their play acting. In that way, and in that more leveled position, I often saw that the child's ad-libbed performance in ongoing play therapy was, if not interrupted, a frequently imitative but quite creative means of communication. It seemed that the very young children related to me through self-revealing "mini-dramas," in which the child functioned as scriptwriter, director, and stage manager at one and the same time. If I watched, listened, and sincerely played the part that the child assigned to me, I was often rewarded with helpful hints and insight into emotionally meaningful material that remained undigested in children's psyches rather than in their stomachs, so to speak. It seemed to me that apparently innocent, spontaneous play was being blithely put to use in portraying emotional struggles with a parent, teacher, or close others with whom the child had unfinished psychological business that day, week, month, or even longer.

Again, it is not my purpose in these memoirs to discuss the theories and techniques of play therapy. Here I wish merely to recall and share with you some of my clinical training years as I personally experienced them. As Shakespeare wrote in Act Two of *As You Like It*, "All the world's a stage and all the men and women merely players. They have their exits and their entrances, and one man in his time plays many parts."

Yes, many parts, large and small, I often thought as I worked in the children's clinic back then. Had Shakespeare, who saw a dramatic world through the eyes of a poet, been born in our time, he would have seen the many additional parts that little children everywhere played in their daily games, and particularly in their play therapy at Philadelphia's Child Study Center in the 1950s.

Group Therapy with Parents

During my second year at the Child Study Center, I had the opportunity to conduct group therapy sessions with fathers. This was a valuable experience in which I learned much as a group co-therapist while assisting some of our more experienced and very skilled psychiatric social workers in their weekly therapy sessions with parents. What was strongly driven home to me was the wide contrast between what the children at the Child Study Center experienced in relationships with key parental figures during their developmental years compared with the family backgrounds of the many violent offenders I had examined during my two years as a psychiatrist at Terre Haute's maximum security penitentiary.

What did the prisoners' markedly different developmental backgrounds and subsequent antisocial behaviors mean, I asked myself. What had been going on neurologically and psychologically in the brains and minds of these different sets of children as they were developing their increasing awareness of their particular circumstances, and sense of identity as individuals?

Back then, we knew even less than we do now about connections between the brain itself, the molecular physiology of our neuroendocrine systems, and the root causes of psychiatry's numerous symptoms and behavior disorders, Even today, some sixty years later, with our new visualization techniques for studying brainwaves, nerve conduction, and cell function at the molecular level, we are still in the infancy of scientific knowledge about the working relationships between the human brain and what we call our mind. Neurophysiology and molecular chemistry were not my forte, and so I felt a need to keep looking for other concepts of psychopathology. This led me to explore psychoanalysis, which was in its heyday in post-World War II America.

Embarking on Psychoanalytic Training

In the mid-1950s, psychoanalytic thinking was prominent in some highly-regarded psychiatric training programs, including those at Yale, Columbia, and the Menninger Clinic. By the time I was close to completing my final residency year at Yale, a small analytic institute was being developed at the Austin Riggs Foundation in Massachusetts, where luminaries such as Robert Knight, Erik Erickson, Merton Gill, and Margaret Brenman lived. As this institute was relatively near Yale, it seemed quite desirable. There were few openings in that early program, however, and I was disappointed not to be granted one.

I applied and was promptly accepted by the Boston Psychoanalytic Institute, but felt ambivalent about the rigidly orthodox psychoanalytic line that was allegedly pursued by them. A friendly psychologist at our Yale-affiliated Veteran's Hospital in Newington, Connecticut aimed me toward the Philadelphia Psychoanalytic Institute, and particularly toward Dr. O. Spurgeon English, a well-known training analyst who was also chairman of the Department of Psychiatry at Temple University's Medical School and Hospital.

After much pondering, and some serious debate about location, I turned down the Boston offer, and chose Philadelphia. So, shortly after arriving in Philadelphia with my new bride, I officially enrolled as a candidate at the Philadelphia Psychoanalytic Institute, and began my so-called "training analysis" with Dr. O. Spurgeon English.

Having found the psychoanalytic technique of "free association" to be interesting and easy, and remembering most of my frequently revealing dreams, I proceeded in my analysis rapidly with that gifted psychoanalytic therapist, who guided us through the paths of unconscious resistance in our psychoanalytic work together. As an instructor in psychiatry at the University of Pennsylvania Hospital, I also picked up additional psychoanalytic insights while working with a highly-regarded analyst, Dr. Leon Saul, as well as from my other training analysts, Drs. Catherine Bacon and Morris Brody, who supervised my several analytic cases required for graduation. Although skeptical about the appropriateness of lengthy classical analyses as a practical form of therapy, my concepts of psychopathology were analytically oriented. Similarly, my case management recommendations at the Child Study Center consisted of dynamic, family-oriented treatment plans tailored according to our evaluations of the child's individual circumstances, level of psycho-social development, peer relationships, clinical symptoms, and patterns of behavior.

By 1956, between the residency training years at Yale, my clinical responsibilities and experiences at the federal penitentiary, the two-year Fellowship in Child Psychiatry, and completion of psychoanalytic training at an approved Institute, I had undergone much of the best psychiatric training that one could find in the 1950s. Now it was high time to go to work and raise a family.

Chapter 6
With Our New Home and Baby, It Was Time to Get to Work

A Full-Time Job or Private Practice?

IN 1956, EIGHT years after obtaining my medical degree and six additional years of post-doctoral training, I finally opened my own office for private practice. Unlike far too many of today's medical school graduates, I was not in debt, but pretty close to broke, with a young wife and child to support. I could now command a substantial fee in the private sector and find numerous consultation jobs in the public sector. As for medico-legal work and court cases, my combined academic years of post-doctoral training and practical forensic experience justified my billing lawyers privately at hourly rates that approached their own fees to the very same clients for whom they sought my services. So, although it took a number of years, I had several things going for me when I started my private practice. I had health, an abundance of energy, good training, and a decent reputation. What more could one ask for, but a bit of continued luck?

In planning to set up my private office, who better to consult with than Dr. Nixon, our Child Study Center director, and former Beverly Hills pediatrician with a huge practice that included Hollywood families? When I asked Dr. Nixon what location he would choose if he were setting out on his own in our Philadelphia area, this very warm-hearted mentor, who had taken a liking to me, pulled out a local street map from his desk drawer, and without hesitation placed his long forefinger down precisely on Philadelphia's City Line Avenue where it crossed the Schuylkill River. Right there

46

stood the Presidential Apartments complex, with new professional offices above the lobby of the newly built Adams House.

Another Child Study Center Fellowship pal, Dr. Ted Cohen, and I were the first in line to sign up for this soon-to-be available floor space. We selected the choicest location overlooking the still green fairways that had formerly been part of the Philadelphia Country Club's golf course. Ted and I agreed to set up offices for two independent practices that would share only a common reception area. To further fill my starting schedule, I spent one day a week as consultant to the Child Therapy Program at Bryn Mawr College. In April 1956, I was appointed as an instructor in the Department of Psychiatry at the University of Pennsylvania, pursuing modest academic interests while working half a day per week in a brief psychotherapy project with Dr. Leon Saul and other analytically oriented therapists.

The bulk of my private practice time, however, was spent in my conveniently located new office close to Philadelphia's Center City and its Main Line suburbs. With a new wife and baby to support, I needed to start making money in private practice. I was soon, however, to embark unexpectedly on a lengthy academic career in forensic psychiatry, which would involve some thirty years of co-teaching third year students at Temple University's Law School, as well as psychiatric residents in our Forensic Fellowship program at Temple's Medical School. This entailed my increasing interest and work in the public sector and the criminal justice system, with its prosecutors, judges, defense lawyers, probation officers, and others laboring in the unavoidable and challenging interface that confronts both the criminal justice and mental health systems in courts, prisons, and mental health clinics.

Before going on to describe that development in my so-called "body of work" and professional career, let me look back at the development of something more important, personal, and intimate—the "work of my body" in providing a home and parental attention for my new family. I remember it starting out with a baby carriage, but of course there was much more.

Beginning Our New Family Life in Philadelphia

Newlywed in June, and leaving Connecticut with our unplanned but eagerly awaited baby well on the way, and a new job awaiting me that September in Philadelphia, a city to which we were strangers, both Jane and I desperately needed to rent a place for ourselves. I still recall the sweltering heat and humidity of late August when my pregnant wife and I climbed up numerous enclosed stairways of look-alike Philadelphia row houses. Little good it did for us to try to heed the advice of our Connecticut friends to relax and not sweat it. Until we found an affordable place to rent, there was no way not to sweat our mid-August apartment hunting in West Philadelphia.

There is a saying in real estate that location is everything. In our case we found an affordable apartment at 43rd and Osage Avenue, just a few minutes from the Institute of the Pennsylvania Hospital's Child Study Center at 48th and Market Street in West Philadelphia. With our expected child, I could not be far off when Jane went into labor. And when she did, we were no longer alone. For a short time, even while getting things ready for the child, it had been Jane and me—until baby made three. It was not that there was such a crowd, but that our little place became so quickly crowded with an infant's seemingly essential care equipment, from diapers and talcum powder to bassinet and baby carriage, that there seemed little room to turn around. And immediately, or even sooner if possible, we were subject to unquestionably entitled and especially welcome visitors.

At age sixty-two, Grandma Freda Heller traveled all alone from Boston to West Philadelphia to be welcomed into our clean, crowded, and humble home, where she exercised her right to inspect her "dear little grandson" David from top to bottom, and to hold him in her arms while pronouncing him to be no less than a "Prince." She quickly explained that Grandpa Herbert was equally thrilled, but could not leave the shop, which was short on help. After being held off by Jane until the following week, her own mother, Grandma Pearl Harris, arrived. She was beside herself with the joy of her first grandchild. David's infant-care equipment, baby presents of cute clothes and the like, had been many, but his personal presence soon swelled to occupy even more than physical space in our new lives.

Watching Our First-Born Eat, Sleep, and Grow

Like most new parents, Jane and I quickly learned together that babies required and regularly occupied much more of our time than space. That was important, realizing anew that time was all we really had, if you got right down to the transient gift of mortal life on Earth. It was simply a bit of time, not physical matter or space that mattered. Miraculous as Nature's breath-taking beauty and physical matter seems to be, we cannot take it with us. With enough planning and patience, however, we discovered that limited space could often be managed, but that when it came to time, our infant's need for a 3 a.m. breast or bottle, like Nature's tides themselves, waited for no woman or man.

Jane and I soon learned that infant care involved not only lots of time, but a lot of extra work, distractions, and sometimes anxiety when unexpected things happened or expected things failed to occur as scheduled in the text or advice books. Several times I needed to consult my old 1943 medical school pediatrics textbook to check a newly appeared rash, while Jane looked for 4 a.m. guidance in Dr. Spock's handbook for perplexed mothers. Only if it was still necessary later in the day did we call the pediatrician. Nevertheless, although it sometimes seemed to have started out that way, our Osage Avenue apartment was not all work and no play.

Infant Dave at Play

David, like most healthy babies, was cute, sweet, and fascinating. When he was not fulfilling his primary duties to eat, drink, eliminate, and sleep, he spent much of his more peaceful time at play and what sometimes seemed like contemplation. We surrounded him with squeeze toys that chirped, as well as colorful mobiles and pinwheels that hung from the ceiling above his crib. His favorite toys, however, were his own fingers and toes, as well as his mouth and mine, which he wanted to probe with his fingers as though to compare and eventually discover, for example, which was his nose and which was mine. He figured it out in time, but as a baby he still retained an uninvited, hands-on, and sometimes drooling interest in my special things, like my favorite neckties, new leather brief case, and his new Mom.

When he began to talk a lot between the ages of one and two, I eventually told little David that his Mom was my wife and that I had seen her first. He simply giggled. He apparently regarded that statement as ridiculous since he had obviously known her far longer than I had—indeed for his entire lifetime. I couldn't argue with him about that, so I let our little miracle win his point. I enjoyed rocking him to sleep while crooning softly through my repertoire of such gentle old tunes as "Coming Through The Rye" or "Just a Song at Twilight," or one of my own Ma's all-time favorites, Irving Berlin's 1927 "Russian Lullaby." So we three got to know each other, in our own special ways, those first two years on Osage Avenue.

Our First Home Sweet Home and Mortgage at Wynnefield Heights

Even before my Child Study Center fellowship was over, Jane and I both knew that we needed more room, and soon. So I was not surprised when one Friday evening Jane said, "Mel, I hear they are building some neat row houses in a new section called Wynnefield Heights. The girls tell me they are very nice. Can we take a look at them this Sunday?" She knew that Saturdays were busy and crowded days for scheduling my weekly therapy appointments for school-age children, whose mothers did not want them to miss classes. So, we made an appointment to go through the sample house right after brunch on Sunday.

Jane suggested that I pack David's stroller in the car just in case he got cranky while we were trying to concentrate on the salesperson's answers to our questions as first-time home buyers. And little David would have endless questions of his own that had nothing to do with buying a house. We had recently gotten him through that most stubborn stage of babyhood known by some parents as "the terrible two's." Actually, David's terrible two's had not been that bad, but he could still make a first-class fuss when he needed to.

Accordingly, while we were waiting out front for our salesperson to show us through the furnished sample house, I quietly gave my wife a message somewhat as follows: "Jane, you are the wife, and you will understandably have many more questions about practical homemaker details than I will. I want you to take all the time you need to ask questions about all the things you want to know about, like the floors, the walls, the laundry, the kitchen appliances— everything. Visualize placement of furniture. Don't let anyone rush you. If the three of us go into the sample house together, after a few minutes, Dave will be climbing on the furniture and wanting to touch everything.

"So here's my idea. I need to take a fast look, but there are only a few essential things I need to ask about now to know if we can make a deal. All I need are maybe ten or twenty minutes at the most to know the basics. So, let me go in first. If the place seems right for us, I'll tell the salesperson that as far as I'm concerned, we have a deal. And Jane, I won't say that unless I think it's really the right place and the right move for us at this time. Then you go in and take all the time you need to decide if this is the place for us to live until we get rich, if ever. And while you're doing that, I will walk or stroller David out back and around the block to get the lay of the land and a sidewalk view of the neighborhood."

Jane smiled and nodded her agreement to the plan, as the salesperson arrived to show us through the house.

Our Parental Assessments of the Wynnefield Heights Row House

The front door of the sample house opened onto a vinyl-floored foyer about four-feet deep and six-feet wide containing a small bench and an umbrella stand. Four steps down led to a full basement with utility room, which held a ducted, hot-air heating system to which could be added central air conditioning. The one-car basement garage and a separate back door led to the outside and rear roadway behind the houses. The remainder of the huge basement could be finished to provide additional living or work space.

Four steps up from the small foyer was a large all-purpose living room. A small powder room and coat closet were at one end. At the opposite end, a dining area was narrowed by an adjoining well-planned kitchen area. Large windows at both ends of the house admitted adequate daylight. One flight up were three bedrooms and a full bathroom with tub and curtain-rod enclosed shower, ideal for scrubbing little children and pets. If one wished to have an "end" row house, its extra open wall at the end of a row contained additional windows that would provide more light and some cross ventilation. It could also, however, add the cost of higher heating and cooling utility bills.

I quickly concluded that this was a brand-new, well-designed, and seemingly well-built house, with family expansion possibilities, in a conveniently located and safe neighborhood, and likely worth its $20,000 base price. So, after my fifteen-minute tour, I said to Jane, "The basic house looks fine to me. If you really like it, and it fits with your plans and measurements as the homemaker, it's our chance right now to pick the best one that's still available today." Jane agreed, and took her measuring tape and personal list of prepared questions in with her to collect details.

As little David and I waited outside, I had been keeping a dutiful eye on him. He was at a talkative stage but seemed, for a change, to have run out of questions about why leaves were green or the sky was blue, and could we not stop for ice cream on the way home? Then I realized that my little son was paying me no attention. That was because his sharp eyes were focused across the street on a crouched cat whose attention was fixed on a seemingly blithe squirrel that had moved tantalizingly, in fits and starts, halfway up a nearby tree. The cat crouched silently while the squirrel hung motionless out an overhanging branch for maybe ten full minutes. With high drama and jeopardy in the offing, Dave let out a whoop and a holler when the squirrel jumped to a neighboring rooftop for a neat getaway. While David was still re-enacting the exciting story of the nimble squirrel and the hungry cat, the salesperson and Jane emerged after her almost thirty-minute tour.

Jane had a smile for me, as well as answers to all the questions she had posed. She said, "I really like it, Mel. It takes care of all our needs until we see what the future brings. Let's buy it." So we quickly returned to the sales office to make our selection before the rest of the best were snapped up. With a large step up from Osage Avenue, we soon moved into the first mortgaged home of our own.

The Real Reason We Bought Our New Row House

There were many good reasons why we bought our new row house in Wynnefield Heights. But the underlying and real reason we bought that house was to make room for another child. Why were we so sure we wanted that? Jane and I had each grown up with a sibling. She had a younger sister with whom she was close, and I had an older brother whom I admired, imitated, and learned so much from when I was little. I knew how good it was to have had an older buddy while growing up. Jane felt similarly grateful that she was not an only child. So, once David was born, a second child seemed inevitable.

It Was Meant to Be

I was there in the delivery room when our daughter was born because the obstetrician was a good friend and colleague of mine. When he invited me into the delivery room, I quickly accepted. Given the chance, instead of worrying in the waiting room, I wanted to be right there with my wife when our new baby was born. It was not a matter of medical curiosity, because as a fourth-year medical student, I had delivered close to thirty babies during our rotation through obstetrics at Boston City Hospital.

Why the birth of my daughter was so emotional for me is because our mom was the only female in our immediate small family. I remembered sometimes thinking when I was a boy how nice it would have been if our Ma had given birth to a daughter like herself, and a sister I might have gotten to know while growing up as children together.

When we introduced his new little sister to David, who would be three in a few weeks, he seemed less than impressed. Recognizing that his reaction was par for the course, I reassured him that it would all work itself out in good time. We named the new baby Joan Elizabeth, so I had a Jane and Joan when we brought her home. She was a calm and easy baby, who soon become the cutest little girl with curly blond hair. When the children were little, and my schedule allowed, I loved spending a few minutes with them before leaving for the office. After a good night's sleep, Joan seemed very cheerful, bright-eyed, wide awake, and pretty. Many little children are, but at age two, her innocent charm often swept me off my feet. For example, I came upon her one day while she was sitting on her toilet training seat pretending to read out loud to her favorite rag doll stories she knew by heart from her favorite picture book, which she held open with both hands while addressing the doll she had perched on her lap. Need I confess that she stole Daddy's heart? What could Jane and I do about that but count our blessings, get to work, and get out to meet our neighbors, whose kids would be our kids' playmates.

Birds of a Feather

We soon made the acquaintance of a number of couples with whom we shared the blessings and problems of rearing similarly aged children. Although we didn't realize it, we had formed a mutual support group without a leader. The mothers were at it all week long. On Sundays, new fathers identified each other as birds of a feather and bonded together while pushing their new offspring in carriages or strollers along the recently poured sidewalks of our newly created neighborhood.

As homeowners, most of us were fully mortgaged and some were further in hock. However, the husbands were each employed with steady jobs, or a nascent enterprise of their own, like a new dry cleaning business. In the post-WWII decade of the 1950s, we were the fortunate young Americans. The Great Depression of the 1930s was behind us. We had been spared, and survived the 20th century's worldwide, homicidal horrors in its barbaric practice of "total warfare," not only against the enemy's armed forces but against its civilians of all ages hunkered down in the basements and bomb shelters of London, Warsaw, or Dresden, or worse yet, in the unknowing, ordinary course of daily life in Hiroshima, suddenly obliterated by a nuclear bomb.

How soon we twenty-five, thirty, and forty-year-olds forgot that it had been only our good fortune to be in the right place at the right time that had spared us. As young fathers, we each were trying to succeed in our own way, and to be able to afford the reasonable things that extra money could buy. Few of us realized that we already had everything that we needed except spare cash or capital. As for capital or equity, our similar, cheek-by-jowl row houses were the first homes that we owned, subject to the mortgage. They were hardly residential yachts, but ensconced in them, we felt we were getting ahead and traveling far above steerage class. Grateful for all that, but young and ambitious, we hoped that these first homes were stepping stones in a path that would grow to further strengthen our families' futures. In short, it was a time to find our relative place in the order of things, to compare, to plan, and to hope.

Defining Ourselves in Comparison to Each Other

In that regard, our similarly situated wives were eager to know each other. It sometimes seemed that the main reason for this friendliness was to find out more about themselves in comparison to what they learned about their neighbors' circumstances and prospects. How else could I explain their curiosity and furtive practice of gossip about their neighbors at that very busy stage of homemaking, with bills overdue, hungry young children to feed, and equally urgent young husbands to satisfy? And yet with all that domestic business pressing hard upon them, it seemed that few could resist the temptation and relief of sharing a few "strictly confidential" minutes of gossip time about their neighbors.

And so, while searching to find out more about who they were and where they stood, our wives grew and learned about themselves by secretly comparing their children, their husbands, their home furnishings, their hair-do's, wardrobes, personal cosmetics, and even their latest undergarments. Sometimes, to our consternation, they told us, their husbands, about where they felt they stood in comparison to others, if only to prod us into keeping up with the Joneses next door or the Goldbergs down the street.

As a newly practicing psychiatrist who respected the powers of unconscious motivation in understanding human nature, I took the long view about gossip, speculating that things must have been the same in Biblical or even in prehistoric times with women and men comparing their family's caves, tents, and best robes with those of their neighbors. I felt that maybe we husbands were not that different, except that we didn't talk about each other that much, if at all. But perhaps we, too, needed close and mutually supportive relationships, and a few additional friendships.

Maintaining Family Ties While Making New Friends in Pennsylvania

Back home, in contrast to in-law jokes, once Jane and I were committed to each other, I felt that our respective parents, hers and mine, were an unspoken part of our marriage agreement. This core family did not spread out to include distant cousins twice removed and far off somewhere, but for each of us, it did include Jane's sister, Sue, and my brother, Saul, as intentionally and emotionally "adopted" siblings by marriage. Moreover, now that Jane and I were not merely a legally designated married couple, but a biologically extended family of four, I knew and appreciated that our little David and Joan were as deeply bonded blood relatives of Jane's parents and sister as they were of my own parents and brother. Although the four grandparents had little in common by way of similar backgrounds, neighborhoods, socio-economic circumstances, formal education, or occupations, they were now an extended family linked by the destinies of their children and grandchildren.

We were raised to believe very conscientiously in the basic decency of maintaining respectful relationships with our parents on both sides. We frequently visited Jane's folks in New Haven, often making the trip from Philadelphia in little more than four hours of mostly highway driving. Laden with David and Joan's small child equipment, we had wonderful holiday-weekend visits joined by Jane's sister, Sue. In due course, Sue's new boyfriend, Harold Baer, Jr., whom we all liked, was a frequent and welcome addition to the family dinners. Harold was completing Yale Law School. He was raised as an only child in New York, where his father was a judge, and his mother was a highly regarded social worker. In addition to Jane's family, I still had a number of medical friends with whom I had trained at Yale, including Don Alderman and my cousin, Ray Yesner, and his wife, Bunny. All these ties were important to me, as Jane's New Haven friends were to her. So, we looked forward to our frequent Connecticut visits.

Accessing Boston was a little more difficult and less frequent, but my parents did come down from time to time, and we maintained frequent contact by telephone and letter. So, what I'm recalling and underscoring here is that I had grown up in a home where maintaining family contacts was very important. It was also an ethnic kind of tradition frequently seen among first-generation Americans, who maintained close contacts not only with their own immediate families, but also with relatives in the old country, be it Italy, Ireland, Greece, Poland, or wherever people could send mail. But all this took extra time. Extra time was a luxury of which I would be in short supply for a number of years, because, in addition to my increasingly busy private practice, my career took a most fortunate and definitive jump with an unexpected phone call.

Chapter 7
Co-Founding Temple's Unit in Law and Psychiatry

IN 1956, ABOUT a year after I completed my Child Psychiatry Fellowship and training analysis at the Philadephia Psychoanalytic Institute, Dr. English's secretary from Temple University phoned me and said that he would like me to meet a young professor named Samuel Polsky, LLB, PhD, from Temple's Law School. We met in Dr. English's office where Sam Polsky and I hit it off almost immediately. Dr. English explained that Dean Bucher of Temple's Medical School and Dean Boyer of Temple's Law School wanted to establish an Institute of Law and the Health Sciences at Temple, beginning with a Unit in Law and Psychiatry.

Sam quickly came to the point and told me what he already knew, that Dr. English and Dean Boyer thought that Sam and I would be highly qualified to embark on this initial interdisciplinary effort as the co-directors of Temple's Unit in Law and Psychiatry. I was flattered and more than thrilled, namely because Sam Polsky and I seemed to be cut from the same cloth. Professor Polsky was a brilliant young lawyer with a full-time, tenured faculty position as Associate Professor at Temple Law School, and he insisted that I call him Sam.

A Bit About Sam

Sam Polsky was a warm and wonderful guy, and this was more important to me than his impressive credentials. About two years older than I, he and I hit it off particularly well, each in need of a brother about our own age, as well as a close colleague. Even our modest backgrounds as first-generation Americans were mutually comforting and compatible. Growing up over his Ma and Pa's grocery store in Philadelphia's Strawberry Mansion district, Sam got scholarships to Harvard Law School, where he excelled both academically and in debating. This was followed by a Rockefeller Fellowship at the University of Edinburgh in Scotland, where he obtained his PhD in Legal Medicine. Sam had started his academic career teaching at Tulane Law School, but he and his wife, Doris, soon had more children than could be comfortably maintained with Tulane's salary. Temple offered him substantially more, and so he had made that switch to Temple Law School. When I met him two years later, he and his wife, Doris, were comfortable citizens of Philadelphia, where they had purchased a large old home in the Germantown area for their five young children.

Why am I telling you all this about Sam? Because he became my very best friend, as he and I went on to share our young and prime-time adult energies while working so well together. He was an unusually impressive, serious-minded, and scholarly person—and yet, beneath it all, a very down-to-earth and regular guy. We ended up collaborating professionally and academically for more than twenty years while becoming closest friends. During our time together, we succeeded in building the best interdisciplinary training facility in Law and Psychiatry in the area.

Working as Co-Directors of Temple's Unit in Law and Psychiatry

Although we had the blessings and backing of our two deans, they had no money to stake us. Sam started the ball rolling by getting our new Law and Psychiatry program a $3,000 grant from the Legal Aid Society of Philadelphia, provided that we matched it. We were then able to convince the Mental Health Association of Southern Pennsylvania to provide the matching grant. So, with that $6,000 and some friendly persuasion, we were able to hire an enthusiastic, bright, and polite young secretary named Pat, who was amenable to working diligently and closely with many of our eligible law students. Her official duties were to answer the phone, greet law students and others who came to inquire about our newly established Unit in Law and Psychiatry, watch the shop, reply to routine correspondence, and keep track of our appointments. Pat was invaluable as the only person on our initial payroll, since Sam Polsky was already salaried as a full-time faculty member of Temple's Law School.

As for me, having long observed the politics, mandatory assignments, and committee meetings of medical academia during my numerous post-graduate years as a house officer in teaching hospitals, I preferred a clinical academic career that provided the freedom of a part-time private practice. Therefore, I opted for a half-time, clinical faculty appointment with private practice privileges rather than a full-time faculty position. In Sam's and my work together, we shared with one another the basic concepts and essence of our respective professions, and in doing so, became each other's private tutors and prize students. Here are some of the ways we proceeded.

Interview Studies: Joint Areas for Lawyers and Psychiatrists to Co-Investigate

Small as their much appreciated dollar amounts had been, the Legal Aid Society and the Mental Health Association of Southern Pennsylvania did not provide us with matching grants in order for us to hire a secretary. That item was not what we had specifically applied for. Rather, we had sent them an attractive and unique interdisciplinary research proposal for a comparative study of the initial fact-gathering office or bedside interviews used by lawyers and doctors when focusing in on the presenting problem of their clients or patients. With this obligation in mind, we boldly undertook our three-year Temple study of the legal interview.

Our study was an all-volunteer enterprise that relied on the generosity of many law students, psychiatric residents, faculty colleagues, and nearby friends in our legal and medical professions. Our first volunteer was Esther Polen, BS, LLB, LLM, a fine lawyer and friend of Sam's. She was not only a most capable colleague, but well-situated to volunteer her time generously since she and her husband owned a successful automobile agency. Esther took on a major role in this project. She frequently worked on an almost full-time basis helping us to coordinate the part-time efforts of the many others who volunteered their professional skills to compare legal and psychiatric interviewing methods and procedures. The project's supporters included Deans Benjamin Boyer and Robert Bucher of the law and medical schools, respectively; Dr. O. Spurgeon English, chairman of the Department of Psychiatry, and Robert D. Abrahams, chief counsel of the Philadelphia Legal Aid Society, among others too numerous to list here. We subsequently presented our findings at the annual meeting of the National Legal Aid and Defender Association, which they published in a forty-two-page, 1960 monograph entitled *An Introduction to Legal Interviewing* by M.S. Heller, E. Polen and S. Polsky.

Co-Teaching Our New Course in Law and Psychiatry

It did not take Sam and me long to get our signals straight as new co-directors. After sharing some initial planning thoughts, in addition to our Legal Interview Study, we immediately started on our new, co-taught course, which was listed in the 1957 Law School Bulletin Boards and subsequent law school catalogs as "Law and Psychiatry." This was an elective course for third-year law students, scheduled for late afternoons so that both evening and day students could attend. Because it was primarily a law school course to which a few of our psychiatric residents also were invited to audit, Sam and I agreed that he would take the lead in planning the class schedule and curriculum. Besides that, both relatively speaking and in actual fact, Sam knew much more about the general concepts of psychiatry and clinical psychology than I did about jurisprudence, the details of legal proceedings, and the guiding principles of case law in legal education.

The Social Significance of Teaching Lawyers

Years before, when I was considering a shift from pursuing further surgical training to a career in psychiatry, my father had asked me point blank: "Melvin, is psychiatry socially significant?" Many times in the ensuing years, that question had reverberated in me. Now, as I contemplated the wonderful opportunity to co-teach a full semester's course in Law and Psychiatry, I could answer my father with a resounding "Yes!"

To begin with, lawyers seemed influential in our society beyond their numbers. When I looked at the make-up of our many community and civic organizations as well as local governments, lawyers seemed to be pretty influential in comparison to public school teachers, college professors, and medical doctors, for example. From our law schools would emerge our future judges, and a large percentage of state legislators, corporate lawyers, business executives, and other influential movers and shakers of our communities. Thus, teaching soon-to-be attorneys the applicable aspects of what I had learned as a clinical psychiatrist would constitute a worthwhile portion of my professional efforts, especially while they were still a reachable and motivated group of students amenable to new ideas.

As for new ideas, after two years of examining more than one thousand maximum security inmates at Terre Haute's penitentiary, I had learned something about the psychopathology of violent offenders as well as the important social challenges, responsibilities, and workings of the huge Federal Bureau of Prisons under the capable direction of James V. Bennett. When subsequently working in 1954 as a senior psychiatric resident with Dr. Lawrence Z. Friedman at

Yale's newly formed Unit in Law and Psychiatry, I was exposed to the ideas of the eminent law professor, Harold D. Lasswell, and others. With these experiences, my view of the importance of the legal profession changed and grew. It seemed to me that working with lawyers and acquainting them with our clinical concepts of mental disorders seemed highly important if we wanted to help many of our patients, particularly persons with behavior disorders encountered in the so-called public sector of psychiatry involving community and state treatment facilities. To whom better than third-year law students could I teach the practical and pertinent parts of what I had learned as a clinician about human behavior, forensic psychiatry, and child development?

With all that in mind, I could answer my dear father's question that had long reverberated in me: "Yes, Dad. Psychiatry is socially significant, especially if one can teach it to law students, an increasing percentage of whom are female these days, by the way." Did I actually believe all that during my years of co-teaching law students? I didn't dwell on it daily, but to have any chance of really loving one's work, as I did most of the time, one had to believe in something.

Teaching Law Students Trained to be Debaters in an Adversary System

In preparing for hearings and courtroom appearances, lawyers gather the facts of a case from their underlying perspective that case law evolved in an adversary system of debate concerning what are the relevant facts. With respect to debated facts, we doctors and lawyers are not that far apart. As a dear friend and colleague Sam Polsky used to say, "At the forefront and cutting edge of science and medicine, distinguished doctors and scientists argue vigorously on behalf of their opposing theories, practices, and procedures." Nevertheless, given our different professional orientations, in each semester's new class, I needed to lay out a bit of common ground between psychiatry and the law for our students before walking them through the names, clinical descriptions, and basic concepts regarding the various mental disorders.

Many of our law students had taken college courses in psychology and social studies. A number of them were somewhat familiar with and openly skeptical about psychoanalytic theory. I was determined to avoid doing battle with these future tigers of adversary courtroom debate. It seemed that some of them were already smiling patiently and politely, while inwardly licking their chops in anticipation of devouring another "alienist," or stranger to the court, as psychiatrists were quaintly called in former times.

Accordingly, I began carefully by stressing that for only a few mental disorders did we have precise notions of their specific causes or etiology, as we usually had with bacterial infections, for example. At the same time, I needed to indicate that psychiatrists dealt with clinical facts and direct observations. Those introductory lectures usually stimulated lively discussion among the class, Dr. Polsky, and myself, which is what we were hoping would happen. Although I did not read from prepared pages, I gave those lectures to our law students so many times that I can remember most of them almost verbatim, as in the following recollected sample.

Sample Portions of Classroom Sessions with Our Law Students

"Let us talk a bit about the practice of psychiatry. In the practice of medicine and psychiatry, as in the practice of law, we deal with both facts and opinions. It sometimes seems that our psychiatric opinions far outnumber our facts, but that is not so. We plan in this course to familiarize you with some of our many facts, and with the ways we obtain and deal with them clinically. In real life and actual practice, we deal with and evaluate three types of clinical facts. These include objective signs like needle tracks in substance abusers; subjective symptoms like alleged headaches, worries, or fears; and an abundance of tests and laboratory findings such as blood studies, x-rays, and complex imaging techniques as well as special studies like electroencephalograms for epilepsy.

"Let's start with signs," I suggested. "Clinical signs such as a characteristic rash in measles, syphilis, or acne are objective facts. Unlike subjective symptoms that are reported or alleged by the patient, clinical signs are directly observable, objective facts. Psychiatrists, like other physicians, are trained to note and describe such observable and characteristic signs as the presence of lethargy, somnolence, agitation, tremors, or disorientation in certain mental disorders. An almost complete lack of manifest emotion, called a 'flat affect,' can often be an alerting and specific diagnostic sign in schizophrenia," I added.

The class seemed to grant me that sometimes psychiatrists dealt with objective, observable facts, but they were anxious to get on with the major mental illnesses that raised key legal questions and issues of competency or exculpatory insanity at the time of an act. Sam, too, seemed eager to move on to our discussion of these classical, long-standing legal issues. I agreed, and why not? After all, it was a well-attended law school elective course that included small numbers of our psychiatric residents each year. So, we moved on in subsequent class sessions to some of the major issues at the intersection of law and psychiatry.

Involuntary Treatment vs. Patients' Rights to Believe as They Wish

Who but a third-year law student would unexpectedly begin our discussion of delusions by asking about the difference between forcefully treating an involuntary patient's delusions and an attack on a U.S. citizen's constitutional rights to think and believe as he or she wished? I should not have been surprised or taken aback by that question. After a moment's pause, however, I replied that persistent delusions and recurrent hallucinations were not manifestations of free thought, but clinical signs of significant disruption of a person's reality-testing ability that were regarded as evidence of the major mental disorders that psychiatrists labeled as psychoses. To illustrate, I described certain overly suspicious, conspiracy-minded patients who were constantly on guard against their paranoid delusions of persecution. I further explained that such paranoid persons are frequently convinced that they are being plotted against, manipulated, and personally endangered by powerful agents or forces that are acting against them through such secret means as thought control or abnormal radio waves.

Delusional systems, I explained, are irrational thoughts that are clinically regarded as rigidly defended false beliefs to which the person clings tenaciously despite all evidence to the contrary. Paranoid delusions of being persecuted on the one hand, or being selected to act as God's personal representative on the other, often have a sinister quality in the adversarial context of the criminal justice system's courtrooms, as well as in clinicians' offices and hospital emergency departments.

Other Hard Issues for the Criminal Justice and Mental Health Systems

Law students sometimes asked such questions as how and when it might ever be possible for the criminal justice and mental health systems to learn to deal with violent offenders or dangerous sexual predators and know when, if ever, it would be safe to release them from maximal security settings with a "reasonable degree of medical certainty." Others raised similar concerns and questions about how to balance a defendant's or an involuntarily committed patient's rights to representation in due process hearings against the safety needs of the community at large. Thoughtful and difficult questions such as these sometimes produced prolonged moments of heavy silence in the class. One of those that I still recall was relieved by loud laughter when one clever student asked humorously if any of these questions to which we had arrived at no satisfactory answers would be included in their final exam.

Good students raising good questions often learned from and taught one another during our classroom discussions. It has been often said that the best way to learn is to teach. Co-teaching with Sam and learning certain things with our students was what we did together for almost twenty consecutive and very privileged years. Our Law and Psychiatry curriculum, however, was not unstructured nor unguided. In the course of their regular assignments, our students were presented with an essential number of long-standing forensic issues to consider academically, as well as for such practical purposes as passing their state Bar examinations. Law schools paid attention to the latter because one of the factors on which our schools were somehow scored was on how well students did on their Bar exams. We sought to prepare them as best we could, sometimes with anticipated Bar exam questions in mind. Few forensic questions were more predictable or "classical" than those concerning mental competency, the M'Naghten Rules, and the so-called Insanity Defense.

Exculpatory insanity and the M'Naghten Rules seemed to be one of Sam Polsky's favorite subjects, and among the very best lectures that he gave to our law school class each semester. I never tired of hearing him on the subject. Some years, it seemed that Sam could hardly wait for me to finish my brief descriptions of the delusions and hallucinations encountered in the various psychotic disorders so that he could then launch into his ensuing discussion of the insanity defense, or exculpatory insanity, as it is termed in criminal law.

Chapter 8
Crime, Exculpatory Insanity, and the M'Naghten Rules

IF YOU ARE not interested in the popular genre of crime and punishment stories, then maybe pick up and read a library or paperback copy of Fyodor Dostoyevsky's classic novel entitled *Crime and Punishment* to get started. However, if you happen already to be interested in crime, punishment, mental illness and the frequently introduced insanity defense, here is the low-down on the M'Naghten Rules for determining exculpatory insanity. Just what is exculpatory insanity and why is it regarded as so important in the law? Well to be brief, it may provide the difference between being found guilty or not guilty. In capital punishment cases, it can make the difference between life and death. Here is what you should know, not necessarily as personal victims of violent crime, but as concerned citizens and potential jurors.

Exculpatory insanity is not a medical diagnosis, but a legal finding that a defendant is without blame and not guilty when a judge or jury decides that the defendant, at the specific time of the crime, suffered from a mental illness or defect that resulted in his or her inability to understand the "nature and quality" of the act and know it was wrong, or could not control his or her actions even though the defendant could plan and carry out the act. This concept and variations of it have provided the basic definitions of exculpatory insanity put by American judges to lay juries, mental health experts, and lawyers in adversary debates and court proceedings since the M'Naghten case in 1843.

Sam Polsky had a scholarly grasp of the development of Anglo-American law pertaining to exculpatory insanity. He had a way of discussing the M'Naghten case almost as though he had been there himself to witness the proceedings. The following is a synopsis of my recollections of how he described it to our Law and Psychiatry course in the 1950s.

The Insanity Defense, M'Naghten, and Sam Polsky

The M'Naghten rules derived from an 1843 British case in which the defendant, a paranoid Scottish carpenter and woodworker named Daniel M'Naghten (pronounced and sometimes spelled "McNaughton") was convinced that his many misfortunes in life were due to an evil plot perpetrated against him by no less an adversary than Sir Robert Peel, the British prime minister. Accordingly, M'Naghten felt obliged to terminate his persecution by shooting Sir Robert. Unfortunately for the prime minister's secretary, Edward Drummond, whom M'Naghten mistook for the prime minister himself, it was actually Drummond that M'Naghten shot and killed instead of Sir Robert Peel.

As for evidence of M'Naghten's state of mind at the time of his bungled attempt to murder Robert Peel, Sam pointed out that the M'Naghten jury had heard numerous fact witnesses testify about the nature of Daniel M'Naghten's mentally ill behavior, leading him to be found "not guilty by reason of insanity." Sam went on to relate that Queen Victoria's displeasure at the news of this verdict was of such concern to the House of Lords that they directed the M'Naghten court to re-examine its proceedings and formulate proper instructions or tests by which juries might find a person not guilty by reason of insanity.

Sam went on to relate that the 1843 court, under considerable pressure no doubt, came up with the concepts and wording that established the M'Naghten Rules for a finding of exculpatory insanity. Thereafter, in most jurisdictions, when mental health experts were requested to testify regarding mental illness in an insanity defense case, they were specifically required by the court to answer whether or not the defendant's mental impairments were such that he or she did not know "the nature and quality" of his or her unlawful act, or if they were unable to resist and control it. Not important to you? The M'Naghten Rules themselves were never satisfactory or that important to me either. What was and has remained very important to me as a child psychiatrist was whether or not a young child should be held legally responsible for his or her harmful behavior, and at what age that exception should kick in, especially in capital cases involving life and death.

What To Do About The M'Naghten Rules

I was always unhappy with the M'Naghten test, not only when testifying as an opinion witness in an exculpatory insanity case, but also as a teacher of mental health law. How could one determine the defendant's knowledge of the "nature and quality" of his or her acts at the time of the crime?

Some judges seemed to require that in order to be found insane, defendants needed to have been so mentally impaired at the time of the crime that they did not know that what they held in their hand was actually a loaded gun, and not a sweet potato, for example.

That was the way the questions sometimes went in the 1950s, when psychiatric testimony could be limited to answering such a purely cognitive question as, "Doctor, did the defendant know it was a gun and that a bullet would be discharged if the trigger were pulled?" If the answer was in the affirmative, then at least the judge seemed quite satisfied that the defendant knew the nature and quality of their act and said, "Thank you Doctor. That will be all." However, getting juries to understand what was required for them to find a defendant to be not merely mentally disordered, but legally insane, was the ongoing difficulty that courts encountered with the M'Naghten rules.

I remember discussing these problems with Sam as we tried to compare and align our individual perspectives on the insanity defense as lawyer and doctor working together on our lectures. Our conversation went something like this: I said, "Sam, the legal concept of 'not guilty by reason of insanity' is not the problem. That is a matter of law and jurisprudence, which is not my field, but something is wrong with the M'Naghten case and its exculpatory insanity rules. Something is missing. How can we find out?"

"Study it," Sam said. That rang a bell.

"But how, where, and when?" I asked.

Sam had given some thought to it. He came up with the idea that we could do an interdisciplinary research study, an exploratory review by university lawyers and psychiatrists of our federal insanity procedures in order to identify existing problems and potential remedies. Teaching and research went hand in hand, he reasoned. Of course, I agreed with him, but how could we get a practical handle on this right now, I asked? Sam replied that since we had already done a reasonably successful interdisciplinary study on the legal interview and presented our findings and recommendations at the annual meeting of the National Legal Aid and Defender Association, why not apply for an NIH research grant to do a study of insanity procedures under federal law? Furthermore, Sam said he thought he knew exactly how to go about getting that grant as quickly as possible. He suggested that all we had to do was take the fast train from Philadelphia's 30th Street Station to Washington, D.C., and call on Judge Bazelon.

"I know Judge Bazelon," Sam said. "I've met him in my travels and he is a great guy. I think he will remember me, and I'll call for an appointment for the three of us to meet." To make a long story short, Judge Bazelon gave us an appointment the very next week.

Judge David Bazelon

I was very impressed and excited at the prospect of meeting the Honorable David Bazelon, chief judge of the U.S. Court of

Appeals for District of Columbia. Judge Bazelon, in his 1954 Durham decision, had set aside the M'Naghten rule and substituted a "Product Rule" instead. With his Product Rule, Judge Bazelon, who had long championed the rights of the mentally ill, proposed that mental health experts be asked two key questions: Was the defendant suffering from a mental illness or defect at the time of the crime? And if so, were the criminal acts a product of that illness? Obviously, the aim of Judge Bazelon's "Product Rule" was to allow more informative and extensive mental health and clinical testimony for jurors to consider at the time of the defendant's trial.

Judge Bazelon was about fifteen or more years older than we were, and was everything that Sam had said about him. Not only was he a "great guy," but a wise, discerning, and erudite gentleman from Chicago, with a warm heart. After we had outlined our proposal and methodology for him, and he had sized us up as couple of capable and trustworthy younger academics who indeed wanted to do a clinical study of insanity defense procedures under federal law, he promised to open doors and make relevant case materials available.

Researching the Insanity Defense

In 1958, we received Research Grant OM 366 and began our long study of Insanity Procedures Under Federal Law. It turned out to be a larger undertaking than we had anticipated, a massive collaboration among our faculty colleagues, professional associates, and senior students at Temple Medical and Law schools. We called upon several psychiatrists and lawyers among our faculty colleagues who were interested in the legal, medical, and philosophical problems which the insanity defense entailed. Along with selected psychiatric residents in our newly established Forensic Fellowship program, they contributed generously in the line-by-line study of the official transcripts of some forty-seven federal trials in which the insanity defense was raised. We understood that lawyers, psychiatrists, and juries of lay persons would all observe an insanity trial from vastly different perspectives.

Where would we find a willing pool of "mock jurors"? An abundance of first-year medical and law students, as well as secretaries and nurses, volunteered to provide their responses as lay persons to materials recorded in the trial transcripts. One question asked our "mock jurors" was whether the psychiatrist made a significant difference in the disposition of each case, and if so, how? We instructed them to report any stimuli or impressions from the transcript materials which influenced their feeling that the defendant was or was not insane in the legal sense.

Our Findings

A team of consulting lawyers and psychiatrists analyzed our trial transcripts and identified a number of reasons why the insanity defense is so problematical to lawyers, psychiatrists, juries, courts, and the public at large. First, the insanity defense failed to provide sufficiently useful, clear, and effective guidelines that lay jurors could apply with confidence in assessing the legal evidence and psychiatric testimony on which they must decide whether or not a defendant was legally insane at the time of the crime. Our findings also revealed that the underlying prospect of capital punishment would lay heavily on the consciences of insanity defense jurors.

In addition, since insanity defense jurors were not provided with the courts' instructions concerning the legal definitions of insanity until after they had heard all the evidence, the jurors' own preconceptions of "insane" as "crazy" in everyday, ordinary usage colored their decisions. Given these findings, we were led to conclude that jurors' decisions in insanity defense trials were based more on the individual juror's emotional responses to the defendant's "viciousness," the victim's "vulnerability," and the circumstances of the crime than on the testimonies of mental health experts brought in by both the prosecution and defense attorneys.

Our 1965 Research Report on Insanity Procedures Under Federal Law

This was a lengthy study and a big piece of work. In 1965, we submitted our NIMH report and findings in a 308-page volume entitled "Insanity Procedures under Federal Law" by M.S. Heller and S. Polsky. It was further recorded as Temple University Research Studies in Law and Medicine. Sam had bound a few hardback copies for Professor Erwin Surrency to hold at Temple's Law School Library, as well as for the two of us as principal investigators, and for one or two others who had given freely of their time. I still have my copy some sixty years later.

Competence to Proceed in the Face of Criminal Charges

Throughout our lectures, Sam emphasized that the competence of a defendant to understand the proceedings and assist counsel was such an important element of due process that it could be raised at any point in criminal proceedings—in bar of trial, in bar of sentence, and in bar of execution of sentence. Our laws required that the defendant must understand what it means to be found guilty, and if sentenced to death, the defendant cannot be executed if he or she were so mentally impaired as not to understand or "appreciate" what is going on. It was the law's focus on competency to proceed that abruptly brought me back to prison psychiatry in 1957, shortly after Sam Polsky and I began working together at Temple. Here is how it happened.

Chapter 9
Developing Our Clinical Teaching Facilities, Back to Prison

I WAS SITTING in our large office at the Law School when our recently hired secretary and the only paid employee of our newborn Unit in Law and Psychiatry told me that Dr. Maurice Linden was on the phone, and could I talk with him?

"Do you mean Maurice Linden, Philadelphia's mental health commissioner?"

"Yes," she nodded. I had never met Dr. Linden, but he was an important person in the public sector of psychiatry at the time. Even before I picked up the phone, however, I knew what the call was about. It was all over the newspapers. Due to an increasing and recurrent shortage of beds in the locked psychiatric ward at Philadelphia General Hospital (PGH,) a large number of mentally ill persons who had been declared incompetent to stand trial while facing criminal charges were being detained in Philadelphia's county prisons instead of a mental hospital.

What was wrong with that? Untried defendants are supposed to be "presumed innocent" until tried and proven guilty. Ask any criminal defense lawyer, constitutional expert, or even second-year law student.

I knew all that as I picked up the phone. After suitable greetings, Dr. Linden said, "Dr. Heller, I think you know the situation at the Courts with PGH patients being held at the County prison system for lack of locked ward, psychiatric bed space at PGH. I'll be brief. How soon can we get together?"'

Since Dr. Linden was an important person with an acutely painful community problem at the juncture of the mental health and criminal justice systems, I postponed or canceled a couple of appointments, and met with him the following day.

Somewhat portly and about ten or more years older and more experienced than I, Dr. Linden leaned forward and said, "Mel, can I call you Mel? I've looked you up. There's no psychiatrist around here with your overall qualifications, training, and special prison experience. I need you to examine these untried defendants, and tell me how many of them there are, and which specific ones, that could be released and treated on an outpatient basis."

Little did Dr. Linden know how eager I was for this chance to step up to the plate. This job seemed right down my alley for a number of reasons. First, for two recent years, as the chief and only psychiatrist at a maximum security federal penitentiary, I had written annual parole progress reports on each of the 1,100 inmates. Second, I also had a substantial amount of practical experience as a prison physician in assessing the actual day-to-day risks of an inmate harming himself or others. The unhappy and worrisome medical task of dealing with a prisoner's suicide threat indeed occurred on more than a few occasions at regular morning sick call. Was it real or manipulative? Or possibly both? Even if it was not my turn as a physician to take sick-call duty that day, whichever doctor did have that duty was bound to ask me to see any prisoner who, it seemed, had come to sick call that day to say expressly that he might commit suicide. That was a threat not to be taken lightly, even by an expert, which at the time I was not.

As these thoughts raced through my mind, Dr. Linden was urging me on to consider the job. Little did he know that I was already "urged" to the maximum, even before he supplied further details. He indicated that his office would arrange for PGH to pay my fees for one-hour examinations and brief consultation reports of no more than one page on each person. As a final point, Dr. Linden added that Ed Hendricks, superintendent of Philadelphia's county prison system, was as anxious as he was get as many of these pre-trial "guests" as possible out of his prisons, and that Hendricks would personally smooth the way for me to get the job done. With that added note, I stood up, shook his hand, and said, "OK, Dr. Linden. I'll take the job and do my best."

"Done," he replied with a broad smile. "If you can get started this week, Ed Hendricks and I would appreciate it. I'll phone Ed and tell him the news. Just call his secretary and let them know when to expect you. Here is the phone number. Hendricks knows who you are. I think he already checked you out with a professional buddy of his at the Federal Bureau of Prisons. He tells me your U.S. prison work got top reviews from the warden at Terre Haute."

Up, Up, and Away

I need not tell you that I was walking on air when I left Dr. Linden's office. He had made me feel wanted, if not needed, and special, if not unique. Truthfully, I enjoyed the flattery, but did not let it go to my head. Those PGH patients were waiting in their county prison cells and there was much work to be done.

How happy I felt that day to have chosen the clinical academic route, which allowed me to devote as much as thirty to forty percent of my time to private practice while spending the larger portion fulfilling my academic duties at Temple's law and medical schools. Had I accepted a full-time, salaried position, such outside work as Dr. Linden's project would have required the prior approval of the department chairman—or, worse yet, that of a faculty committee—to consider the pros and cons of taking it on. How great it felt to be able finally to earn my way, and chart my course as an assistant clinical professor and co-director of Temple's new Unit in Law and Psychiatry, I thought.

My co-director and increasingly close colleague, Sam, and I shared not only our interdisciplinary academic tasks and professional interests, but increasingly our personal and family situations as well. In our joint mission to develop Temple's new Unit in Law and Psychiatry, it seemed that Sam and I were each experiencing a rather rare sense of becoming brothers-in-arms, so to speak, rather than sibling rivals or competitors. Sam was both thrilled and amused about Dr. Linden's rescue project for Superintendent Hendricks' uninvited mentally ill "guests," who were temporarily misplaced by the courts in our county prison for lack of locked ward bed space at Philadelphia General Hospital. Sam said this was an example of the need for our mental health and justice systems to get their act together. He assured me that he would hold down the fort while I attended to our city's "mental health emergency."

The next day, driving up Roosevelt Boulevard on my way to Philadelphia's Holmsburg Prison, the sky was clear, and it seemed that the sun and I were both shining. "Here I go, back to prison work," I thought. I wondered with an amused smile if my returning so willingly to prison made me some kind of "recidivist," a term referring to a repeat offender with a pattern of returning to prison. But enough of such extraneous thoughts as I drove along, because there I was at the visitor's parking lot outside the high stone-walled enclosure, and there was much work awaiting me behind the heavy steel door at the prison gate.

I was greeted by a polite guard who, seeing that I had no briefcase or other packages that might need inspection, simply asked if I were carrying any contraband. Satisfied in that regard and that I appeared indeed to be the Dr. Heller that was expected at 8 a.m., he brought me to Superintendent Hendricks' office, in which a table was stacked with a dozen or more records of the prisoners I was scheduled to see. Superintendent Hendricks and I shook hands and chatted briefly as I thumbed through a few of the folders, several of which were quite thick with extensive medical records, prior criminal histories, and sometimes both.

I was not dismayed since I had requested that their Record Department supply me with everything they had on each case. Superintendent Hendricks told me that they had cleared out a small examination room on a cell block from which the block officer would bring me patients as I called for them. So grabbing a half dozen of the less bulky records, I quickly got started with what I hoped might be the least complicated ones, and dug right into the first batch of the approximately seventy or more cases awaiting my attention. I wasted little time in getting familiar with the task. Things actually went so smoothly, and I felt so comfortable in relating to these prisoners and their guards, that I had completed the first nine cases on the first day.

Superintendent Hendricks Took an Interest and Kept a Close Watch

Admittedly, I started with what seemed like the easiest cases rather than the ones with the thickest, telephone-book-size files. Superintendent Hendricks, good administrator that he was, had been keeping a supervisor's eye on Dr. Linden's new psychiatric consultant. I was more pleased than surprised when two of my next day's patients told me that the superintendant himself had been checking up on my work with them. Obviously, one or more of them had overheard the guard's end of Hendricks' phone call to the noisy cell block. Prison news sometimes traveled faster on the inmates' grapevine than it did by telephone back then. Actually, I was both impressed and personally grateful that Mr. Hendricks took personal interest in how I was working with this special subset of his prisoners.

The Forensic Psychiatrist's Role

It was not my place to state in so many words whether or not these mentally ill persons were competent to stand trial. That was a ruling for the Court to decide. What my case evaluation needed to determine was whether or not the defendant was currently so impaired by mental illness as to be unable to understand the proceedings and nature of the trial, and could not really assist counsel in his defense. These concepts constituted the legal tests for competency to proceed in the face of criminal charges. Where were their lawyers, one might ask? Few of these defendants could afford private legal fees. Most of them were indigent, represented by an under-staffed public defender system. Many of those I was scheduled to see in the following days had languished "temporarily" for months in the limbo of their jail cells, caught in the cracks between the mental health and criminal justice systems.

So, the first question I needed to address was whether or not the untried defendant was still mentally ill, and if so, was the defendant so mentally ill that he presented such a risk of harm to himself or others that he required custodial supervision and safe management in a secure environment. It was really my assessment of that clinical risk that was my essential task in this matter. I proceeded carefully, but confidently, insofar as I had done literally hundreds of such assessments in my prior work in preparing parole progress reports and other clinical evaluations that called for my consideration of an inmate's potential risk of harm to self, others, or property, for that matter. Was the person, for example, a potential arsonist habitually fascinated by fires?

Predicting the Future Dangerousness of a Given Individual

That psychiatrists were called upon to make such assessments raised many proper questions as to whether or not a psychiatrist, or any other specialist, can reliably predict the future dangerousness of another human being. From my prior work with offenders, I had learned that the short answer is "No." But since the question of these defendants' future dangerousness was either implied or openly raised by the Court, I had learned to proceed both cautiously and humbly with my clinical prognoses and predictions of future risk.

Thus, in court testimony, when judges had directly asked me, "Dr. Heller, in your professional opinion, is this person dangerous?" my very polite and respectful reply would go something like this: "Your Honor, with all due respect, I am no better than the weatherman. The best I can provide is my five-day forecast. Our statistical predictions and probabilities of risk in large groups of persons can have scientific validity. But in predicting the future dangerousness of a specific individual, I can do no better, if as well, than weather forecasters with all their charts and instruments. Neither the weather forecaster nor I have complete information about the risk of a future storm, or what its exact proportions might be a month from now."

Often, when all the evidence that could be forthcoming was in, courts, parole boards, probation officers and others needed to make decisions, and their best recommendations were based on less than complete information. Under such circumstances, when facts are inadequate or conflicting, courts considered the opinions of persons whom they recognized as "expert" witnesses based on their individual qualifications. I knew that in such situations, courts, like the rest of us, needed any help they can get. And so, when Philadelphia General Hospital ran out of locked ward bed space for their increasing case load of mentally ill persons facing criminal charges, decisions needed to be made regarding their potential risk of harm to themselves or others.

I Was In The Right Place at the Right Time

Unfortunately, when mentally ill persons are charged with crimes, but not yet tried and found guilty, they tend to be regarded categorically as potentially dangerous until proven otherwise. "Safety first" was the motto with prisoners. And who, especially back then, would object? Who would protect the defendant's rights? As was often the case, few of these mentally ill defendants awaiting trial in jail, but who had been legally found to be incompetent to stand trial, had the money to afford a private lawyer. Almost all were indigent, with few family resources, and dependent for legal services on the Public Defender Association, which was hopelessly overstretched at the time. As time dragged on, all that these persons had going for them were a few outraged citizens and a free press that persisted in repeatedly publicizing the matter and demanding that something be done about it. And in that way, it landed on the shoulders of Dr. Maurice Linden, the city's mental health commissioner, and Superintendent Ed Hendricks of the County Prison System

Fortunately for these "temporary" prisoners, Dr. Linden did not postpone things even further by appointing a committee. Passing on to a group of others the complicated issues involved in seventy or more cases would likely result in several months of added deliberation and a fifty-page committee report with recommendations. Instead, Dr Linden found in me a relatively young psychiatrist with intensive and recent prison experience, along with a new academic rank and title, and the time, energy and motivation to step right in to clinically examine and sort out these unfortunate pretrial detentioners.

How I Evaluated Risk of Future Violence in Prisoners

In my former experiences as a prison psychiatrist, I had found that the offender's past history and record of prior violent behavior were the most important predictors of future violent behavior. There were no blood studies, litmus tests, or other measures for the reliable prediction of future violent behaviors in individuals, and there still are none. The best we could do was to look at the individual's track record. In plain English, and as unprofessional as it may sound, we approached the practical matter of an inmate's future dangerousness much like a handicapper of horses. All too often, this is the way things can be in making medical predictions of future complications or untoward developments. Be it in cardiology, oncology, psychiatry, or any other clinical specialty, we assess various factors. In my own specialty, when asked to assess the risk of violent behavior in a given individual, I carefully considered the following variables.

What was the inmate's back story? What has been the condition of his or her home environment? What personal circumstances and stressors will he or she likely be carrying upon release from custody? Is he or she capable of making practical and rational plans? What are his or her relationships with others likely to be upon release from custody? Will he or she likely be returning to a slippery track as a recurrent alcohol or substance abuser? Does he or she have an emotionally supportive family or a significant other to share the ride and help them go the distance?

These seemed to me to be the right questions to ask myself about the person I was assessing. If I composed them in professional language and terms, I found that I could often provide the Court with a clinical opinion that was reasonably helpful. It was that kind of practical working approach that had often put me on the same page with parole officers and others in the criminal justice system who sought my opinion.

Becoming Friends with Ed Hendricks

I found myself saying these things to Superintendent Hendricks, who had invited me to meet privately in his office while sharing a sandwich and coffee for lunch. I had met him only a few days earlier. I don't think either of us had expected to spend a full hour with one another, but we hit it off. Prison wardens and superintendents sometimes need someone to talk to, and psychiatrists are supposed to be good listeners. As we warmed up and the coffee grew cold, we trusted each other to share some things about our own backgrounds, our work, and how we each came to our respective professions.

The superintendent kept calling me "Doctor." He was maybe ten or twelve years older than I, not like Paul Madigan, a warden who had been old enough to be my father, and of whom I had been most fond back in my days at the Terre Haute federal penitentiary. So, thinking back at how much I had learned from Paul Madigan, whom I had since missed, I remember saying to Ed Hendricks something like, "If you keep calling me 'Doctor', I'll have to keep calling you 'Superintendent'. No disrespect intended, but when we're in private as we are now, wouldn't 'Ed' and 'Mel' be easier?"

Laughing, the superintendent replied, "OK, of course. You are right. Mel and Ed would be a more relaxed and better way to talk about our work and our views. And that's what I'd like to do. So tell me something. I hope you won't be insulted. You seem like such a regular guy. How did you get to be a psychiatrist?"

It was my turn to laugh. "Well, I didn't intend to be a psychiatrist. I started out in surgery, and spent two years as a surgical intern and resident." Then I told him the long story of how I struggled over that decision, and how and why I eventually switched to psychiatry. I felt that he listened very intently and patiently. Then he said, "That is something else we have in common, beside our interest in prisons. I, too, struggled over changing what I thought I wanted to be."

He went on to tell me that he had studied to become a priest, and had been within seventy-two hours of taking his vows and being ordained when he changed his mind.

"That must have been a very difficult time," I offered. "Yes. I prayed," he replied. I asked him if he had any regrets. "No. I did the right thing. I still have my faith, and am blessed with a fine wife and six healthy kids, a large family, good friends, and a very responsible and challenging job that I like."

Because we were each so busy at opposite ends of town, I was to see Ed only a small number of times on occasions when our work brought us together. Yet, we felt in that brief time a potential kinship as two who had struggled and dared at a personal crossroad to set out on different paths than the ones we had initially pledged ourselves to pursue.

Chapter 10
Extending Our Contacts in Forensic Psychiatry

The Pennsylvania Prison Society

SAM AND I agreed that it was essential to expose our Law and Psychiatry students to real clinical experiences, not as observers, but as active participants in the actual work of courts and prisons with real prosecutors, defense lawyers, and justice system personnel. Seeking to link our students with these experiences, I met with individuals from the Pennsylvania Prison Society, which was founded in 1787 "to diminish the excessive and undue misery of prisoners." In due course, I was invited to join their Board of Directors and had the privilege of working with a number of truly remarkable and distinguished members, such as Judge Edmund Spaeth and Nellie Bok, as well as Drs. Norman Johnson, James McKenna, and Marvin Wolfgang, fellow academics with long standing interests in penology. A number of my articles on prisons and prisoners were published in the Pennsylvania Prison Society's journal.

Calls From Eastern State Penitentiary

My clinical background as a Yale-trained psychiatrist, board certified in both adult and child psychiatry, with the unusual professional experience as chief psychiatrist for a federal maximum security penitentiary, made me a relatively rare commodity in the mental health market of the 1950s. As such, my phone repeatedly rang with calls from the nearby Eastern State Penitentiary in Philadelphia.

I had known that Eastern State Penitentiary was no ordinary prison. It dated to 1829 and was still standing solidly where it was built, on a location that subsequently became 22nd Street and Fairmont Avenue in contemporary Philadephia.

The old prison had been the subject of much interest to early penologists. Constructed like a wheel, its cellblocks radiated out from a central security station or hub. Most inmates were in single cells, which were thought to encourage solitary reflection and deep personal penitence. Hence, it was a "penitentiary" rather than a prison, but a rose is a rose, and it was a prison to those who experienced such solitary confinement in the unyielding enclosure of its bars.

William Banmiller was the warden at Eastern State Penitentiary. Serendipitously, Dr. Michael Morello, director of treatment services at Eastern State, had heard "good things" about my prior prison experience from Superintend Hendricks and others.

Developing Further Facilities: A Contract With Eastern State Penitentiary

In 1957, Warden Banmiller and Dr. Morello were very interested in recruiting a Chief of Psychiatry at Eastern State, which had been recently renamed as the State Correctional Institution in Philadelphia. There were few whom they regarded as qualified, and apparently even fewer who were both suitable and particularly interested in the position. Truthfully, I might have been tempted to undertake the professional opportunity and challenges of Eastern State Penitentiary had I not been so happy at Temple's Law School and the Medical School's Department of Psychiatry. Sam and I knew that Warden Banmiller and Dr. Morello needed to find better ways to provide psychiatric services at Eastern State Penitentiary, and we came up with an idea.

We knew that our supervised senior residents and forensic fellows could provide the best available services, and that a working relationship with Eastern State would reward our Temple Unit in Law and Psychiatry with a much needed additional clinical training facility for them. Sam had never been inside the famous Eastern State Penitentiary, although he was very familiar with its historical significance and present situation. It seemed only natural when I suggested to Warden Banmiller and Dr. Morello that Sam might join us at my next meeting with them. They were delighted. Mike Morello, who had heard Sam speak at one of his lectures about the interface of the mental health and the justice systems, offered to take Sam on a quick tour of the prison's treatment facilities on 3 Block while I further discussed with Warden Banmiller the details and scope of the prison's needs for psychiatric services. We agreed that these were substantial.

In short order, Sam returned and cheerfully announced that he found the tour of the facilities "utterly fascinating," and favorably compared the penitentiary's massive construction to several ancient strongholds and edifices that Sam had seen in his student days at the University of Edinburgh in Scotland. Looking much like everyone's favorite uncle, Sam then listened sympathetically, quietly, and with an air of considerable professional understanding while Warden Banmiller spelled out Eastern State Penitentiary's pressing psychiatric needs.

After a bit, Sam asked if he could speak. I did not know exactly what he was going to say, but trusted that he would say it well and according to our plan. Sam and I knew that very few people, including psychiatrists, have the endurance, motivation, and sheer will to study real prisoners and their keepers in an actual maximum security penitentiary environment. In this instance, Mike Morello and Warden Banmiller needed psychiatric services for Eastern State, and lawyer Sam was ready to present and close our deal. Our proposal was straightforward and in Sam's words went pretty much as follows:

"Warden Banmiller and Dr. Morello, thank you for letting me sit in on this meeting. I can fully understand why you would like to find someone like Dr. Heller to provide psychiatric services at Eastern. Well, you can't have him. We need him at Temple. Even as much as we would like to have Dr. Heller full time at Temple, we currently do not have him full time That is because he has chosen to provide us with little more than half time as a Clinical Assistant Professor so that he could retain the right to pursue a private consultation practice in addition to his academic career. So, Mel and I have come to an idea. We are each busy, jointly teaching both Temple law students and psychiatric residents about common concerns and frequent problems encountered at the juncture of the mental health and criminal justice systems, with which you, working in Corrections, are all too familiar.

"Mel and I want to interest and train more psychiatrists in our forensic fellowship programs. To train such residents, we need forensic facilities. If we set up a program to do this at Eastern State Penitentiary, we can give you better than Mel. We can give you many Mels."

Sam then laid out our plan for Temple's Unit in Law and Psychiatry to provide the services of supervised psychiatric residents and fellows in forensic psychiatry to what would be its major clinical facility, Eastern State Penitentiary. He pointed out that Eastern State Penitentiary's proposed salary for a highly qualified, full-time academic psychiatrist would be divided to cover the modest annual stipends of several full-time psychiatrists in the forensic fellowship program.

Seeing Warden Banmiller's growing interest, Sam added that we had already gotten the "okay" from Temple's administration, as well as from Dean Boyer at the Law School and Dr. English, Chairman of the Psychiatry Department at the medical school. Sam assured Warden Banmiller that as part of his academic duties,

Professor Heller would personally supervise the forensic fellows through regular group sessions, which would be held in our modestly renovated clinical facility to be established on 3 Block at Eastern State Penitentiary. And we could start right away.

Warden Banmiller, who had been trying for months to find suitable psychiatric help, could hardly believe his ears, but Mike Morello knew that we really would make it happen. Three weeks later, the contract was signed. This brought a large additional clinical teaching facility to the Forensic Psychiatry Fellowship program at Temple.

Hello From the Citizens Crime Commission

Following my brief prison project concerning the overflow of Philadephia General Hospital's untried, mentally ill criminal court patients who had been improperly held in cells at Philadelphia County's prisons, I received a call from Ephraim Gomberg, executive director of the Citizens Crime Commission of Philadelphia. He invited me to attend a meeting of their Board of Directors and present a brief talk about my former experiences with mentally ill offenders among federal prison inmates.

Ephraim Gomberg, who soon befriended me in many ways, was a remarkably capable executive with a background in newspaper work and public relations. It was instructive and indeed wonderful for me to see him work the aisles so effectively and persuasively in meetings with various groups of people, including influential persons on his own Board of Directors. The political strength of the Crime Commission Board of Directors came primarily from well-situated citizens drawn from the commercial and industrial base of the community. I soon learned that Board members of Citizens Crime Commissions in large cities like Philadelphia included CEOs, corporate presidents, and highly placed vice presidents of the community's major industries and employers. In addition, the Board of Directors included a modest sprinkling of community-concerned academics with impressive credentials in sociology, penology, and criminology.

Temple's Diagnostic Services to the Court of Common Pleas

In the early 1960s, the Citizens Crime Commission of Philadelphia sponsored a series of judicial seminars on sentencing. I was asked to participate on the panel of speakers based on my experiences with the Federal Bureau of Prisons and sentenced prisoners at the U.S. penitentiary in Terre Haute.

Following one of these seminars, the Honorable Vincent Carroll, president judge of the Philadelphia Court of Common Pleas, approached me most kindly by saying with a smile that he had heard "mostly good things" about me. He asked if I would be interested in reorganizing and providing psychiatric services for the Court. Based on the contract arranged between Temple and Eastern State Penitentiary, I suggested that Temple's Unit in Law and Psychiatry could provide forensic fellows, which included supervised senior psychiatric residents with special interests in forensic psychiatry, to supply diagnostic and clinical evaluation services to the Court of Common Pleas.

President Judge Carroll and the Board of Judges were most enthusiastic. They arranged a contract with Temple University for its Unit in Law and Psychiatry to provide psychiatric evaluations of defendants and pre-sentence offenders for Philadelphia's Court of Common Pleas. This contract was adjusted according to the Court's increasing caseload, and was renewed annually for an additional twenty-some years through the successive president judgeships of the Hon. Donald Jamison and the Hon. William Bradley.

The Children's Aid Society

Alongside my academic work, I encountered several couples in my child psychiatric private practice who became involved in legal adoption issues. Through one of these couples, I met Dr. Elizabeth Lawder, the director of the Children's Aid Society (CAS), which was then the Commonwealth's largest adoption and foster care agency. Adoption and foster care had been prominent features in the backgrounds of juvenile and young adult offenders with whom I had been working in the correctional system. Knowing that foster care and adoption involved child psychiatric concerns that were replete with legal issues, I had applied to work with CAS to gain more direct clinical experience with foster child and family forensic issues. In my work with CAS, I was exposed to such issues as the birth mother's informed consent when giving up her child for adoption, as well as adverse child developmental matters connected with physical, emotional, and sexual abuse in foster care.

Dr. Guy and Our Psychiatric Services at the County Prison System

As Sam's and my relationship with Philadelphia's county prison system developed and my own scope of work also grew, we were very much in need of and fortunate in recruiting a well-trained and unusually capable psychiatrist from another medical center across the city. He was about my own age, and was looking for "a change of scene"—a new job, a new neighborhood, new associates, and a new start. Dr. Edward Blair Guy turned out to be one of our most valued forensic colleagues and good friends.

Sam Polsky and I quickly oriented Ed Guy to the newly developing field of forensic psychiatry. We familiarized him with the basic issues and exposed him to the enormous challenges and needs of so-called "correctional psychiatry." I eagerly shared my own prison experiences to help jump-start him on his path to becoming one of the most capable and dedicated forensic psychiatrists. For many years, Dr. Guy served us and Philadelphia's County Prison System admirably as their chief psychiatrist under our Temple University contract to supply mental health services to the prison system.

Our Temple University Fellowships in Forensic Psychiatry

I shall mention only a few of the many fine individuals who came to study Forensic Psychiatry with Sam Polsky and me in the late 1950s and 1960s when few if any other Forensic Psychiatry Fellowships with extensive clinical and academic facilities were being offered. Drs. Norman Anderson and Fred Herring III were among the very first who signed on for our new fellowship program. Some of our very brightest and well-trained psychiatrists were from abroad. Such doctors as Brij Sethi from India, and Juan Pedro from Puerto Rico enhanced our perspectives about comparable mental health laws and procedures in their own countries

Through our several state and county service contracts, we had ample funds to add two additional Forensic Fellowships for child psychiatrists whose clinical time was split equally between the Children's Aid Society and Temple's forensic program. In successive years, we gained two of our most worthy and interesting Forensic Fellows, Dr. Paul McQuaid from Ireland and Dr. Martin Gay from Scotland, who added their distinctive accents, professional viewpoints, and diverse perspectives on the American and British Mental Health Acts and legal procedures. As these are my memoirs and not an official or complete history of Temple Unit in Law and Psychiatry, I recall and acknowledge only very few of the many people who were personally noteworthy in my recollections.

Academic Lawyers and Psychiatrists in Our Criminal Justice System

My personal interests remained focused on exploring the further prospects for increased interdisciplinary efforts by doctors and lawyers working in partnership within the framework of our mental health and justice systems at national, state, and local levels. That was what our Temple Unit in Law and Psychiatry was all about— to serve as an interdisciplinary academic and clinical vehicle that enabled doctors and lawyers to study and work together on mutual problems encountered in law and psychiatry, or the interface of unlawful behaviors and mental disorders. One of the smallest, best, and early interdisciplinary forensic groups on which I was asked to serve was a committee of lawyers and psychiatrists appointed in 1958 by the Commonwealth of Pennsylvania's Attorney General.

The task of the committee was to discuss and make recommendations for the management of mentally ill persons encountered in the criminal justice system. This had been a longstanding and recurrently acute problem in Pennsylvania as well as in most states nationwide. The basic cause, as I saw it, was our historic and cultural ambivalence, not so much about crimes, but about the kinds of persons that committed them—criminals. Were criminals mentally ill, or simply bad? Mad, bad, or both was the question that remains. The practical problem was in the management of varying degrees and types of mental illness regularly encountered in the state and county prison systems.

So I was gratified and flattered to find myself appointed to this small committee, which included the highly regarded Philadelphia psychiatrist and analyst, Dr. Philip Quentin Roche, and Dr. William Camp, a much respected psychiatrist with extensive clinical and administrative experience in the state mental hospital system of that time. The expert lawyers included the Honorable Judge and Criminal Law Professor Joseph Sloan, as well as several additional lawyers with special interests in mental health law. These included Russell Levin, Esq. and, of course, Sam Polsky, LLB, PhD.

Among the various committees on which I have served, this initially small, friendly, and good-natured group was distinguished for its lack of subtle rivalries and big egos. We each had enough personal credentials, confidence, and practical experience to feel privileged to listen to each other's viewpoints rather than to compete and argue about minor differences that could be blown into major disagreements. Consequently, despite many differences in our professional orientations and academic backgrounds, we enjoyed each other's company so much that after our committee submitted its report, Dr. Phil Roche proposed that we continue meeting monthly for supper at a private dinner club to which he belonged on Camac Street in Philadelphia's Center City.

After a few more such meetings, someone asked what we should call ourselves. I think it was Judge Sloan, while getting into the spirit of things, who first suggested that we call ourselves the Camac Street Irregulars. With the motion seconded and passed unanimously, we continued monthly supper sessions as the Camac Street Irregulars (CSI) until we outgrew the club's cozy quarters. Word of our monthly meetings had gotten around and soon colleagues would ask if they might attend a meeting. And then, could they come back for another? Of course we'd be delighted to have them come, but where to meet and where to put forty or fifty lawyers and mental health professionals that had expressed repeated interest?

Our Camac Street Irregulars Became the Community Services Institute

With the enlarged group now including such additional luminaries as Judges Beriberi, Beryl Caesar, and Lisa Aversa Richet, as well as Jim Crawford, chief of the Appeals Division of the District Attorney's office, we had no trouble securing the evening use of a suitable and commodious meeting room in Philadelphia's City Hall. Growing further by word of mouth, the expanded group soon included numerous faculty from neighboring universities and law schools, as well as both prosecutors and defense lawyers, and a number of experienced mental health professionals with shared forensic interests.

As for me, I was at the top of my game and in my glory with this interdisciplinary group of mental health professionals and lawyers whom we had somehow welded together from scratch. No longer a novice, I felt at home in their company and secure in my own expertise and accomplishments. Through good psychiatric training, energy, enthusiasm, a bit of luck, and being in the right place at the right time, by 1967, I had achieved the rank of full professor, as well as director of the Forensic Division of Temple's Department of Psychiatry, and continued as co-director of our now decade-old interdisciplinary Unit in Law and Psychiatry.

With our newly enlarged large group of colleagues meeting in our new location, we could no longer retain the sentimental but undignified name of the Camac Street Irregulars, nor use it when inviting such distinguished guest speakers as the Hon. John Biggs Jr. of the Third Circuit Court of Appeals. So, I suggested that we keep the original initials of the Camac Street Irregulars (CSI) and simply change them to stand for Community Services Institute as our new official name. In response to this and other unspecified qualifications, I was somehow nominated and elected, among much laughter and applause, to serve as the newly named Community Services Institute's first president in 1969-70. It was my subsequent pleasure and honor to be succeeded by Alan J. Davis Esq., the chief trial lawyer at one of Philadelphia's most prestigious law firms, where the fees were so high that Alan claimed he could not afford them himself were he to need a lawyer.

The Clinical Work of Our Temple University Forensic Fellows

Temple's forensic psychiatry clinical efforts within our state and nearby county criminal justice systems consisted of professional evaluations and consultations performed in courts, prisons, and penitentiaries. Our court reports and testimony, although highly individualized on a case-by-case basis, were more structured and formal between relatively congenial professionals, even during highly adversarial, and sometimes heated, cross examinations.

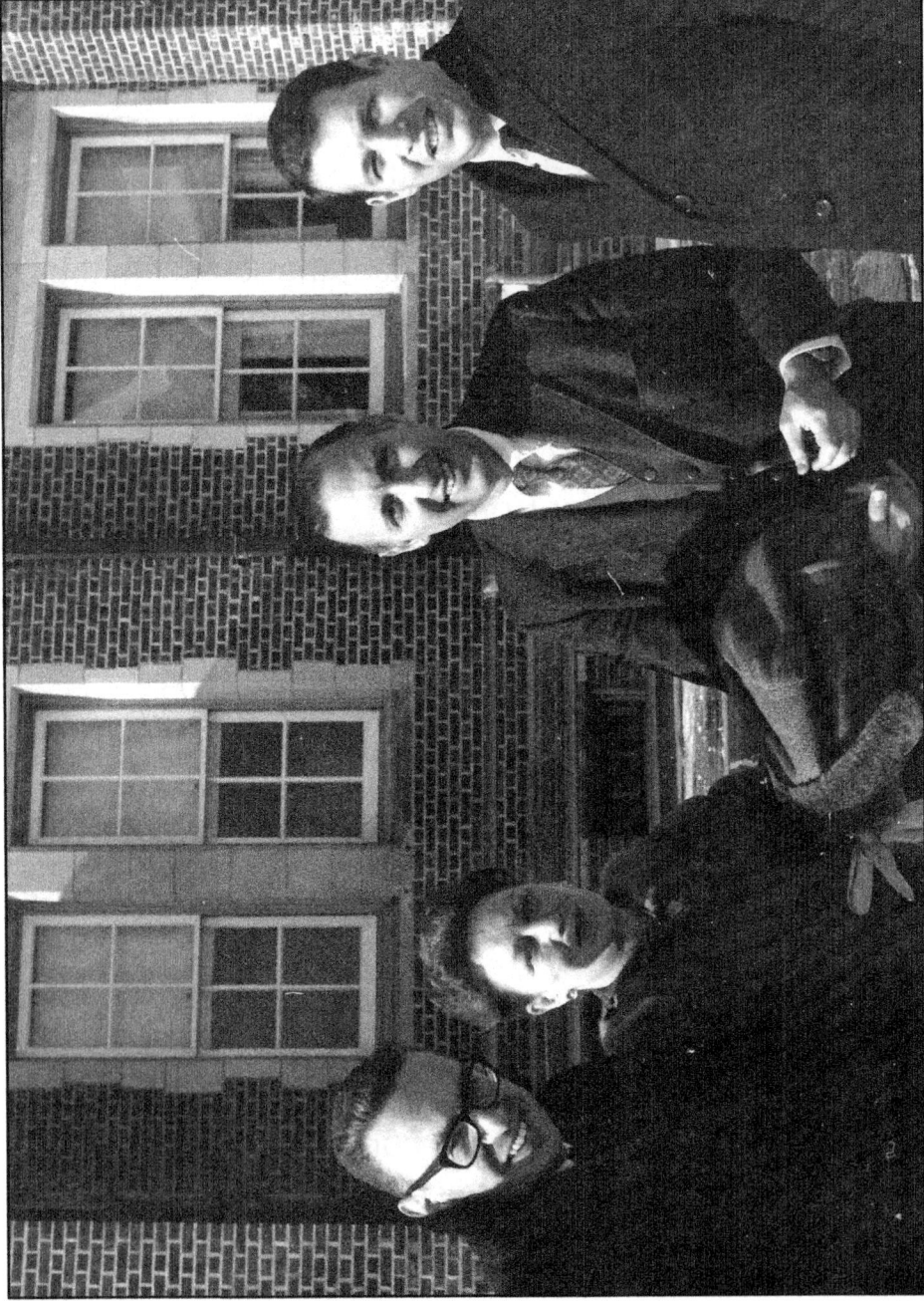

Forensic Fellows at Norristown State Hospital where Author sought to recruit mental health professionals to work part time in prisons. (From Left to Right): Forensic Fellows Drs. Bob Sadoff, Sheila Scott, Author, and Dr. Norman Jablon.

Our forensic work in prisons, on the other hand, often involved the more challenging, less promising, and troublesome clinical prospects of dealing therapeutically with forcibly incarcerated and frequently frustrated inmates, who were often subject to punitive discipline within the justice system's detention faculties, where interpersonal conflicts and violence erupted with regularity. What kind of an unpromising place was that for a mental health professional? Or for any human being for that matter, inmate or staff alike? Was it not somehow significant that I rarely, if ever, encountered among our prison visitors any of the busy judges who pronounced the prison sentences that our prison inmates were ordered to serve?

It bothered me that the judges themselves did not conduct regular spot checks to see how things were going in the places to which they sentenced prisoners, but I knew better than to ask back then. Who were we, as co-directors of Temple's Unit in Law and Psychiatry, or even if we were the deans of the Law and Medical Schools, to do battle with our politicized prison system? When I shared my concerns with my partner, Sam Polsky, he rejoined: "What did you expect? What public sector enterprise is not politicized? The whole public sector is an adversary political system. And properly so," he added.

Rallying The Troops

So, instead of taking on the political system directly, I appealed to the scientific curiosity and research interests of our small group of forensic recruits most of whom, were only ten to twelve years younger that I was at the time. I confessed to them that some ten years earlier, when I had almost completed two years as a surgical house officer, during a rare off-hour, I happened to drop in on a psychiatric conference at Yale's adjoining Institute of Human Relations. It was 1950, only a few years after the end of World

War II, and already the newly brewing Cold War had heated up to the very dangerous Korean conflict. The session was one of Yale's frequent psychiatric conferences on topics of special interest in human behavior. I did not know the names of the prominent guest lecturers, but unlike our few psychiatric instructors in medical school during the forties, they were dynamic and fascinating.

I confessed to our students that I, who by then had performed a fair number of hernia repairs and appendectomies under supervision, as well as many hemorrhoid operations, experienced a deep moment of insight—an epiphany. It seemed clear to me that we were not going to be wiped off the face of the Earth by hernias and appendicitis, not even by heart attacks, malaria, or cancer. But we might very well blow each other off our lonely planet. This powerful thought was by no means original with me, but it must have sunk in while I was stitching up a hernia or hemorrhoid, which can be a painful ordeal if you have one, but not a threat to Mankind.

Excessive human violence and total warfare were more imminent and long-term threats to human survival than any others we perceived. Coining a term, I asked our crew, "Why not study the psycho-biology of violence? And where, for starters, might we find better subjects to work with than violent offenders in the criminal justice system?"

Noting that one hardly ever encountered among regular prison visitors the busy judges who pronounced the prisoners' sentences, nor the legislators who prescribed prison sentences as just and lawful treatment, I asked our psychiatric residents and forensic fellows, "Should not our legislators who prescribed these lawful punishments and the specific judges who sentenced these inmates take note of our increasing recidivism rates, and order individual follow-up studies to find out why prison sentences serve to punish and detain the prisoners, but rarely serve to rehabilitate our increasing numbers of violent criminal offenders?"

With particular respect to the relatively neglected field of prison psychiatry, I went further and asked, "Would not our detailed studies of the early life circumstances, developmental backgrounds, and causes of violence in individual offenders be as interesting and worthy a way of spending one's medical career as the study of cancer, for example?"

So much for the earlier teachers who sought to rally the clinical troops in the trenches of our criminal justice system's "correctional" institutions. We were not politicians, but we and our forensic colleagues published a variety of multiple-authored papers by Heller, M.S., Polsky, S., Sadoff, R.L., Traylor, W.H., as well as Guy, E.B., Ehrlich, S.M. and Lester, D., as research associates. Seeking to reach not only psychiatrists, but a larger groups of psychologists and associated mental health professionals, we published some of our articles in various such journals as the *American Journal of Psychiatry*, *The Bulletin of the American Academy of Psychiatry and Law*, the *Journal of Social Psychology*, the *Prison Journal*, the *Journal of Social Psychology*, the *Journal of Forensic Sciences*, *American Journal of Social Psychology*, and the *Journal of General Psychology*. These efforts did not bear immediate fruit. There was no rush by mental health experts to enter prison work. It took years and new generations of mental health professionals to enter the growing fields of forensic psychiatry in courts and prisons and agencies for neglected, abused, and troubled children.

Sam Polsky and I taught our Forensic Fellows as much as we could about what we knew from our own professional experiences and viewpoints about the best ways to handle their courtroom situation and themselves in dealing with the needs of their clients and the Court. Although our Forensic Fellows had substantial clinical experience with patients during their prior residency training, working with defendants in courts and prisons was different from seeing patients in one's private office or public sector clinic. In matters of competency and pre-sentence examinations, as well as probation and parole evaluation, our Forensic Fellows and their patients needed to understand that third parties were involved—namely, justice system personnel as elected or appointed representatives of the public. And so we discussed and hashed out these crucial exceptions and limits to traditional concepts of doctor-patient privacy.

New Forensic Fellows in an Old Historic Prison

A growing group of psychiatric residents, forensic fellows, and helpful legal colleagues like the frequently involved and energetic lawyer, Ike Pepp, from the Defender Association, began joining our weekly meetings with Sam Polsky. Sam referred to these meetings as our Medico-Legal Clinical Conferences. These were usually held in our own psychiatric section on 3 Block of the Eastern State Penitentiary, where our doctors now occupied a number of former prison cells that had been scrubbed and repainted to serve as small offices and examination rooms.

Sergeant Ronald Marks

Working with us as our "host" in this massively built, ancient penitentiary was a young State correctional officer, Sergeant Ronald Marks, who had been placed in charge of Block 3, the Hospital Block, by Warden Brierley who succeeded Warden Banmiller. Ron Marks was recently back from the Korean conflict, as I recall.

I soon learned to be most grateful for the warden's fine choice of Ron Marks because Ron was an extremely bright, well-organized, calm, capable, and very conscientious correctional officer. Sergeant Marks was about a dozen years younger than I, but very mature in his judgment and comportment.

I eventually took a special "older brother" interest in Ron's future, and remember urging him to take a college course or two to increase his prospects for further advancement. I still recall repeatedly telling Ron that he had leadership potential.

"Ron, you've got what it takes. Enroll in a college course or two. You could become not just a lieutenant or a captain, but even a warden.

"You really think so, Dr. Heller?"

"Absolutely, Ron. No doubt about it."

Ron apparently took my advice, because not only did he become a warden in time, but he went further to become Pennsylvania's Commissioner of Corrections.

Some Psychiatric Residents and Forensic Fellows Who Worked with Us at Temple

I am proud and gratified at having introduced a number of very fine physicians to forensic psychiatry, both directly and indirectly, in response to the ongoing need for mental health professionals to work in the criminal justice system's courts and correctional facilities. Forensic Fellows who subsequently continued to include the practice of forensic psychiatry in their careers included Drs. Arthur Boxer, Edward Guy, Norman Jablon, Larry Rotenberg, Robert Sadoff, and Ralph Wolf, to mention but a few of the "old originals" who worked with our Temple Unit on Block 3 of Pennsylvania's Eastern State Penitentiary for a time of mutual interdisciplinary learning in law and psychiatry more than fifty years ago.

These pages are simply my memoirs and not an official history of our Temple Unit in Law Psychiatry. With that note, let me say a bit more about some of those who came to work with Sam Polsky and me and then went on to spend a substantial part of their professional lifetime in forensic psychiatry. Proceeding alphabetically, I want to particularly mention Dr. Arthur Boxer, who came to our Temple forensic program shortly after completing his psychiatric residency training at Norristown State Hospital. Dr. Boxer went on to became one of most experienced, compassionate, and capable clinicians who devoted a major portion of his psychiatric career working with prisoners. After the historic Eastern State Penitentiary was closed at Philadelphia's Fairmont Avenue in 1971, Dr. Art Boxer continued his work at Graterford and other prisons in Pennsylvania and New Jersey. I am gratified in note that as of 2015, Dr. Arthur Boxer, a newly arrived octogenarian, only a dozen or so years my junior, is still actively treating and writing prescriptions for state and county justice system prisoners in need of psychiatric care.

Next alphabetically were two equally dedicated and capable prison psychiatrists, Drs. Edward Guy and Norman Jablon. Dr. Ed Guy skillfully supervised our Temple University forensic services at Philadelphia's Country Prison system, and Dr. Jablon subsequently headed our State Maximum Security Diagnostic Facility that we established at nearby Holmsburg at the Commonwealth's request.

Dr. Larry Rotenberg had been another outstanding Forensic Fellow, who went on to become chairman of the Psychiatry Department at Reading Hospital in Pennsylvania. I was subsequently told by a colleague that Larry's forensic consultations were especially outstanding, comprehensive, and appreciated.

Another very fine psychiatrist who completed his Forensic Fellowship training with us at Temple is Dr. Ralph Wolf, still very much in practice as a forensic psychiatrist. Dr. Wolf had conducted a medical practice as an internist prior to his subsequent career in psychiatry. Ralph developed a special interest in substance abuse, and has had extensive clinical and administrative experience in managing a group of government-supported substance abuse treatment centers along the East Coast. Dr. Wolf, who was one of our later Forensic Fellowship recipients, is the only forensic psychiatrist I have trained who regards the widespread incidence of drug-related crime as a legitimate and urgently-needed sub-specialty of forensic psychiatry. I have little doubt that a number of criminal court judges would agree with my positive assessment of his difficult forensic work with alcohol and substance abusers encountered at the frustrating interface of the mental health and criminal justice systems.

Drs. Bob Sadoff, Jonas Rappeport, and the American Academy of Psychiatry & Law

One of the many fine psychiatrists that Sam Polsky and I were privileged to mentor during their initial forensic fellowship training was a remarkable young man named Robert Sadoff. Of all the forensic fellows and psychiatric residents that we taught at Temple, none showed a greater degree of academic interest and scholarly potential than young Bob Sadoff. From his very earliest days with us, Bob confided to me that his eventual goal was to teach forensic psychiatry. Accordingly, Sam and I took a particular interest in Bob.

As time went on, Bob became personally special to me. I began to regard him inwardly and hopefully as a potential successor or heir in the further academic pursuit of our shared and much-needed subspecialty of forensic psychiatry. Although I was only about a dozen or so years older than Bob, and maybe more of an older brother than a father figure for him, I felt fortunate that Sam and I had found this very personable and promising psychiatrist who wished to pursue an academic career in forensic psychiatry. Accordingly, I began bringing Bob to special meetings and introducing him to my own contacts and friends at key clinical facilities and agencies with which our Unit in Law and Psychiatry had developed cooperative and ongoing working relationships.

One of the most fortuitous gatherings to which I invited Bob in 1969 was a founding meeting of what would subsequently become the American Academy of Psychiatry and the Law (AAPL). This was initially organized almost entirely through the personal efforts and leadership of Dr. Jonas Rappeport, a prominent forensic colleague in nearby Baltimore, who most deservedly and capably went on serve admirably as AAPL's first and founding president.

As for myself, in 1969, I was firmly established academically after more than a decade of co-developing Temple's forensic psychiatry program with Sam Polsky, as well as my own, part-time private practice. I had limited time for attending more than the essential number of our many national and regional professional meetings. I had no ambition to seek office in the American Psychiatric Association (APA) or American Psychoanalytic Association (APsaA) nor in our newly-formed AAPL.

At the initial organizational meetings of AAPL, our Temple psychiatrists represented the largest single voting bloc. I encouraged them to vote in favor of establishing the American Academy of Psychiatry and Law (AAPL) and to back Jonas Rappeport's candidacy as the Academy's first president. I felt that Jonas was a great guy, and exactly the right person to be honored as AAPL's founding president. But another motive underlying my own modesty was that I had brought along with me the single most promising academic prospect in our Temple Forensic Fellowship program, Dr. Bob Sadoff, whom I hoped to subsequently promote as AAPL's second president when Dr. Rappeport completed his own two-year term.

Certain that Bob Sadoff would do a great job, I took great pleasure in pursuing his nomination and his subsequent election to succeed Dr. Rappeport as AAPL's next president. Frankly, this was an easy call because Bob had done such a fine job as chairman of AAPL's Membership Committee during Dr. Rappeport's presidency that he was by then a shoo-in to succeed Jonas.

I was much rewarded and gratified to watch Bob as he went on to develop his own distinguished career in forensic psychiatry. Unfortunately for Temple, it was at Penn, our neighboring university, where Bob Sadoff went on to attract and nurture his own groups of very capable and devoted forensic psychiatrists, as a new generation of professional "grandchildren" during my most fortunate and lengthy lifetime. When all is said and done, what greater reward can teachers have than to be succeeded by truly productive and highly regarded scholars?

Chapter 11
National Concerns about Violence and TV

WHILE DEVELOPING THE forensic psychiatry program at Temple from 1957 through the 1960s and beyond, our political, social, and international worlds were shifting and changing. In 1968, I felt that the closely adjoining worlds of mental health law, public-sector psychiatry, the criminal justice system, and politics were beginning to shift under our feet. Some big and disturbing things were happening post-WWII during the Nixon, Kennedy, and Johnson presidential years. In the ongoing Cold War with the Soviets and their allied satellites, the American public viewed with growing alarm Russia's 1957 leap ahead with Sputnik in the race toward outer space. In 1960, similarly disturbing had been the sight of Nikita Khrushchev, leader of the nuclear-powered Soviet Union, belligerently banging his shoe against the podium at the U.N. while threatening to "bury" us, literally and figuratively. Viewers of TV's nightly news were further troubled by increasing prospects of a military stalemate in our unpopular, prolonged, and costly involvement in Vietnam, not to mention our Cuban Bay of Pigs fiasco, and the long-brewing civil rights showdown at home in Selma, Alabama.

Street Violence, TV, and Senator Pastore of Rhode Island

Frequent depictions of violence in TV entertainment programs seemed to culminate in national dismay and outrage over the sequential assassinations of Reverend Dr. Martin Luther King Jr. on April 4 and Senator Robert Kennedy on June 6, 1968. Numerous teachers, pediatricians, and mental health professionals claimed that our children were at risk of being psychologically harmed by their continued exposure to the TV networks' overdose of violence in entertainment programs, and declared that the American public and its children had seen more than enough of such television fare. So had the powerful and politically astute U.S senator from Rhode Island, John O. Pastore. In Senator Pastore's mind, the risk of harmful effects on children posed by frequently depicted violence in network television's entertainment programming needed to be investigated forthwith. Whereupon Senator Pastore succeeded in having the Surgeon General of the United States mandated to spend a million dollars of research monies to study the effects of television-portrayed violence on children, and the causal relationships, if any, between television-depicted violence and street violence.

What had TV and the mass media to do with the law, the criminal justice system, psychiatry, and the mental health professions? Since laws were attempts to regulate and control human behavior, and since psychiatry claimed to have some professional understanding of human behavior and its disorders, the two fields encountered a common territory. Among the mass media, the ability of television to inform, instruct, persuade, motivate, and influence human behavior through advertising products, shaping styles and attitudes, and promoting political campaigns and candidates for election was formidable—if not a bit frightening in matters of social significance. As for TV-depicted violence harming children and stimulating aggressive tendencies and behaviors in certain viewers, mental health professionals, educators, child behavioral specialists, and a variety of newly minted experts on TV scrambled to get aboard the million dollar research train envisioned by Senator Pastore's Congressional Committee. The major broadcasters themselves felt a need to respond to Senator Pastore's mandate to study the effects of TV-depicted violence on children and youth exposed to so-called "action-adventure" programs.

Busy as Sam and I were in our Law and Psychiatry program, we made little note of all this until October 1968, when we received an unexpected phone call from the National Association of Broadcasters (NAB) in New York. I had never heard of the NAB or their so-called Code Authority, but their call turned out to be an invitation that considerably broadened my personal interests and perspectives in law, the mass media, and forensic psychiatry during the years that followed.

How We Got Involved With Network TV

What happened was that the director of the NAB, Stockton Hellfrich, and his associate, Jerry Lansner, had somehow heard of Temple's Unit in Law and Psychiatry and the interdisciplinary work that Sam and I were doing in courts and prisons with violent offenders. Perhaps looking for a different angle or approach, they invited us to consult with them in New York about the networks' problems in editing violent content in TV entertainment fare. It certainly sounded interesting to us as a couple of university professors working together at the interface of law and psychiatry.

Where Sam and I Were Coming From That Day

What child psychiatrist had not wondered about the effects of violent TV programs on children's development, and particularly a forensic expert who had spent much time in courts and prisons evaluating perpetrators of violent crimes? So admittedly, I was more than interested. Nevertheless, at our end of the phone call from the NAB, we quickly asked ourselves what, if anything, did the broadcasting of violent TV images on police and crime shows, and other so-called "action-adventure" entertainment fare, have to do with our combined work in law and forensic psychiatry? Perhaps a lot, at least according to Senator Pastore's view of the broadcasters' legal obligations for licensing renewal according to the Federal

Communications Commission's regulations. Did we want to get involved with that political controversy? Certainly not officially as co-directors of Temple's Unit in Law and Psychiatry. For myself individually, however, viewing the situation as a clinical professor rather than a full-time University employee, I was clearly entitled to conduct a part-time private consulting practice on my own.

As for Sam Polsky, after a dozen distinguished years as a full-time law school professor, he explained that his personal contract allowed him to devote as much as one full day per week in pursuit of a professional project of his own special interest. Why not explore a pilot project on the subject of "FCC Regulations and The Risks of Broadcasting TV Violence in Network Entertainment Programs," for example? To both Sam and me, NAB's phone call seemed, at the very least, like a pleasant invitation for a paid-up trip to New York plus a generous consultation fee and—most important of all— perhaps a rare chance to obtain an inside view of commercial TV's highly competitive and profitable programming practices. So, we readily agreed with Stockton Hellfrich's suggestion that we meet with him "and a few NAB folks" at their New York office on the following Wednesday.

Meeting With the NAB in New York

When we arrived, we found that the NAB had set up a small group to meet with us. This included Stockton Hellfrich, who appeared to be in his late fifties or early sixties at the time. I still recall him to this day as a most gracious host who resembled one of my favorite liberal arts college professors. He was both warm and polished as he quickly introduced us to Jerry Lansner, his very knowledgeable and capable younger associate, and then to two colleagues from the American Broadcasting Company, Alfred R. Schneider and Grace Johnson.

Grace Johnson, Schneider's associate at the NAB meeting, quickly impressed me as a likable, intelligent, and level-headed lady with much TV editing experience in working with prime-time programmers and producers of ABC's TV entertainment fare. But it soon seemed clear that it was Al Schneider who found himself frequently and personally in the hot seat during the recurrent legal concerns and public relations battles between ABC's top brass and Congressional committees, reinforced recently by the constant carping of critics that swarmed to support Senator Pastore's accusations that violent programming on television was potentially harmful to America's children.

I stated that in our professional experience, viewing violence on TV was not a significant cause of real-world violence, but that viewing violence first-hand at home or the streets, and experiencing it personally were frequent factors in the developmental backgrounds of violent offenders. That flat-footed statement, to which Sam nodded in approval, did much to relax our new NAB acquaintances.

Alfred R. Schneider was the vice president in charge of ABC's Department of Broadcast Standards and Practices. As such, he was ABC's chief censor or "gatekeeper," as he called himself in a book he eventually would write about his work. I soon found myself liking these four NAB people. Despite the tensions that they might have felt then, as pressured representatives of an industry currently targeted by Senator Pastore's Congressional committees, these four people were more frank and candid than defensive in talking with us. And why not? They sought to establish a consultative relationship with us, rather than an adversarial one.

Neither Sam nor I were in the habit of watching TV's numerous action-adventure programs. As concerned and observant parents of young children, however, we had each found much to criticize in television's depictions of violence in routine action-adventure programs. Nevertheless, in our view, TV was not a major, or even a minor, cause of crime in America, but it could indeed shape the behavior of persons predisposed to crime by glamorizing it, instructing, and making it seem easy. I knew what Sam and I were thinking, but was not sure about what the others were thinking, and if we could find common ground with these high-powered television people.

Finding common ground with strongly opinionated lay people could sometimes be a problem for psychiatrists, I had learned. Not so with lawyers like Sam, however, who seemed laid back with almost everyone everywhere we went. Newly met people seemed very comfortable with Sam. There was apparently something reassuring about Sam's presence. Although a large man, scholarly and distinguished in manner and speech, Sam's personal warmth made him seem somehow type-cast "like everyone's uncle," as Al Schneider would later describe him in his fine book, *The Gatekeeper*.

Finding Common Ground at Harvard and Yale

Things got even more relaxed between Sam and Al Schneider when they discovered that they were both Harvard Law School alumni. Not that Harvard was so unique, but they were pleasantly surprised to see themselves not as newly-met strangers finding middle ground in the midst of a political and public relations battle about TV violence, but as fellow law students who had missed being actual classmates by merely a few years difference in age. That seemed no longer to matter because they soon were chatting like fond classmates about their younger days, and chortling about memorable professors whose famous courses they had taken within a year or two of each other. Sam then brought me into their conversation by referring to my "less fortunate background" as a Yale-trained psychiatrist rather than a Harvard one. However, he quickly added that I had more than compensated for that disadvantage by further training as an analyst and Board-certified child and adolescent psychiatrist, as well.

I knew what Sam was up to with his Harvard versus Yale routine. He was using that as an easy opening to inform the group that he knew of no child psychiatrist with Dr. Heller's top-notch training who also had as many years of real and practical experience in evaluating the behaviors and backgrounds of violent offenders. Sam pushed it further by adding that Dr. Heller could more than hold his own when discussing adverse effects of viewing TV violence in comparison to the more harmful results when children actually witness real violence being inflicted on another, or experience it themselves as victims of repeated beating and worse abuse at home and in the streets.

My Turn to Talk About Violent Offenders

So, when this NAB group turned to me and asked what I thought about TV violence as a child development concern, my opening remark was that neither Attila the Hun, Jesse James, Al Capone, nor Willie Sutton and generations of lesser known armed robbers and violent offenders had grown up with TV in their homes. Nor had Hitler, Stalin, nor the rapists of Nanking children been exposed to television prior to perpetrating the slaughter of millions, including their own citizens, in the twentieth century's most violent outbreaks of mass murder and destruction. So should we blame television? Or should we undertake a serious study of how people become a Hitler, a Stalin, or develop the ability, personality, and desire to become known and feared as a dedicated and practicing sadists in a Nazi concentration camp or gulag?

"Do we really know what makes people like that—or should we blame it on television, and go back to sleep?" I asked. Because I truly believed from our ongoing work with hundreds of violent offenders in courts and prisons that TV was not the real culprit in child-rearing, I came right out and said so. I told them I did not have complete answers, but that my clinical findings as a forensic psychiatrist strongly suggested that antisocial behavior had more to do with angry, fearful, forlorn, and resentful feelings of personal impoverishment, emptiness, and alienation from society than viewing television. I also noted the diminution or complete absence of mutually gratifying parent-child interactions during the child's ongoing formative years.

Al Schneider then asked in lawyer-like fashion, "Why don't more child psychiatrists seem to share your views about TV's relatively small influence as a major cause of criminal violence?" Having been cross-examined by prosecutors and defense attorneys in numerous court cases during the past dozen years, I had anticipated such a question. Reminding the group that I was speaking only for myself as a private consultant, and not for Temple University as one of their professors, I readily granted that psychiatrists, like lawyers, were rarely if ever of one opinion. As for divided professional opinions, I noted that even our Supreme Court was often known to split five to four on key decisions. In like fashion, I added that a similar group of nine psychiatrists would probably provide varying views concerning contested mental health issues. That brought forth an approving smile from both Schneider and Polsky, which I appreciated.

I then proceeded to answer Schneider's question about why my viewpoint about TV causing violence was a minority one. I stated as humbly as I could that I knew of few, if any, child psychiatrists, besides myself, that had any lengthy experience in working clinically with large numbers of known violent offenders. I then gave them a brief synopsis of my career in forensic psychiatry, beginning with my introductory years as a uniformed officer in the U.S. Public Health Service assigned for two ongoing years of full-time medical duty as the chief and only psychiatrist for an 1,100 bed maximum security federal penitentiary, followed by the completion of my specialty training in adult psychiatry at Yale, then further sub-specialty training in child psychiatry and psychoanalysis, which was followed by a decade in academia working closely with my esteemed colleague, Professor Polsky, as co-directors of Temple's interdisciplinary Unit in Law and Psychiatry. That brief discourse along with Sam's academic credentials and reassuring presence seemed to sew it up for the NAB folks, who invited us to serve as their consultants.

Chapter 12
Moving On To Broadcast Standards at ABC

FOLLOWING SUBSEQUENT CONSULTING sessions with the NAB, Al Schneider requested that Sam and I work directly with him in reviewing edits for proposed broadcast materials. We were happy to do so because this quickly introduced us to the practical work of broadcast standards editors. More important, in the course of working directly with Schneider, he, Sam, and I came to know and relate to one another as individuals. Sam and I truly liked what we saw in Schneider. We felt that he was sincere, honest, and very bright. As well as being a most knowledgeable TV executive, Alfred R. Schneider was a straight shooter with whom we could communicate candidly and cordially. For his part in relating to us, Al knew that Sam and I were also straight shooters, and not private investigators employed to uncover hidden agendas or wrongdoing at ABC.

As consultants hired by ABC, we sought common ground in which we could professionally study—together with network Broadcast Standards and Practices (BS&P) personnel—the problems, risks, and prospects in depicting violence and other important and controversial subjects in TV entertainment programs. As a shrewd, very decent, and insightful lawyer, Al Schneider understood that Sam and I were not TV employees, and that ABC was not buying our opinions, but merely purchasing our time and expertise. To their credit, no one at ABC ever suggested, assumed, or behaved otherwise. Something better happened. Mutual trust developed, and we were brought into the kitchen.

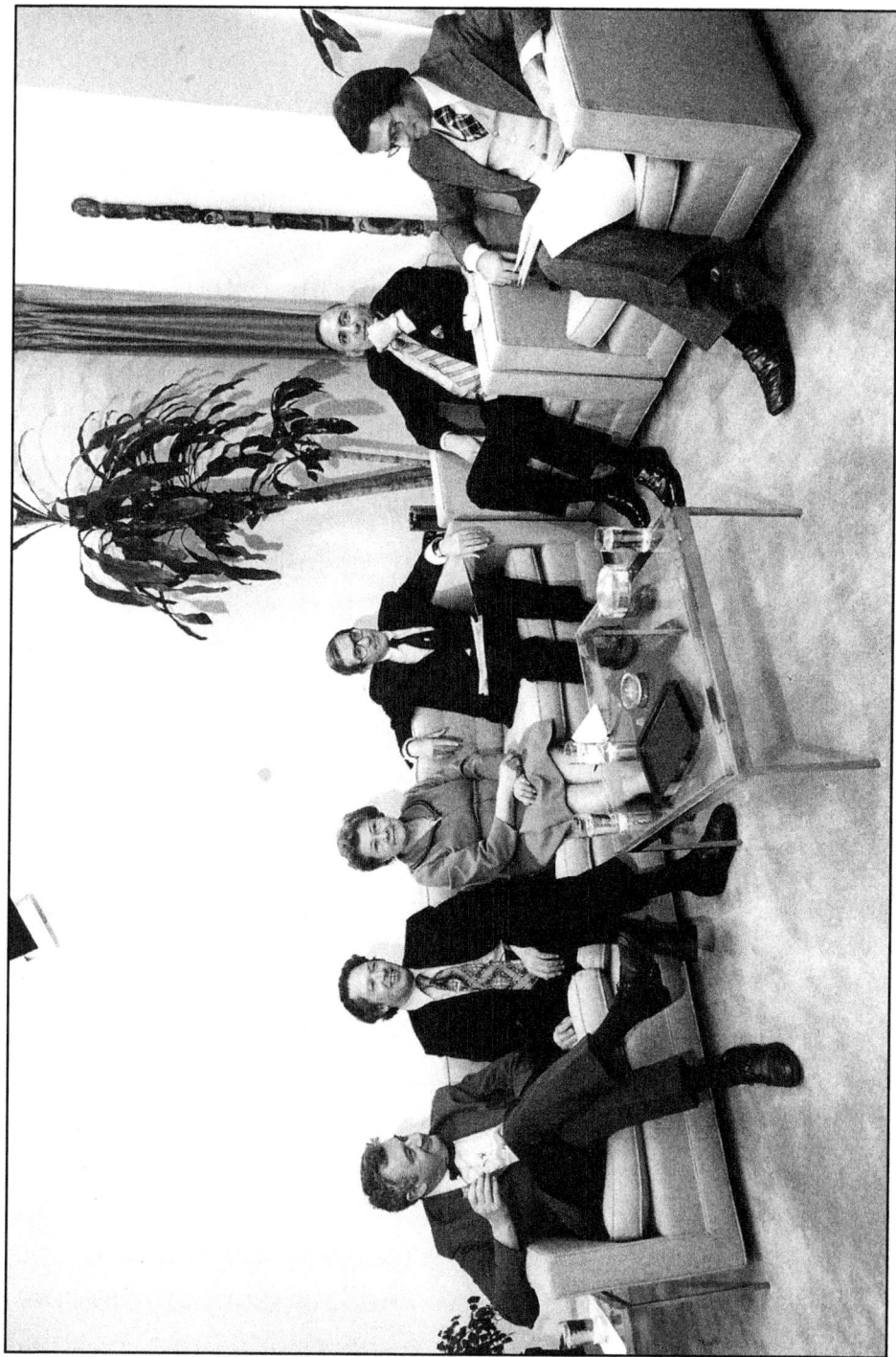

Early meeting at ABC with consultant Sam Polsky, ABC's Marvin Mord, Grace Johnson, Al Schneider ABC's Director of Broadcast Standards & Practices, Consultant Author, and ABC's Rick Gitter (from left to right).

The Hot and Busy Kitchen of Broadcast Standards and Programming

As trust developed, Sam and I were introduced to the frequently hot kitchen where top programming cooks made out their new recipes even while planning their weekly schedule far ahead for the next season's prime-time broadcasts. There was much at stake in fierce competition between the three major networks. In the ongoing battles for dominance in airtime and advertising revenue, each programming decision was painstakingly calculated to provide a network with the most viewers and highest ratings. If ABC were to be successful, its programmers would need to be resourceful and push the envelope of public and their affiliate broadcasters' acceptance. If there were no need to push the envelope, there would be no need for BS&P editors. That was the first and last thing BS&P editors needed to understand in their weekly course of modifying scripts or rough cuts and working things out together. But that was often too easy to forget in arguing over personal points of contention.

BS&P editors were engaged in the trenches during recurrent struggles with more powerfully positioned programmers and producers. Consequently, they were in need of objective and practical guidelines, if not a prescription for Prozac or a stiff drink at times. Why all the stress and tension? It was because the stakes were so high. Commercial television included such a huge and lucrative advertising business that its programming content was ultimately determined by economic factors—the bottom line of every commercial enterprise. Needless to say, once we were brought aboard, we found this consulting work with BS&P editors, and occasionally programmers at ABC, to be really interesting, often informative, and at times quite fascinating. And Al Schneider was comforted that a couple of medical and law school professors with extensive professional experience in courts and prisons were not too quick to share the popular and simplistic view that excluding violence from TV entertainment fare would solve America's worrisome problems with crime and guns in the streets, nor diminish the number of children who misbehave, steal, and bully each other in their schoolyards.

Some Dynamic Things We Learned About Commercial TV and its Viewers

Programmers, producers, and network executives understood that commercial television was catering mostly to that large category of viewers who turned to TV in an attempt to gratify their various needs for passive diversion and entertainment. Depending on their moods, feelings, and situations, viewers can select entertainment programs that are either stimulating and arousing, or relaxing and sedating, Others have special uses for TV. Consider the widespread situations and needs of many parents of young children for whom TV may provide a readily available babysitting function. In certain children's programs, serialized characters seemed at times to serve as members of the child's "extended family," conveniently summoned or invited by the push of a button. Unlike hired baby sitters, they do not need to be picked up, brought home, paid, or supplied with Coke and potato chips. The only thing that TV wanted of its viewers, whether children or adults, was that they watch and listen to its programs and its sponsors' messages.

TV Networks as Profitable Billboards for Advertising Products and Services

As the commercial networks became increasingly effective and profitable electronic billboards for advertising products and services, they substantially succeeded in influencing the public's opinions, styles, manners, fads, and purchasing preferences or habits. Perhaps of even greater significance, was television's emergence as a powerful factor and paid agent in promoting political candidates and causes through professionally-crafted broadcast messages that were produced and rehearsed as high-cost advertisements in well-funded election campaigns. Like any large commercial enterprise, TV could benefit the public, but we understood that the primary goal of network TV was to benefit its owners or shareholders. It seemed that commercial television's primary purpose was not to serve the public, but to serve the public up to the advertiser—like fresh fish caught in a barrel. The biggest catches usually went to those who produced the most attractive and popular program, or bait.

Digging In As Consultants—Violence In Children's Play and Games

Despite the general outrage over TV violence, which has only gotten worse with the more recent advent of cable TV and other mass entertainment venues, any constitutional lawyer, as well as Sam, knew that violence could not be totally expunged from TV. Moreover, as a child psychiatrist and analyst, I felt that there was a prosocial aspect or "place" for certain depictions of violence in TV entertainment fare that showed children (as well as adults) their harmful consequences in meaningful human terms. So how, and at what times, if any, should what kinds of violent depictions be broadcast to America's homes via network TV? Those were the big questions for television programmers and broadcast standards editors.

In such matters, my own focus as a child psychiatrist was on "the best interests of the child." But how might one determine the child's best interests amidst the loud clamor and conflicting views in the public and Congress? As with any appliance, tool, or toy, not to mention weapons, purchased or brought into the home by adults, the Networks argued that it was the adults' responsibility to observe and supervise TV usage by children.

All those considerations called for much discussion between Sam and me. Both of us surveyed and were familiar with the wide body of professional literature and research studies on the subject. I drew, as well, not only on my own training as a child psychiatrist and my forensic clinical experiences with violent offenders in courts and prisons, but on my own personal development as a child and teenager. Few of us are blank slates in such matters. As a teenager myself, I had been much entertained for a time by reading some extremely violent content in the pre-TV action-adventure fare of such pulp magazines as *Flying Aces*, *Doc Savage*, *The Spider*, *The Shadow*, *Weird Tales*, and yes, *Spicy Detective*, as well as *Buck Rogers* with his far-off rocket ships and death-ray guns in the comic strip section of our Sunday newspapers.

From even earlier on, closer to home as small boys in our own backyards, we frequently acted out our heroic fantasies of violence as cops and robbers, cowboys and Indians, or good guys and bad guys. We dispatched each without mercy and would lay there on the grass or back porch where we had been shot or scalped, dead or dying, but still in the game until mother called us to hurry and wash up for supper. Our death-dealing games of violence were emotional, intense, and very exciting to us as little boys, long before TV beckoned us to watch and participate passively, without all that running around and exertion.

Would the Emotional Impact of All TV-Depicted Violence Be the Same?

As for Al Schneider's request for us to identify and provide ABC with Broadcast Standards guidelines for depicting violence, Sam and I asked ourselves whether its emotional meaning and impact would be the same and rated equally in all its contexts and circumstances. Would the violent slapstick of *Charlie Chaplin* or *The Three Stooges*, for example, carry the same emotional impact as the violent physical contact of professional football or hockey players, or wholesale gunplay in gangster films? Would the devastating destruction meted out by the death ray guns of six-legged creatures from an outer space fantasy carry the same impact as a wild cowboy shoot-out? Or would the bloody clashes of armored knights or the violent sword play of *The Three Musketeers* carry the same emotional impact as the violence of an FBI skirmish with machine-gunning gangsters in familiar-looking streets? It was obvious that not all violent depictions were the same and could not be assessed or counted in the same way. In our view, the emotional impact of portrayed violence on any given TV viewer would vary according to what that viewer brings to the screen by way of life experience, and the manner and circumstances in which the violent material is portrayed.

Circumstances, Storylines, Contexts, and Portrayal Variables

Some circumstances and portrayal variables heightened or intensified the emotional impact of television-depicted violence while others diffused or dampened its impact. Broadcast Standards editors needed to identify and discuss the different circumstances and portrayal factors with the help of standard and rational guidelines in their editing work. Television allowed an episode of violence to be portrayed through a broad variety of modifying technical effects that are available for shaping and determining the context and impact of the portrayed materials. These technical resources include an almost infinite repertoire of emotional modifiers available to the director, such as the selection of background music, the choice of lens, camera position, zoom effects, close-ups, use of color or black and white, or shutter speed for slow-motion or ultra-fast depictions of the action. Additional combinations of individual story lines and contextual factors can be minimally modified to allow programmers and broadcast standards editors to creatively and cooperatively solve portrayal problems of almost any TV content. Thus, television provides the director with an instant and almost infinite technical palette with which to color or shape any piece of action.

Planning and Implementing Editing Guidelines

At our ongoing consultations, we laid out our deliberations for Al Schneider. Ordinarily reserved in his judgments, he became increasingly enthusiastic and exclaimed, "Great! These kinds of distinctions and details are just what we need in editing violent content. If you two can take the lead in helping us to outline a uniform set of practical and dynamic decision points, we'll fly you out to our West Coast group to schedule a set of seminars for you to discuss your guidelines and help train our editors to apply them."

So, Sam and I began our series of adventures in Los Angeles and meetings with Tom Kersey, Al Schneider's very capable West Coast deputy in Broadcast Standards, and his staff of dedicated BS&P editors.

ABC's West Coast Editors and Programmers

The editors were a relatively young and quite vibrant group of people, almost all of whom were college-educated as well as a few with post-graduate degrees in education or literature. They were not a bunch of thin-lipped doctrinaire critics with red or blue pencils. I generally found them to be a very congenial group of conscientious, thoughtful, and polite people who could quietly hold their own during protracted arguments with more highly paid programmers. In our monthly work with ABC's BS&P editors, which eventually went on for years, both Sam and I found ABC's editors to be every bit as stimulating and challenging as the law students and psychiatric residents that we met with academically in our clinical and classroom work at Temple.

Our seminars and discussions with ABC's West and East Coast Broadcast Standards staffs led in 1978 to ABC's publication of my book entitled *Broadcast Standards Editing*. It was, as far as we knew, the first book of its kind. As such, it was distributed to TV editors, programmers, and producers in the industry. Stockton Hellfrich of the National Association of Broadcasters had recommended the book for writers and communication students at the time, and sent me a very kind letter of appreciation.

Long before that, however, and quite early in our consultation work, in 1970, Al Schneider came to us with immediate and pressing concerns. Senator Pastore's Congressional Committee had demanded that the Surgeon General's Scientific Advisory Committee on Television and Social Behavior investigate the potential harm to children posed by their exposure to violent content on TV. What was ABC to do about that? Ignore it, stand by, or fund additional studies to demonstrate its concerns and commitment to the welfare of its child viewers?

Senator Pastore's Congressional Concerns and Demands for Research

Al confided that Leonard Goldenson, ABC's chairman and CEO, and his top brass were concerned about Senator Pastore's push for research on the effects of TV violence on children and the causal relationships between TV violence and street violence. Goldenson felt that ABC should respond to the challenge with its own study. But how? CBS and NBC had been in business longer, were more secure than ABC, and had long employed their own research psychologists. Not so at the time with ABC, which had joined the other two older, established and financially secure networks in 1953 as a "junior" needing to survive and grow. Leonard Goldenson had given Al Schneider the responsibility of selecting academics to carry out ABC's share of the massive research activities that had been stirred up by Senator Pastore's demand that the effects of violent content in TV broadcasts be studied.

Al told us about ABC's position and circumstances because he wanted to convince Goldenson and ABC's leadership that Sam and I should be independently funded to do the major share of ABC's contribution to that research. He tried to convince us, as well. Initially, Sam and I respectfully declined because our limited and independent consulting relationship was fine, but all the time Sam had. We were each thoroughly involved and happy at Temple University with our academic Unit in Law and Psychiatry, and with our efforts in establishing clinical facilities for our pioneering fellowship program in forensic psychiatry.

Although we indeed valued and enjoyed our regular consulting work with ABC, we did not wish to undertake the additional responsibility of a major, long-term study. Sam Polsky further explained that, although his own contract as a full-time tenured professor allowed him to pursue his own choice of research one day per week, his consulting work with ABC's Broadcast Standards editors already took up the bulk of that time.

Al did not give up. Pressing on, he said, "OK, I understand. You two have your University programs and teaching obligations. Look, Mel, what if you two just lay it out and design the study. Then, you and Sam can farm it out to capable people that you know. Surely, you two can do that. ABC has budgeted a million dollars to match the Surgeon General's funded studies. I can promise you complete independence, our full support, and no restraint or interference from ABC." How could we resist?

We Agreed to Design, Supervise, and Write ABC's Funded Research Study

Understandably, before committing all that money for its outside, independent research study, ABC's chairman and CEO, Leonard Goldenson, and his top brass wanted to hear and see for themselves just who these two professors were, and why it was that Vice President Schneider had so much confidence in them. And so, when Sam and I were asked to present our recommendations to ABC's top executives for carrying out the research, Al Schneider advised us that they would like to hear mostly from me as a child and forensic psychiatrist. Explaining that ABC employed enough lawyers, and that Goldenson himself was a Harvard Law graduate, Schneider suggested that they would especially like to hear about my ongoing clinical work with violent offenders in courts and prisons. This work had led to my views and hypotheses that antisocial violence in children and youth had multiple and longstanding causes, rather than blaming it on the latest suspected culprit, television programming.

Al suggested that Sam should begin with perhaps a three to five minute explanation of the study's rationale and approach to the problem, and that I should then take over and talk for approximately fifteen minutes about how we proposed to study the effects of TV-depicted violence on children's behavior. So, that was how we proceeded.

Presenting Our Research Proposal to CEO Goldenson and Staff at ABC

Sam began and did an excellent job by very briefly and concisely describing Temple's Unit in Law and Psychiatry, and our university-affiliated clinical work in courts and correctional facilities, where we had examined the case histories and developmental backgrounds and criminal behaviors of literally thousands of violent offenders over the previous decade. We had found that the actual witnessing of real violence inflicted on another person, or experiencing it as victims themselves in real time, were the most significant factors in the developmental lives of recurrently violent offenders in comparison to non-violent offenders. With their appetites whetted by Sam's well-received introduction, I was able to spell out for ABC's executives our hypotheses, research plan, and where we were coming from in non-technical language, pretty much as follows:

Our Hypotheses, Research Plan, and Where We Were Coming From

I began by posing the question: "If viewing violence in TV entertainment fare harms child viewers, in what ways might such depictions harm them? And if harmful, let us focus particularly on those children that might be especially vulnerable to any adverse effects of viewing violence in TV entertainment fare." I went on to say that TV violence cannot harm people in totally mysterious ways, like some new virus that suddenly appeared and began devastating our children and youth. If TV portrayals of violence caused particular harm to certain viewers, it could do so only in specific ways. These included the familiar psychological mechanisms of identification, imitation, and modeling, all of which might promote and encourage aggressive styles and violent means of problem-solving.

I suggested that exposing children to graphic depictions of violence on TV might risk that some of them could be emotionally stressed and overwhelmed to the point of having nightmares about violence. Other viewers might become habituated and inured to up-close "hard-core" violence, thereby blunting their compassionate regard for victims of real-world violence. Distinct harm also could result from antisocial learning, by simply demonstrating novel and potentially replicable antisocial behaviors or new criminal techniques shown on TV. In other words, "Monkey see, monkey do". But it is not always as simple as that with our children.

I added further words to the effect that, "As with our individual responses to literature, paintings, poetry, music and more, our human reactions to TV portrayals depend on what we, in our specific situations and circumstances, bring personally to the stories that we see on the screen." That much I knew as a child psychiatrist who had chatted with many dozens of young children in play therapy about their favorite Mother Goose rhymes, their scariest fairy stories, and remembered parts of strange dreams the night before.

I spoke for about ten or fifteen minutes, outlining what we would do in farming out our individual studies among a group of experienced mental health experts and clinicians working with children and youth. Then, following a nod from Al Schneider, I stopped for questions. There were a few, but most responders offered expressions of interest and approval. One gentleman, however, asked about our research experience, Sam stood up to take that one, explaining that, although our academic careers did not depend on research grants, we had done a few studies, including our five-year project on "Insanity Defense Procedures Under Federal Law," described in our NIMH research report of 1965. Then another somewhat older person, whom I took to be Leonard Goldenson himself, stood up, looked at his watch, and with a small smile and faint nod of approval, departed. Schneider spied the nod, meant for him no doubt, and seemed delighted. ABC's CEO and Chairman Goldenson and his top staff had given us well over half an hour of their very busy time and undivided attention in order to check us out, and apparently were satisfied with what they saw and heard. Sam and I received the contract for a five-year research study on TV violence and the vulnerable child.

Chapter 13
Our Research on TV Violence, Children, and Youth

Starting Our Studies on TV Violence and the Child

AS FOR THE detailed tasks of proceeding with our ABC-funded independent research studies, Sam was both frank and to the point when he said, "Look Mel, this is essentially a mental health and child psychiatric study. This project is not like our prior research on the insanity defense, which was always more of a criminal justice system problem than a basic issue in clinical psychiatry. The question of TV violence and its effects on children is primarily your field and your project. John Pastore's Senatorial committee did not call for a political or scholarly investigation of our broadcasting laws or the legal rights and responsibilities of broadcasters." Sam continued on a more personal note, pointing out that while I, as a clinical professor, was entitled to spend as much as half-time in private practice, his professorship was a full-time position that allowed only limited leeway and time to engage in private professional pursuits. So, for these very practical reasons, we both needed to realize that the on-site monitoring and coordination of our independent, sub-contracted, research studies would fall largely to me.

By way of sharing the load more equally, however, Sam proposed that it was an easy matter for him to take over the bookkeeping, financial, and administrative end, as well as to put together and write the major portion of our final report to ABC when the five-year study was completed. These were substantial jobs that he could handle from his desk while I pursued our on-site monitoring and coordination duties with our individual project supervisors and their research personnel. Wasting no time, Sam started us off by forming a private non-profit corporation to receive ABC's research funds and disperse them to the individual project members.

We called our entity the Education Research Fund (ERF), which sounded impressive. Neither of us, however, had the ambition, talent, or taste for the world of corporate finance. Our designing, sub-contracting, coordinating, and completing ABC's million dollar research study of children and television violence was as far as we ever got in the business world. We were both pretty excited, however, about our ABC research grant and the chance to prove once again that we had what it took to design and carry out another five-year research project. So, in 1970, we were ready to begin.

Having consulted with the National Association of Broadcasters (NAB) and increasingly with ABC for the two prior years, Sam and I felt that if TV entertainment programs with violent content were indeed harmful to children, then our best chances of finding evidence of that would be in focusing on groups of especially vulnerable children. Focusing on children with known emotional and learning disorders, as well as children from broken homes, would likely yield more data about the potential for harmful effects of violent content in TV's entertainment programs than would studies of well-adjusted youngsters with passing grades at school while living at home with at least one, if not two, attentive parents. Where would we find such groups of children?

We had contracted with ABC to design and oversee the research, but not to implement the study ourselves. Rather, we planned to farm out individual projects to highly qualified mental health colleagues who had clinical experience with children with emotional problems and learning disorders, as well as vulnerable children from broken homes and known juvenile offenders with antisocial behavior problems. Because of my early focus on the combined sub-specialties of child and forensic psychiatry, and my ongoing clinical work with child agencies, courts, and prisons for the past fifteen years or more, I had developed close working relationships with those kinds of mental health professionals, several of whom who now agreed to serve as independent project supervisors in our TV study.

Finding Appropriate Groups of Study Subjects

For our research about the effects of TV-depicted violence on children, I needed to find representative groups of especially vulnerable children as study subjects. As a practicing child psychiatrist, I knew most of the mental health programs and special schools that catered to the needs of children. These included facilities to which I had referred families, and from which I had sometimes received patients. I knew just where to find the groups of vulnerable children that we sought, because I had been there many times before.

I had known Lou Bernstein for a number of years when I had been a consultant at the Greentree School, formerly known as The Sklar School, on Philadelphia's Schoolhouse Lane. Lou was a kind, soft-spoken child psychologist with extensive experience and knowledge of the many kinds of psychological tests and scales used in measuring children's abilities and characteristics. Dr. Bernstein and the Greentree School's staff were pleased to participate in our TV studies. Dr. Bernstein served as the independent project supervisor of his team. I knew their special teachers and was familiar with their emotionally troubled and learning disordered students, who might be especially vulnerable to any untoward effects of viewing violent content in TV entertainment programs.

Our Study at Greentree with Emotionally Vulnerable Children

An initial group of thirty of these children were randomly selected as eager volunteers to watch a number of regular TV programs during special recess sessions. The children ranged between the ages of ten and fifteen. Five were girls and twenty-five were boys. All of them had manifest learning disabilities and difficulties in school achievement as functions of their personality problems and unfavorable environmental conditions. Although learning-disordered, none was mentally retarded. In their classroom and schoolyard behavior, some were verbally disruptive but not physically aggressive. If any children were likely to have trouble handling violent content on TV, their teachers believed that these were prime candidates.

During sixteen successive weeks, these children were shown some fifteen regular TV shows, which ABC supplied on 16mm films. Project personnel, teachers, and staff collaborated in evaluating the programs' violent content and dividing them into three categories according to their intensity and degree of aggression and violence. According to their determination, the programs ranged from such minimally violent series as *The Flying Nun* to such maximally violent series as *FBI*, *Combat*, and *Felony Squad*.

Before and after each television viewing session, the children in the study were given a number of standard psychological measures and scales dealing with variables relevant to aggression to evaluate each child's reaction to the particular program. These psychological tests and measures were in addition to the clinical assessments of the psychologists and psychiatrists, as well as the observational reports of the children's own counselors and teaching staff.

Dr. Francis Duffy and St. Joseph's Home for Boys

To include a population of vulnerable children from broken homes, we enlisted the services and clinical resources of Francis Duffy, S.J., PhD. Dr. Duffy was the director of St. Joseph's Home for Boys. This formidable and now historic edifice was built in 1929 as St. Joseph's House for Homeless Industrious Boys on Philadelphia's

West Allegheny Avenue. Dr. Duffy was a scientific colleague and Jesuit priest with a scholarly background in sociology, whom I knew to be dedicated to the service of orphaned children in need of a father, a mother, or both. I had seen a couple of youngsters from St. Joseph's Home, and regarded Dr. Duffy as a remarkably experienced clinical colleague in the long-term care and treatment of homeless children and adolescents.

Dr. Duffy agreed to be the project supervisor for a pilot study of homeless boys ranging from ten to fifteen years in age. He and his staff psychologists, Bernard Meehan and John Doney, closely coordinated their work and procedures with those of Dr. Bernstein and his staff at Greentree. Let me now hasten to briefly introduce the three other independent project supervisors in our closely coordinated and interrelated studies of the influences of TV-depicted violence on learning disordered schoolchildren.

Edward Guy MD, Project Supervisor at Philadelphia's County Prison System

Sam and I regarded ourselves as fortunate to have as well-trained and clinically-skilled a psychiatrist as Dr. Edward Guy to serve as Director of Psychiatric Services for Philadelphia's County Prison System, for which our Unit in Law and Psychiatry provided psychiatric services by contract between the County and Temple University. Dr. Guy built our county prison mental health services, ably assisted by Sheila Scott, PhD and Claude Harms, PhD, among a very dedicated and unique cadre of university-affiliated professionals with substantial experience in working with prisoners, including large numbers of youthful offenders whose developmental backgrounds and television experiences we were anxious to investigate.

Janet Hoopes, PhD, our Project Supervisor at Bryn Mawr College

Dr. Janet Hoopes, professor and director of the Psychology Department at Bryn Mawr College, conducted independent, but coordinated studies of cognitive style and its relationship to the child's perception of violent aspects of TV entertainment programs. This was a significant study of not only what children learn from TV, but how they learn it. What and how they took things from TV depended on whether they were "levelers" or "sharpeners" of the stimuli or "data" they absorbed from TV. "Levelers" tended to take in their stimuli quickly, all in a scoopful or bunch, so to speak. "Sharpeners," on the other hand, tended to focus on the stimuli in more detail, more slowly and critically, piece by piece, "sharpening" their view on individual aspects of the violent content. Our TV studies by Professor Janet Hoopes and Randal W. Wimberley exploring children's cognitive styles added the significant psychological dimensions of "levelers" and "sharpeners" to our information about what and how children learned from their TV stimuli—or what their parents might pick up as "levelers" and "sharpeners" from the perusal of their daily newspaper, for that matter.

J. Alexis Burland, MD as Project Supervisor

Last but not least of our projects included in-depth studies of children from the emotionally-troubled and learning-disordered subjects in our research sample. Professor Polsky and I chose Dr. Burland as a long-experienced clinician and highly-regarded child psychoanalyst whose perspectives on the vulnerable child's balance of ego strengths and aggressive instincts added a further dynamic dimension to the varieties of inner psychological strengths and weaknesses with which individual children viewed violent content on TV.

A Synopsis of our Results in TV Violence and Children Studies

Results of our studies of these children indicated that exposure to violent content in such TV shows as *FBI*, *Combat* and *Felony*

Squad did not lead to an increase in violent behavior. Neither the extensive battery of psychological measures and standard tests for aggression, nor the direct observations of the children's classroom teachers, counselors, and the project's research staff showed any relationship between the intensity of violent content in the TV shows and a subsequent increase in the children's aggressive behavior.

On the other hand, observing television programs with relatively more violent content produced more aggressive fantasies and thoughts in these children, as demonstrated by their picture-drawing and story-telling tests. The results of the pre-post testing and clinical evaluations in response to TV program materials indicated that inner emotions and attitudes, such as negativism, resentment, and increased suspicion of others, were stimulated by exposure to violent television content. Exposing the emotionally-impaired and learning-disordered children at Greentree School to TV-depicted violence did not, however, increase their behavior problems, nor did it decrease them, in the opinion of the raters.

In our TV studies of young adult offenders, our rationale was that young persons charged with crimes of violence, and prisoners whose institutional adjustments were marked by pugnacity may be readily identified as a youthful population that had been vulnerable or predisposed to violence. Clearly, their various forms of aggression had brought them into forceful conflict with the law. Our lengthy research on youthful offenders in the Philadelphia prison system began with an initial pilot study of thirty-five young inmates. Dr. Ed Guy and our independent TV research team at the prison studied all of the criminal justice system's information available on each offender, plus their standard psychological evaluations and clinical interviews.

As for a brief glimpse of their young prisoners' experiences with real violence, in contrast to TV-depicted violence, sixteen of the thirty-five youthful offenders had stabbed or seriously cut people, and fifteen had shot at least one other person, indicating an impressive propensity for actual violence. None of the initial group felt that television had played any causal role in the development of their antisocial and criminal behaviors. This finding, however, was in marked contrast to the instructional role that certain TV shows played in their detailed illustration of how to, and how not to perform criminal acts. Twelve of the thirty-five youthful offenders were consciously aware of acting out techniques of a crime they had seen demonstrated on television.

The time spent on the pilot study was rewarded by the development and refining of our clinical investigating techniques and data collection guides for our study of youthful offenders' experiences and responses to viewing violent content in television programs. The data collection guides served as uniform worksheets for each interviewer, and consisted of two major sections. The first section dealt with the prisoner's developmental history, antisocial background, and record of violent behavior. The second recorded his television-viewing patterns and experiences. Following the pilot study, one hundred additional subjects were chosen at random from volunteers in the younger groups of prisoners, since these were the only ones with a full lifetime of exposure to TV.

By way of a brief summary for readers interested in the makeup of the one hundred, randomly selected youthful offenders who volunteered as subjects for our TV study, the majority were African American, and the rest were of other racial minorities. Seventy-two were incarcerated while awaiting trial; twenty were sentenced, and eight were awaiting sentencing. The mean period of incarceration for the pre-trial prisoners was five to six months. Eight had been waiting trial for over a year.

As for their manner of violence and individual kinds of crime, the criminal court's breakdown of the subjects' primary charges were approximately as follows: Homicide, 32%; assault with intent to kill,

14%; burglary or larceny, 12%; robbery or aggravated robbery, 32%; rape or assault with intent to rape, 7%; assault and battery, 3%. All of these violent defendants grew up with TV in their homes.

As for their developmental backgrounds, half the subjects came from intact families. Thirty-three were raised by just their mother, one by just his father, and fourteen grew up in one or more foster homes. Most were from large families. Thirty-eight were from families receiving partial or total help from the Department of Public Assistance. Sixty-nine of the subjects, by their own rating, grew up in a high crime area. Seventy-three belonged to a gang, forty-seven of whom had more than three years of membership. Gang membership correlated higher with their level violence than any other variable in our study.

Regarding television's influence on their criminal behavior, twenty-six of these subjects reported trying criminal techniques they had seen on television. The main TV source for twenty of these young men was a series called *It Takes a Thief*. This was a show in which the fictitious criminal succeeds in daring and well-thought-out criminal plans. Only three of the youthful offenders reported failing or getting caught while using television-inspired techniques.

Along with our TV studies concerning emotionally-troubled children with learning disorders, and matching studies of children from broken homes, Dr. Guy expanded our investigations of violent youthful offenders with an additional study of one hundred and thirty-five randomly selected, youthful prisoners ranging in age from sixteen to twenty-seven (mean age of twenty-two),with findings consistent with those of his first group of young offenders.

My View of How Things Stood in My Work at Age Fifty

The first two years of our five-year project had been especially productive and busy ones for me since I needed to do weekly site visits at each of the independent project locations. As time went on, the independent project managers coordinating their work and findings with each other were increasingly on their own. Sam's and my work was done except for ongoing monitoring, and the major task of organizing and writing up the final report. And so, in 1972 at age fifty, how was I situated in my career?

I was at the top of my game academically as a clinical professor of psychiatry, co-directing Temple's Unit in Law and Psychiatry as well as our new Fellowship Program in Forensic Psychiatry, with its well-integrated clinical teaching resources in Philadelphia courts and correctional facilities. In addition to my private practice with individual patients, I was the psychiatric consultant in Broadcast Standards and Practices to a major television network. What more could I have asked for in my body of work? On that note, let's leave my body of work and look now at the ongoing work of my body— my family, our domestic life, and friends.

Chapter 14
Family Snapshots in the Home, 1960s and 1970s

WHEN I LAST described our family life in these pages, Jane and I were in our newly built Wynnefield Heights row home with our three-year-old son, David, and our infant daughter, Joan. It was that busy and happy time in life when the days seem to fly by. Suddenly, our sweet infant Joan had grown into a blond, curly-haired, three-year-old chatter-box, and her big brother Dave was in first grade at his neighborhood school in Belmont Hills. What about Jane, their busy young mother?

Jane and Her Agenda

Jane was putting the final touches on her happy job of tastefully furnishing and decorating out new little row-home. While doing so she had made a number of new friends with whom she shared recipes, and bits of choice news about their young married and child-rearing worlds. She was also taking an art appreciation course with the highly regarded and strongly opinionated Ms. Violette de Mazia at the famous Barnes Estate nearby. We had found a number of compatible couples with whom we shared our few weekly hours of essential leisure time. What next? I knew what I wanted to do with my life, and was doing it. Jane did too.

Although she had thought she ought eventually to obtain a postgraduate degree and pursue some kind of professional career, nothing seemed quite right. One day, she stopped debating with herself and announced to me that she had decided there was nothing more she'd rather do than to have a third child, and would I cooperate to make that happen? Of course, I'd even be more than willing to cooperate, but are you sure that's what you really want? I asked. What about law school and sharing my forensic interests as husband and wife? No, she did not want to go to law school like Tim Beck's wife, Phyllis. And no, even though she enjoyed interior design and architecture, she did not want another degree. What she definitely wanted now was another baby.

Who was I to argue, or shirk my marital duty of pleasing a wife in urgent need of service rather than my male need for love-making? Writing these words at age ninety-three, after a long life, it seems that the most passion I had was with a woman who somehow felt I could give her something that money could not buy—like a happy home and a baby. Unfortunately, achieving that human dream takes a lot more work and ongoing devotion than getting pregnant. But pregnant she got.

It was after three months of her patiently determined ardor that Jane greeted me with a kiss and a contented smile from ear to ear. Glad to see a happy wife, I washed up and poured myself a scotch. When I returned and the kids were upstairs, Jane stage-whispered, "Guess what, Daddy. I saw the gynecologist today, and I am completely, thoroughly, and officially pregnant!" Somehow she looked as gratified and satisfied as the proverbial cat that swallowed the mouse. It was no mouse that her contented belly contained, but our baby Paul, off to a great start in what would become a most successful, interesting, and broadly gratifying life. My reproductive efforts, as well as academic career, and private practice, were doing well. It was time to sell Wynnefield Heights and move up.

Jane's Cuisine

Jane tried, but was not successful at breastfeeding. So she switched to formulas and warmed bottles served with love. This interest in formulas and food preparation seemed to have spread beyond breastfeeding and was somehow carried over to the dining table. The result for all of us was that Jane became an outstanding cook of good food, tastefully prepared and attentively served. I came increasingly to appreciate the diligent and artful interest that my wife had taken in cooking.

Gourmet cooking was initially a hobby that Jane enjoyed for many years, but which she later pursued part-time professionally when she catered such limited but elegant affairs as omelet parties. These were for a chosen clientele of people to whose homes she would bring a small amount of her own equipment and ingredients to create, demonstrate, and serve the most delicious and aromatic choice of omelets that could be found on Philadelphia's Main Line. This was not a large business and was mainly known only to her increasing circle of friends. The result for our children was to grow up in the care of a devoted homemaker and mother, and a memorable cook who learned her first food skills from Alva, Jane's mother's cook in New Haven.

Continuing to Grow With Our Kids on Flat Rock Road in Penn Valley

By the time Paul, our youngest, was born in 1961, we had found our definitive family home. It was in an upscale Main Line neighborhood called Penn Valley, where it stood nicely on the corner of Sprague and Flat Rock Road. It was a well built, two-story farmhouse-colonial to which the prior owner had added an additional large living room with a pan ceiling and a huge picture window that overlooked the distant lights of Philadelphia's Center City high-rises from its green suburban hilltop lawn some four miles away. The attached garage and back driveway were shielded from the large rear yard by a tall white fence, which featured an espalier apple tree and other plantings. Jane and I loved the place, which compared favorably with her parents' impressive home, and was far above the middle-class apartment rentals in which I had grown up in Boston's Roxbury and Jamaica Plain neighborhoods. Although we had the many adjoining fields of Boston's Franklin Park in which to play ball when I was a boy, here in Penn Valley I now had a beautiful flat front yard on which to toss footballs and baseballs with my young son, David, from the time he could catch and throw a ball until he went off to college at University of Rochester.

Pushing Dave

David was a fairly good athlete and I pushed him to be even better. Pushing Dave in every way I thought might advantage him was one of my larger faults, as I look back on these snapshots of him and me. I bought him a piano and drove him weekly to Mt. Airy in Philadelphia for a piano lesson with Mrs. Levingood, a very skilled classical pianist who worked patiently with David. He did well for a time under Mrs. Levingood's tutelage, and in due course was able to play violin-piano sonatas with me.

By 1972, David had turned seventeen. Having kept at least one foot on the ground during the youth-troubled sixties, he was bright, strong, healthy, a good reader, but not a top student at the Haverford School. Despite my efforts to interest him in Tufts, my alma mater, he chose to go his own way and signed up for the University of Rochester, which had been recommended by one of his Haverford School advisers. It would take David a while to find himself, and even longer to open up and confide in me.

Joan and Paul

Our two additional blessings were Joan, then age fourteen, and Paul, age eleven. Joan was cheerful and always had a wonderful imagination with a dramatic flair. She also had a sweet singing voice that grew to sound a bit like Joan Baez when she became a teenager and played the guitar. She was a born songster who reminded me of my Ma when I was little. With two sons, and only one daughter, need I tell you that she was the apple of my eye?

As for Paul, he seemed to have grabbed the best genes from both sides of the family tree. He was a cute baby and everyone loved him when he was little. When Joan was six or seven, she adored her three-year-old brother, and like a little school teacher, she dressed him in various dramatic costumes to enact heroic or magical roles from children's stories. I remember coming home one evening to find Jane laughing as she prepared dinner. Joan had made a beard of white cotton batten and pasted it quite expertly over Paul's chin and cheeks. With a pillow stuffed into the waist band of his red pajama pants and his normally bright pink complexion, he made a cheerful Santa Claus for the evening. All our adult friends took kindly to Paul. At eleven, he was a bright and capable youngster with enough mechanical skill to enable him to earn after-school money in a bike shop. Where did the time go and what would become of them, I sometimes wondered as I left for the office in the morning. But they were healthy, and were doing well enough at school and at play with friends. What more could a father want by way of life's dividends?

Chapter 15
Friendships, Acquaintances, and Further Developmental Years

Circles of Friends

IN ADDITION TO old friends who predated our marriage, Jane and I made new friends among mutually compatible couples, as well personal friends of our own with whom we shared special interests. Among all my adult friendships, Sam Polsky was by far my closest friend, trusted confidant, professional ally, and colleague. We not only taught and thought alike, but shared almost everything else as working buddies with mutual interests and values that bound us together.

Different circles of friends that grew from my shared professional interests in law and psychiatry provided additional perspectives and variety in our social lives. Because of my subsequent and growing faculty relationship with Dr. O. Spurgeon English, he and his wife, Ellen, became academic friends. Jane and I looked forward to their annual Christmas parties, which featured much music, libation, and laughter. Spurge, as we all called him, was a born and versatile musician who played a number of instruments surprisingly well, including the accordion, banjo, piano, and guitar. Our friend, Dr. Kenny Gordon, another young analyst of note, and a talented sculptor, played both the clarinet and flute. The holiday crowd included many of our fine Temple faculty in the Department of Psychiatry, in which Spurge English served as chairman, friend, and mentor during what we felt were its best years. Within the Department's cordial frameworks, there sometimes developed smaller, even closer groups of friends, who would share special interests and clinical research projects.

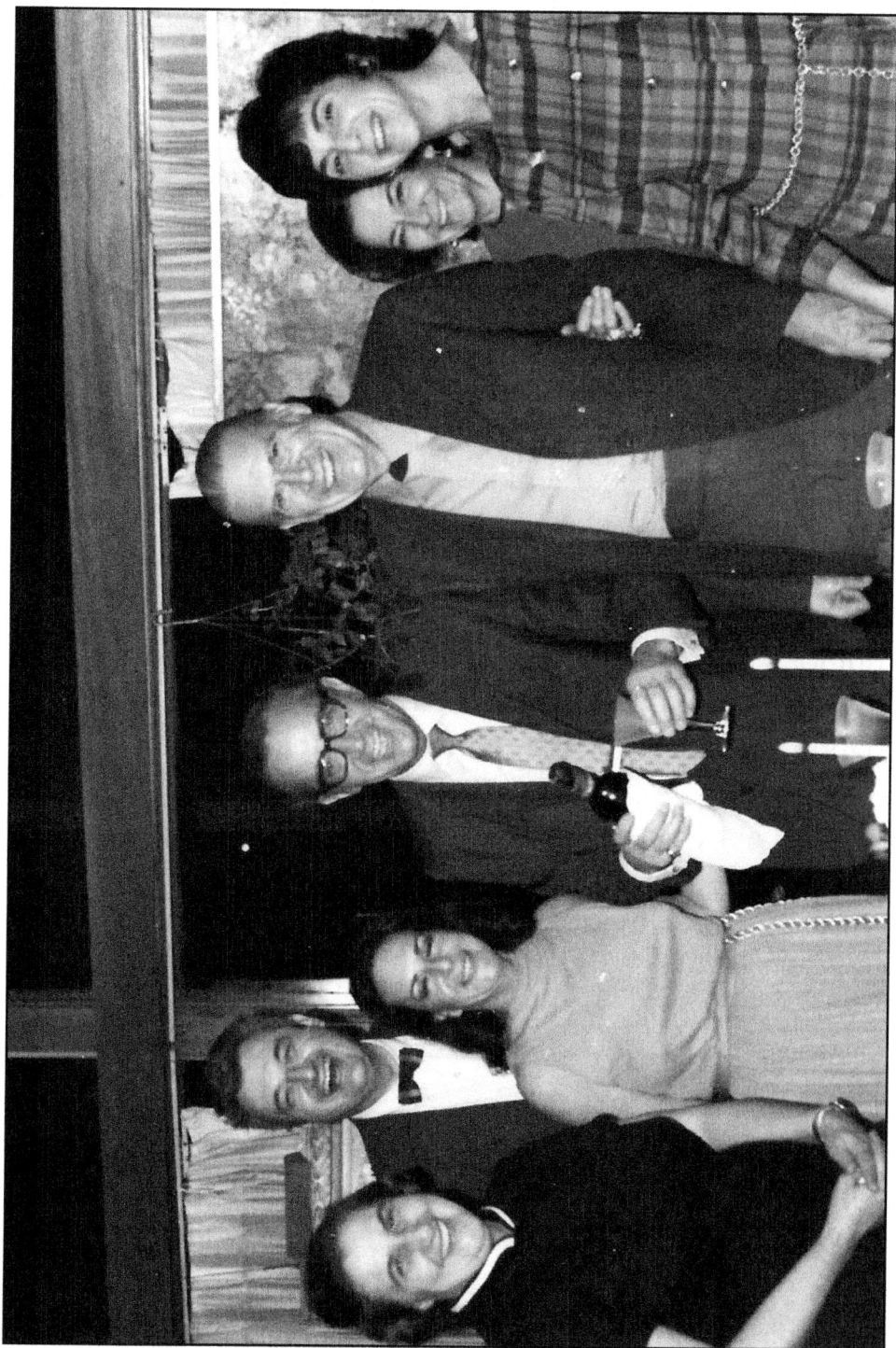

Partying with (from left to right) Doris and Sam Polsky, Joan and Gene Crane, Dr. O. Spurgeon English, wife Ellen, and Author's wife, Jane.

Marty, Rita, and a Special Circle of Friends

Perhaps like ripples in a pond, this small circle of social friends began with our acquaintance with a compatible couple, like Marty and Rita Eisenberg, whom Jane and I met when we brought our children to learn something about the spiritual lives and religious legacy of their forebears at Temple Beth David in Wynnefield. Jane and Rita shared many interests as mothers of young children and homemakers for busy husbands, while Marty and I found each other sufficiently interesting for us to hit it off with each other as a foursome.

Marty was a business man, which was a change of pace for me and my professionally-oriented groups of doctors and lawyers. However, Marty had an equal and insightful interest in people, not as patients or clients, but as customers and consumers. Moreover, in my eye, Marty bore a strong physical resemblance to Woody Allen, in addition to displaying a similarly insightful and philosophical sense of humor. Also, as an unneeded but welcome bonus, Marty enjoyed pouring a generous glass of scotch on the rocks with perhaps a splash of club soda or water. If I sipped and graciously commented that it was a rather good scotch, he'd cock his head quizzically and ask, "Tell me. Have you ever had a bad scotch?" How could one find a more pleasant pal than that for a relaxing evening?

Marty was similarly adept at his work. He owned and personally managed a large furniture and appliance store in South Philadelphia, His success was due in no small part to his keeping up with styles, customers' needs and shopping habits, as well as economic trends, and current events, all of which impinged on my overall interests in human behavior, which, in turn, intrigued Marty. He was particularly interested in our attending certain movies together, and asking me afterwards for my psychiatric and analytic insights about the characters and situations. I think that was about as close to therapy as Marty ever came. So how did this grow into a circle of friends for Jane and me?

Marty had referred Dr. Ed Guy to me for potential employment at

Temple University's program in forensic psychiatry at a time when Dr. Guy was in search of a new direction and change of scene in his psychiatric practice. Dr. Guy, who was already an experienced clinician, had such leadership potential that Sam Polsky and I hired him, and placed him in charge of the forensic psychiatric program at the County Prison System, where he grew rapidly to become one of the most capable and gifted physicians working in the difficult and challenging field of correctional psychiatry. Ed soon became not only a valued colleague at Temple, but a personal friend in a small new circle of special acquaintances and interesting people, beginning with his new wife, Pat.

Dr. Ed and Pat Guy

Pat and Ed Guy each had been married before, with growing children from their marriages. Pat had two teenage children, who chose to live with Pat and Ed at the breakup of her marriage to their father, the details of which I knew nothing. It was rumored that she had been a patient of Ed's and that the breakup had been messy, but I never probed or made judgments about their pre-marital lives. As Jane and I understood and observed their situation from the time we first met them, it was our opinion that it was an intense and mutual love affair that brought them to their second marriage, which, as the years went by, turned out to be a successful, happy, and fortunate union. I am told that both Pat and Ed have predeceased me at this elder point in my life. I remember them fondly, among a now departed and sorely missed circle of special friends that also included George Thompson, Adelaide Bry, and Gene and Joan Crane. So a few more recollections of this special group of friends might be in order, continuing with George Thompson and Adelaide Bry.

George Thompson and Adelaide Bry

George Thompson and Adelaide Bry co-habited more peacefully and pleasantly than sinfully they felt. George, a golfing buddy of Ed

Guy, shared such a remarkable resemblance to the famed movie actor, James Stewart, that people would boldly approach him for his autograph at airports and restaurants. He handled it with aplomb and grace. George was an extremely likable and bright person, who sold real estate for a living.

Adelaide Bry was both an introspective and very sociable person, and a writer who could interview people without their realizing it, and write about them as thinly disguised characters in her stories. Adelaide was a tolerant but shrewd observer of human nature, while she pursued a broad range of personal interests, as did the others in this small group. Accordingly, there never seemed to be a shortage of things to talk about, and we met frequently, mostly at Pat and Ed's interesting house. Pat was a rather creative interior decorator. She was also a creative cook, and both she and Ed enjoyed entertaining our group of friends in their newly shared home. Jane and I also enjoyed hosting these friends in our recently purchased Penn Valley home.

Our meetings at each other's abodes were frequently augmented by occasional mini-vacations, shared trips to the Jersey shore at Cape May, as well as Jamaica and other Caribbean resorts. Jane especially enjoyed travel; unlike me, she loved to read guide books and make detailed plans for our trips. Travel seemed to be a way that Jane celebrated life, and so perhaps a note about our not infrequent family travel seems to be in order in these memoirs.

Some Early Travel Times in our Heller-Harris Generations

I was not a widely traveled or tourist-minded person by nature, except perhaps for wandering leisurely through the pages of good books about other places and times. Lest you think, however, that my busy office days had been all work and no play, we actually did more than a bit of traveling, too. Jane succeeded in getting me to take her to Europe as soon as Dave and Joan were old enough to spend some summer weeks in Connecticut with her parents, before our youngest child, Paul, was born. And Jane's continued enthusiasm for foreign travel was such that in 1965, she got us to enroll in a memorable Temple University-sponsored faculty tour of the Greek Isles, with the choice of several subsequent days in either Israel or Jordan.

Equally memorable had been Bob and Florence Abrahams' invitation to spend a week as their guests in their historic former sugar plantation on the Caribbean Island of Nevis, adjoining St Kitts. Robert Abrahams was chief counsel for the Public Defender Association, which had partially funded our research study on the legal interview back in 1957. Nevis was known mainly as the birthplace of Alexander Hamilton. Known by fewer persons, but of great interest to Florence Abrahams, Nevis and other Caribbean Islands had been inhabited by Sephardic Jews in early colonial times. It was Florence Abrahams' hobby to collect evidence of this Jewish migration, and she delighted in discovering Jewish ritual menstrual baths called mikvahs, which resembled miniature swimming pools, in the excavated remains of former Jewish settlements in the Caribbean islands. So travel, I learned, sometimes provided as much or more of an education as it did a vacation for me.

I think that my wife inherited her love of travel from her father, Dr. Benedict R. Harris, a clinical professor of medicine and cardiologist at Yale. He had taken himself to Europe as a young man for additional medical training with the famous cardiologist, Dr. Johan Mönckeberg. Later, in 1940, at the age of forty-one and too old to be drafted, he felt it was his duty as a doctor to volunteer for the Navy, where he served as a lieutenant commander on the hospital ship USS Haven, stationed in the Pacific. He was subsequently promoted to Commander. His ship was assigned to go into Nagasaki and Hiroshima right after the nuclear bombs fell there. Much later, my then father-in-law and the maternal grandfather of my children again left his successful private practice as a middle-aged cardiologist to take himself off to Japan for two years (1967 to 1969) to serve as medical director of the U.S. Atomic Bomb Casualty Commission in Hiroshima.

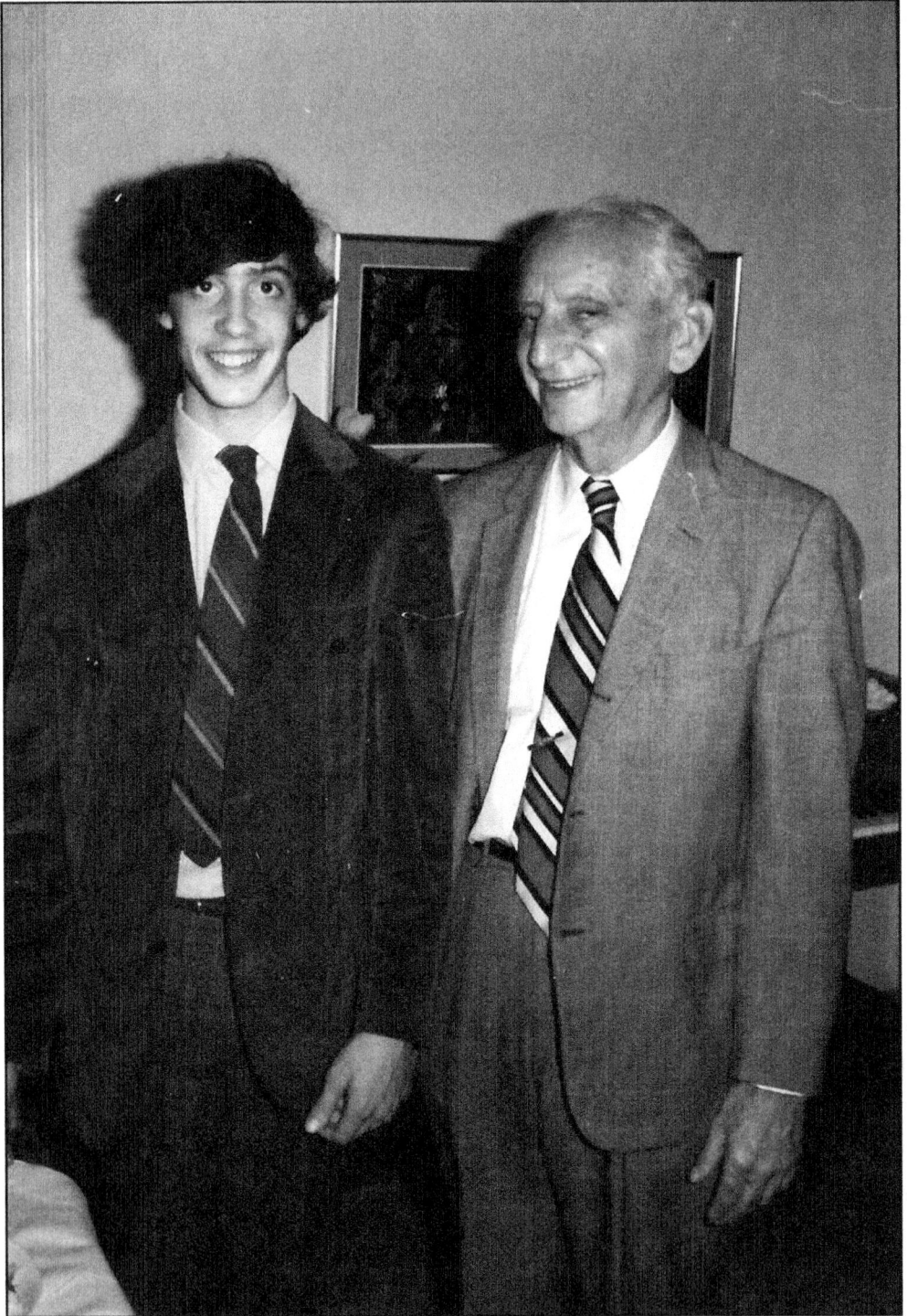

Benedict R. Harris, MD and his first grandchild, David Harris Heller at age thirteen (1967).

Jane's mother was aghast at the prospect of leaving their lovely suburban home in Woodbridge, Connecticut to live halfway up an unknown hillside in Hiroshima. Neither would she allow her good husband to run off without her to live by himself for two years, U.S. Atomic Bomb Casualty Commission or not. Would you believe that this sweet and very wise woman, who would be my dear mother-in-law for some twenty years, came back raving about Japan and Hiroshima, where she had found an old potter, locally famed, who invited her to study his craft with him for a time. She then urged Jane and me to send our two older children to her for the summer to share an adventure with their Grandma and Grandpa Harris in Hiroshima instead of an overnight camp in Pennsylvania. So Jane packed them off to Hiroshima for what I hoped would be a fabulous opportunity for our thirteen-year-old son David to play Little League baseball with Japanese boys while our ten-year-old Joan created Japanese pottery with her Grandma Pearl. What a story for Joan to tell her girlfriends in Penn Valley when she got back—or even now in Baltimore, where some of her friends are now grandmothers themselves.

What about Jane and travel to Asia with saké or tea and me back then? Not to be outdone, Jane subsequently booked a Far East trip for us to explore Japan, Thailand, and Hong Kong for ourselves. And so, by 1967 or so, we all had traveled some considerable distances from home during the first dozen years of our marriage while making babies and friends, and as I pursued my academic and private practice careers.

Eventually, my father-in-law's favorite and recurrent destinations would become the more limited and closely circumscribed putting greens of the Woodbridge Country Club's lovely golf course. But as he aged, he got increasingly waylaid in its many sand traps and gave up golf for good to watch baseball or golf tournaments on TV in the cool and quiet comfort of his private study at home. A similarly diminished, but fortunate elder fate would await me, as I type and ponder these words in a retirement facility. However, as for our own travels circa 1970, Jane and I were soon to take a memorable and very privileged Mediterranean cruise aboard an elegant private yacht. This was a result of our growing friendship with Gene and Joan Crane, and Joan's close friendship with Simone Korchin.

Meet Gene and Joan Crane

It was through Pat and Ed Guy that we met Gene and Joan Crane, Pat's former brother-in-law and sister-in law, with whom Pat maintained a close and ongoing relationship following her divorce from Gene Crane's brother, who was the father of Pat's two early-teenage children. To add seemingly further insult and injury to Gene Crane's brother, both of his and Pat's children chose to live with their mother and her new husband, Dr. Ed Guy. Gene Crane appeared to handle all this recent family drama quite calmly, perhaps because he was professionally unflappable as a popular TV anchorman on Philadelphia's CBS news and weather programs.

Gene's wife, Joan, also had a professional background in television. She had done roles in popular children's programs, and she and Gene knew numerous people in Philadelphia's arts and entertainment community who were not part of Jane's or my particular crowd. Let me hasten to add that Gene and Joan were blessed with an only child, David Crane, who was in his early teens when Jane and I met him. David Crane went on to do his parents proud by achieving huge success and lasting acclaim in his own right as a writer, director, and producer of the long-running NBC television series, *Friends*. On that happy note, let me get back to the time when Gene and Joan were still raising David and pursuing their own friendships that might have made for slightly different episodes than the ones depicted in their son's subsequent sitcom.

Gene and Joan Crane were Friends with Barney and Simone Korchin

Now our circle enlarged through Gene and Joan Crane's links to another couple, Barney and Simone Korchin. What Jane and I learned about the Korchins was told to us by Gene and Joan Crane. As I understood things from Gene, Barney Korchin had retired as a vice president at Penn Fruit a few years earlier, in good shape both financially and physically. Barney enjoyed traveling in Europe and became increasingly interested in purchasing contemporary European art from French and Italian painters who were not yet commanding top prices.

Joan Crane told us that Barney's wife, Simone, was her good friend, and was French. As a Jewish teenager adrift in the streets during the German occupation of France, Simone had survived by good fortune and her wits in such enterprises as filching unfinished cigarette butts from idle ash trays and then re-rolling their remaining tobacco in new cigarette paper to sell to people desperate for a smoke in Nazi-occupied France. Joan also described how Simone developed into a beautiful and talented young woman, for whom it would be only a matter of time before she would meet and marry the "right kind of man." He turned out to be an American service man, Barney Korchin, who whisked her home with him to America. Not only was Barney handsome, quick, and smart, but Jewish, too. You can picture the rest, as I needed to, while Joan skipped happily ahead to more recent times when the Cranes and Korchins became such good friends that Simone and Joan easily convinced their husbands that the four of them should start an art gallery business.

And why not? Joan explained that Barney was comfortably retired and enjoyed traipsing through Europe in search of promising new painters. Simone and her close friend Joan were both at home, much interested in art, and available to open an art gallery. Gene Crane's broadcast schedule also would allow him some time to participate. So, the four of them in partnership opened two galleries at high end locations: one in Bala Cynwyd, Pennsylvania, to be run by Joan, and the other in Manhasset, Long Island, to be run by Simone. Their circle of friends would soon widen once more.

It so happened that Simone's gallery was next door to the hairdressing establishment frequented by the wife of William Levitt, who, not long before, had sold his famously successful home-building business to IT&T, a huge American conglomerate run by the very capable Harold Geneen, making William Levitt the largest single stockholder of IT&T and one of the richest men in the United States. No longer running his own business, and with a bit of time on his hands while awaiting his wife at her hairdresser's shop, Levitt wandered out of curiosity into the recently opened Crane-Korchin Art Gallery next door. And there, among all those beautiful, interesting, and hopefully irresistible works of art on display, what caught his eye the most, and unsettled him, was Simone herself.

William Levitt, Navy veteran, experienced and successful business man, had been unsettled once, many years before, by a long affair with his present wife, who had been his secretary and much more during his first twenty or thirty-year marriage. It would take a Simone to unsettle William Levitt a second time. He now had everything a man might want that money could buy: an impressive thirty-room estate on well-tended acres, complete with a new tennis court and elegant swimming pool, as well as a huge, well-kept, private yacht with crew, and respected friends in high places. But with all this in his enviable domain, Bill Levitt fell in love. As Joan told us Simone's story, it would take more than a yacht and William Levitt's super salesmanship to entice Simone into an affair and unhinge her from Barney.

Joan's Story of Bill and Simone

William Levitt, in love with Simone, courted her avidly. Joan explained that it was not just Bill's wealth that unhinged Simone.

She and Barney were hardly poor. Rather it was Levitt's ardor and persistence in pursuing his love for Simone after she hurled away and rejected his initial proposals for less than a marital commitment. Joan, as Simone's close friend, ally, and art gallery partner, was understandably concerned for her, but must have relished her own role as Simone's trusted female confidante, as when Simone confided to Joan critical moments in her high stakes drama with Bill. For example, after his courting her for a number of passionate days and nights of cruising under the stars, while under way and alone on the fantail of his yacht, Bill presented Simone with a most impressive ten-carat diamond ring from the famed New York jeweler, Harry Winston. Joan related that Bill had not, however, placed it on her finger, but in her hand. Simone held it in her open hand for several moments while looking both at her lover and the $30,000 rock he had handed her, and then this beautiful woman and former refugee from France, spun on her heels and hurled his sparkling gem into the sea. Joan told me, as though she had actually witnessed it, that Simone stood there unblinking and steadfast as Bill watched in disbelief the disappearance of the diamond and its box into the deep, dark sea.

I can mention these very human, dramatic, and psychologically meaningful matters, as told to me by Joan and Gene, because neither the Cranes, nor Bill or Simone, nor any of the people mentioned here have ever been patients of mine, nor consulted with me professionally. As we age well into our nineties, I hear from none of them, and I was told that Bill died in 1994. As for Bill, a nationally prominent person, much of his lifestyle and biography are public information, to which I wish to add nothing more than my fond and respectful recollections of the short time I knew Bill Levitt personally. He was a quickly passing friend, and a prominent person in the socially rarified atmosphere so infrequently encountered close up in most people's everyday lives, including our own. But for the Cranes, Jane and I would never have met Bill and Simone, nor been invited aboard their yacht. This is how it happened.

Meeting Bill and Simone Levitt at Gene and Joan's Party

Jane and I met Bill and Simone Levitt at a small party at Gene and Joan Crane's house, which was a short distance from ours in Penn Valley. We had been there several times before with our small circle of friends, who frequently entertained each other in our homes, as I mentioned earlier. This time, Gene and Joan's lovely home was literally festooned with excellently framed new paintings, which impressively stretched from wall to wall, covering every bit of available space. It was, of course, the overflow of impressive art with which Barney Korchin had stocked the Crane-Korchin galleries in Bala Cynwyd and Manhasset. Gene was busy pouring drinks while Joan went about introducing Bill and Simone to our circle of friends. Pat Guy may or may not have met Simone a time before with Joan at their Manhasset gallery, but I am not certain. What I am sure of is that it was the first time Jane and I met the Levitts, that they were each charming individuals, that Gene kept the wine flowing, and that it was one of the best parties that Gene and Joan had hosted for our group.

Bill and Simone sparkled while speaking with us and our friends, as though they had known us all for as long as they had known Gene and Joan. Bill took the time to spend more than a few minutes with Jane and me, talking mostly about my work in law and psychiatry and how I got into it. I explained it a bit, and told him that the country desperately needed him to build a specially designed Levittown for the correctional system, instead of wastefully constructing high-cost federal penitentiaries and state prisons. He almost choked on a stuffed olive, laughing at my suggestion, and returned the compliment by saying that he wished we had met before he sold his company to IT&T and, had he stayed in his own business, that we would have made good partners. Bill Levitt was not quite old enough to be my father, but I guessed he was a good fifteen years my senior. I was flattered that he liked my joke and spent a few more minutes alone with me talking about his appreciation of his good health.

A Surprise Invitation from Bill Levitt for a Cruise

I was surprised about ten days later when a lady phoned to ask if I had time to talk with William Levitt. Since I was not with patients, but reading reports at the moment, I told her it was a good time to talk. So, he got on the line and said he was planning a small party and would Mrs. Heller and I like to be guests on his yacht, with Gene and Joan Crane and perhaps another couple or two, for a ten-day Mediterranean cruise this coming August? Knowing that Jane would be thrilled, I cannot remember accepting an invitation more quickly. Jane was not only thrilled, but in immediate need of more input about dress and other essential information, especially when travelling with the likes of William Levitt. So Jane quickly called Joan Crane, who had cruised with Levitt before, and had been tipped off, she said, that we would be invited to complete a party of eight for the cruise. I shall spare you the details of Joan's tips to Jane, except to note that aside from casual, relaxed cruise wear, Joan advised that an evening gown and tuxedo would be wise additions for this particular trip. How wise, practical, and essential, I thought, were such wives in social situations like this when all I had wondered was what reading material and which camera and what lenses I should bring.

Our Mediterranean Trip on a Magic Carpet

Because it is too good a story to keep you waiting any longer, let me get you as quickly aboard with us as I can. We flew to Rome where we were picked up by one of Levitt's crew and transported to the harbor where Levitt's boat was docked when cruising the Mediterranean. It was an impressive-looking yacht which bore the name *Les Amis*. I guessed her to be about one hundred and fifty feet long, and had never seen a neater looking boat. One of the crew subsequently told me that Levitt had purchased it from the president of the Johnson and Johnson corporation a few years back, that he had done it completely over from stem to stern, and that you couldn't find a more ship-shape yacht (his very words) anywhere along the Mediterranean. I rarely took a sailor's story about a boat or a fish at face value, but it was clear that he was most impressed with the owner's policy of sparing no expense in maintaining the quality of his ship and its crew.

Sailor's stories aside, I knew only what I saw with my own eyes or heard with my own ears, such as the engines purring like a kitten when idling, or thrumming evenly at high speeds. My eyes saw a well-managed boat and its crew being supervised by a former U.S. naval officer with enough Seabee experience and executive ability to build and manage large sub-divisions or small villages (called Levittowns) for America's returning WWII veterans. Levitt's little project called *Les Amis* was just a wealthy man's nautical hobby for relaxing with his friends.

Meet the Captain and the Crew

Be a friend, come aboard. Meet the Captain and the crew. The first persons to politely welcome us board were two huge crew men, who I was told were from Samoa. They were smoothly built like heavyweight wrestlers, but they could have passed for massive sumo wrestlers at the early stages of training for the Japanese super weight championship. When aboard *Les Amis* with his guests, Levitt maintained his full crew with nautical and mechanical abilities as well as stewards with housekeeping skills, and even a fine French cook whom he apparently tempted to leave a hot inland kitchen on city streets for a more relaxed, cooler, and well-paying position aboard a luxurious private yacht.

Captain Heinz

The most unusual and unexpected person I encountered among Levitt's crew was its captain, called Heinz. I never knew whether Heinz was his first name or his last. And now, writing these words so many years later, I do not know if there is anyone still alive to ask for more details about him. I remember being absolutely astonished when Levitt's crew members told me that Captain Heinz had been a WWII German submarine commander, and the only U-Boat skipper in Hitler's Mediterranean submarine fleet to survive that naval war. I felt tempted, but did not feel in a position, as Levitt's guest, to ask him about why and how he came to hire Captain Heinz, of all people. But I do remember wondering if the good Lord had indeed arranged for this former Nazi U-Boat commander to be the only submarine captain to survive the destruction of Hitler's Mediterranean submarine fleet only to serve as captain of a luxury yacht owned by a self-made, very wealthy Jewish-American builder of homes for returning WWII veterans.

As I say, I do not know the facts, but I lived with Heinz and Levitt for a week or more aboard the yacht and got to know them both. I remember them as though it were yesterday. Captain Heinz was a very alert and highly intelligent gentleman, of average height, with pale blue eyes. He was an objective and self-disciplined person, but seemed also to be given to introspection and self-examination. This latter tendency was enhanced perhaps because of his knowledge that I was a psychiatrist. We had a number of contacts under various circumstances. For example, it was a nautical courtesy for a ship's captain like Heinz to be invited when we visited other people's yachts for small parties with drinks and music, and a chance to dance with the ladies.

Heinz loved to dance very politely with all the ladies, and had nothing against a few drinks, which he downed less politely and rather quickly on the side. This seemed to make his eyes get red, and his mind wander to matters of courage. And as the couples danced to the slow, dreamy music we preferred, Heinz would glide with his lady dance partner toward Jane and me to briefly whisper the word "Courage," and then dance away, only to circle the room and re-appear to whisper in his German accent, "Courage, Doktor, is a vooman vid-out hair (a woman without hair)." And then he would once again dance off, only to reappear with a different dance partner and another drink to suggest that, "Courage is a vio-leen vid-out shtrings (a violin without strings)," and dance away once more.

Maybe what he was trying to come to grips with was that "courage is a German U-Boat without torpedoes, lying submerged with little remaining air, under a threatening sky controlled by Allied aircraft, and a stormy sea patrolled by the enemy's destroyers." I don't know if that was a cause of his obsession with the rare and valued coin of courage, or its opposite side of cowardice and fear—but I liked Heinz. There wasn't a Nazi bone left in his body. I wished I could have been his analyst, and helped him with his obsession. But maybe he didn't need me. He had met the enemy, and it wasn't the Bill Levitts of America's and Europe's' Jews. It was the ancient human poison of collective paranoia, re-absorbed and spread by various Hitlers through centuries of ethnic slaughter, and bubbling again currently in the heads of skinheads, extreme religious radicals, and the murderous racial supremacists and ethnic cleansers recurrently encountered in the history of our so-called human civilizations. But let us turn to more pleasant matters, like our cruise on the Riviera in Levitt's yacht, and his fellow yachtsmen.

The French Riviera, Portuguese Counts, and Daughters of French Admirals

Levitt had befriended a small but rather amazing group of French Riviera yacht people that included a Portuguese count who was married to the daughter of a French admiral. She was a statuesque blond, who measured perhaps half a head taller than the count, to whom she had presented the gift of his life, their infant daughter, some eighteen months earlier. Also aboard was his wife's equally tall and attractive girlfriend. The three of them often stood together, with the broadly smiling and contented count in the middle, cradling their precious infant daughter in one arm, while the other remained free for a cocktail, or whatever. Just what the arrangement was I never knew or figured out, but the count seemed to have found a way to live peacefully and gratefully with whatever blessings and other developments that married life had brought him.

Let me hasten to note that, in addition to his royal credentials, the count was a trained and certified naval architect who had designed his own yacht, which happened to cruise a knot or two faster than Levitt's *Les Amis*. This advantage posed no difficulty for Levitt when racing for "fun and honor," as he put it, against the count's yacht to a mutually agreed pleasant destination perhaps an hour or two away from their starting point. That was because of Captain Heinz, who knew every nook, current, tide, and navigable channel in the Mediterranean, where he had had to out-fox and hide from Allied aircraft and naval destroyers. At the wheel of Levitt's *Les Amis*, Heinz always managed to beat the count's yacht by a few minutes, despite its small speed advantage over Bill Levitt's boat.

La Belle Simone at Carrara Boatyard: A Lesson in Yacht Building

The most exciting reason that *Les Amis'* size and cruising speed posed no problems for Bill Levitt was that he was already far along in building a brand new yacht in nearby Carrara, Italy. It would be called *La Belle Simone* and would be about one hundred feet longer than *Les*

Amis. La Belle Simone would have everything on it that seven million dollars could buy. It would include the most up-to-date engineering and marine electronics, as well as an elegant interior décor, with baths of Carrara marble, no less, Last but not least, it would feature a unique, quite remarkable section of its hull that would swing wide open from the owner's suite to provide a broad, fresh-air view of the sea, plus private access to its waters for an early morning dip. Bill Levitt, master builder that he was, and so in love with Simone, was anxious for us to see what his labor of love could produce.

We guests were most enthusiastic for a preview of *La Belle Simone* while she was under construction. So off we went in *Les Amis* on a bright sunny day for a pleasant cruise from the southern shores of France to Carrara, Italy. We soon arrived there, too soon, I thought, because the waters were so calm, the sky was so blue, and the day was delightful. For nautical me, however, a trip to a commercial boatyard in Carrara, famed for its fine marble that was prized, carved, and sculpted by the likes of Michelangelo and Bernini, was not to be sneezed at either.

That the Portuguese count would be there to explain things would be very helpful, I thought with a smile, just in case I could ever find time to build a sailing dinghy in my crowded garage at home. I had always loved boats, and had sailed small dinghies on the Charles River as a twelve-year-old in Boston years ago.

As for my own yachting prospects, if any, Levitt's and the count's lofty circumstances were so far above our financial means and so far beyond our regular social circles that I wondered for a moment what I was doing there, listening as they considered one costly alternative versus another. "Simply having a vacation and enjoying it," my inner voice reminded me, "Don't let it go to your head." I would need to listen to that voice soon again, as the Riviera's social season was about to reach its late summer crescendo and peak at Monaco's Annual Red Cross Ball.

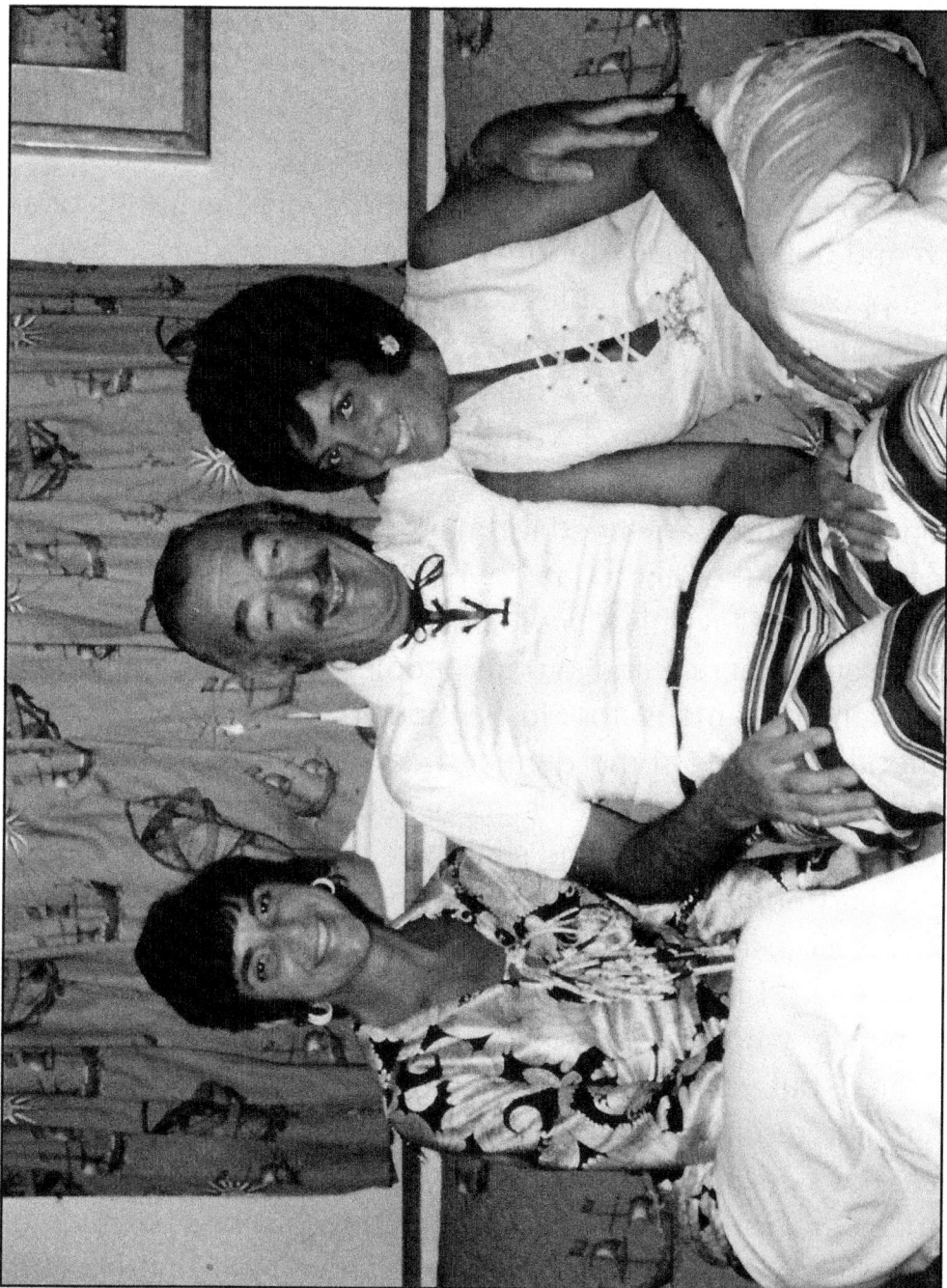

Author's wife Jane, Bill Levitt, and Simone (left to right).

Prince Rainier, Princess Grace, and Gregory Peck at the Red Cross Ball

As guests of William Levitt and under his guidance, we sat at a prominent table that he had reserved for our group at the Red Cross Ball. It was an annual gala affair to benefit charity, and from where I was sitting, it didn't seem to hurt the socially elevated image of Monaco as a place for the rich and the famous to play back then. So what were we doing there? We were the guests of a very rich and quite famous American whom I counted as a recent friend. I supposed that other tables contained a few ordinary people like me as guests of other rich and famous people whom I might not recognize. But which was which and who was who, and how could you tell the difference, I wondered as I casually scanned the room. I amused myself by thinking that for me, it was like being at a masked ball without any need for masks.

I whispered my thought to Jane, who laughed as she continued to gaze across the lavishly decorated room while I wondered if some of the guests of rich and famous people might not be thinking that I was rich and famous, too. Just a thought while getting myself in the mood for doing some dignified and serious dancing with Jane, who almost always looked so cool and reserved at any party, but on this night looked slim and slightly regal in a special evening gown she had purchased for our trip. Speaking of regal, several times in the course of the evening with this amazing group of people, Jane and I found ourselves dancing elbow to elbow with Princess Grace, who looked fabulous and radiant in the arms of a sophisticated, but very real and apparently relaxed Gregory Peck, who bore little resemblance to Melville's Captain Ahab.

Grace and Gregory had innate star quality, I thought, even as they danced graciously among their attractive, but less handsome earthlings on the dance floor. It was not Peck's fault that he was born to look like everyone's hero. I was, however, a bit slow to forgive him as Jane stole furtive looks across the room at him when we were sitting down between dances. As for Princess Grace, she was stunning, and it was to my credit that I never leaned toward her and Peck to say I knew her brother, Jack, with whom I had worked out a few times when we both had frequented the Philadelphia Athletic Club a few years earlier. We were friendly and gracious, but strangers at a ball, and even with a few drinks, I respected that. But Bill Levitt was no longer a stranger to me.

A Quick Look at Bill Levitt's Feet

As I said of Captain Heinz, it is hard to spend a week or two with a person in the close quarters of a boat without getting to know him, especially if he was the least bit sociable. It seemed to me that Bill Levitt was born to be sociable. He seemed to enjoy meeting new people. He was interested in them, and loved to talk with people everywhere, although, as the saying goes, he did not suffer fools gladly. I felt that he was very sophisticated and forceful, but basically a sincere and friendly man, who could be surprisingly boyish and relaxed for a mogul. For example, at ease with our few guests in the ship's lounge of a late afternoon, Levitt would kick off his stylish loafers or deck shoes. which he wore without sox, then wiggle his toes, and announce with more satisfaction than modesty, "You know, I've got pretty feet," as though his "pretty feet" were a gifted asset worth millions.

And as the other men laughed, my medical eyes and psychiatric ears understood that inside this very wealthy man was a truly lovely, very human, and basically humble person. Like a peasant, he quite properly prized his still-healthy and serviceable, sixty-five-year old feet far more than he did his new Rolls Royce, which, unlike his bare feet, I had never seen, but had heard others speak of with admiration. I had no experience with Rolls Royces, but as a physician aboard Bill's boat, my eyes took in, at a single glance, a pair of feet with high arches, good skin color, straight toes without bunions or other manifest deformities, as well as trim ankles with no evidence of discoloration, dermatitis, or edema. This diagnostic acumen was not an inborn talent of mine. I had developed it many years earlier as a surgical intern at Boston's Beth Israel Hospital, when required on frequent night calls to perform numerous physical exams and complete workups on someone who just happened to be passing by the emergency ward entrance with a week-old blister and thought he ought to see a doctor.

With that background and my subsequent experience of seeing an even larger number of sixty-five-year-old feet of some of the older members of the Philadephia Athletic Club in the shower room after their various workout routines, I could see Levitt's calling attention to his feet not as the narcissist bragging of a silly old man, but as a good-natured and witty gesture of a somewhat philosophical person, who quite properly appreciated his feet, which appeared pretty in his eyes as a beholder. So much for medical eyes, psychiatric ears, and intuitive impressions of the remarkable and likable man I found Bill Levitt to be during the relatively few and fascinating days I was privileged to know him.

Getting to Know Much More About Bill Levitt

There were many other things I saw in Bill as we got to know each other. His views of life were more expansive than narrow, and his tastes were more expensive than frugal. He lived high. Although he was a most generous host aboard his boat, when we dined ashore a few times at especially choice restaurants, it was routine for his guests to pick up the bill for our regular table of ten, and subsequently split it among the four husbands in our group. We were not poor men, but the tabs for ten people, including the Levitts, were pretty hefty, especially since Bill would order a bottle or two of Dom Perignon as the meal progressed, which was entirely fair since it was what he served at our regular dinner aboard his yacht. Other things I noted about Bill was that he was perceptive, compassionate, and sentimental. He noticed that I always turned to the right when someone spoke or called my name, no matter what direction the sound came from, and he asked me in private if I had a hearing problem. I told him that a few years back, in 1963, I suddenly developed a buzzing, called tinnitus, in my left ear and within a few weeks could hear nothing with that ear. It was caused by something called sensorineural deafness. It was common and could be from a virus, a toxin, or exposure to loud noises. But there was nothing to be done for it, even with powerful hearing aids. I could still hear perfectly out of my right ear, and I felt I could get along with my one good ear as well as Moshe Dayan could with one good eye. Bill listened to my brief explanation with interest, and said, "I like your attitude. Good for you!" and added off-hand that he knew Moshe Dayan and had met him after the Six Day War—as though everyone knew him too.

Then, perhaps to make me feel hopeful and better about my left-sided hearing loss, he confided that he had been a heavy smoker some years before, and had lost his voice following surgery to remove growths on his vocal cords. Could I imagine, he wanted to know, what this affliction did to his life, as well as to his business. in being unable to communicate except by writing notes? Yes I could imagine, and was stunned. Bill was not one to give up easily. He persisted in searching for a remedy, and finally found a surgeon in Switzerland who allegedly used Bill's own tissues to re-build his vocal cords, and it worked.

The first thing that this builder of Levittowns then did was to place a call from Switzerland—not to his office, but to his aging mother, who had not heard his voice in three years. Out of the blue, she heard him say, "Hello Ma. This is Bill." And then he went on to describe to me that all he heard was the sound of his mother crying. He waited for a minute and then this wealthy builder of

Levittowns said, "Hey Ma. This is long distance from Switzerland. It costs a lot, so please say something."

He stopped and looked at me as he took off his glasses and said, "You know, Mel, all I could hear was her crying from happiness, so I cried too. Can you understand how I felt?" he wanted to know. Yes, I could understand. Then I knew another reason why Simone loved this very powerful, strong willed, yet sentimental older man, who had been the first-born son and the apple of his Jewish mother's eye, and hopefully, I thought, would never give up trying to please "La Belle Simone," this beautiful woman he now so prized and loved.

When Barney Korchin Showed Up

I had never met Barney and was surprised to see him show up for a few minutes in Monaco one day. He appeared to feel quite welcome and relaxed about being there. He seemed to behave more like an old family friend than Simone's ex-husband. The problem was mine in assuming there would be the kinds of blame, resentment, and animosity I had seen in so many of my newly divorced patients. So why shouldn't he have felt comfortable among all these sophisticated and civilized people? After all, had he not spied Gene and Joan standing out there by Levitt's dock? And had Barney not known Gene and Joan Crane for years, and been partners in their recent art gallery business? Silly me, I thought. Why shouldn't Barney have felt comfortable on Bill Levitt's dock? But it was more than that. Bill Levitt was an emotionally as well as financially secure mensch. He could afford to be generous with Barney, who needed no financial help, but must have appreciated feeling like a former family friend rather than a dishonored and unwelcome loser. In that regard, I was told that when the Levitts were away and not using *Les Amis*, Bill had told his crew to allow Korchin to relax aboard when the yacht was unoccupied and tied up at its dock. So Levitt maintained a distant but amicable relationship with Korchin, which, I thought to myself, was another nice thing he did for Simone. I had never encountered Barney before or since, and all I can recall of him is exchanging a brief "Hello" with a confident and pleasant-looking man, who appeared in no way to feel deeply forlorn, depressed, or unhappy. How could I explain Barney not feeling heartbroken?

As I write about all this at the age of ninety-three, it is not my job to look back and judge others forty years later, but to try to understand them if I can. These were not my patients, but need I tell you how many patients I had seen whose marriages had cooled, and they had been living through mutual years of forbearance and endurance? If those were indeed Barney and Simone's not uncommon circumstances, it would seem that when they were married, Barney enjoyed the marital freedom of wandering without his wife through France and Italy, for weeks on end, to meet promising and interesting young artists. I had no idea if Barney wandered in other ways, but apparently that possibility did not concern Simone sufficiently to insist upon accompanying Barney in his travels. As I say, I never spoke with Korchin, but sometimes wondered if he had felt at times like Henny Youngman, the British-American comedian of the 1950s and 1960s, who often appeared on *The Ed Sullivan Show*. Youngman was famed for one-liners. For instance, when talking of his wife, he would say, "For example, take my wife," then stop and look around at the audience, and add, "Please!"

Flying Home and Flying High in 1972

After Jane and I flew back to our home, and Bill and Simone flew back to theirs, we saw little of them thereafter as we busied ourselves in our regular routines of raising our children. They were teenagers before the Vietnam War ended, with its political turmoil, protests, and unrest among our youth. By the time I reached fifty in 1972, the war was winding down, and Jane and I, who had watched our children like hawks when they were teenagers, felt fortunate that they were not into drugs or worse. Drugs could be purchased, not only in inner city neighborhoods, but also in suburban schools, where more affluent students were armed with larger resources and allowances. So, we escaped that.

As for my work, our academic program in forensic psychiatry at Temple, which had developed university-affiliated clinical facilities in courts and prisons, was the best in the tri-state area. Sam Polsky and I had created the first fellowship program in Forensic Psychiatry that we knew about. We had a wonderful staff on whom we could rely to meet with us regularly to discuss the legal, clinical, and case-law issues of their weekly caseload.

Our part-time private work as ABC's consultants in Broadcast Standards was an increasing source of professional interest, with psychological, legal, and government regulatory issues that posed ongoing ethical and licensing challenges for the broadcasting industry. As for studies, we were heading into the third year of supervising our five-year research projects on the effects of TV-depicted violence on vulnerable children and youth. We weren't as rich and successful as Bill Levitt, but we were perched on the top of our little world, just as he felt perched on top of his loftier financial and social worlds. Everything seemed to be going wonderfully well. Little did we anticipate that in the changing affairs of mice and men who were at the top of their game, there was one direction that the passage of time could take, and that is down. We can fall like leaves if and when our time comes.

Chapter 16
Round One: Tinnitus and Anxiety About Hearing Loss

Bumps in the Road

NINE YEARS EARLIER, in 1963, at the age of forty-one, I had hit a medical bump in the road with the onset of hearing loss. This setback began with a strange hissing sound and feeling of fullness in my left year. When the hissing sound, called tinnitus, did not go away in the next few days, I felt it was essential to see an ear, nose, and throat (E.N.T.) specialist. I was fortunate to be examined the next day by Dr. Harold Wilf, MD, a neighbor who was a highly regarded E.N.T specialist. He diagnosed a hearing loss due to inner ear problems in the cochlea. It was called sensorineural hearing loss, for which there was no specific treatment. Within two weeks I could hear nothing in my left ear but the hissing sound of tinnitus.

Hearing loss was not my specialty, and after consulting several additional specialists, it seemed there was not much that could be done about it. Although upset to be left with only one ear in working order, I could hear perfectly well in my good right ear. If the handsome young man with the eye patch could sell Hathaway shirts on TV, and if Moshe Dayan could plan winning battles in the Middle East as a one-eyed Israeli general, then I could make the best of things and carry on as a one-eared psychiatrist. And so I did, until nine years later in 1972, when I heard the ominous sound of tinnitus in my good right ear.

I dreaded that new hissing sound in my right ear because it was the same tinnitus I had heard in my left ear some nine years earlier, and that left ear went on to become completely deaf within two weeks. Now with tinnitus suddenly hissing in my right ear, would that ear now follow the same course that the left one had? If so, was I on the brink of becoming totally and permanently deaf? The idea of a psychiatrist, an analyst, or psychotherapist going completely deaf might not seem to others as dramatic as a surgeon going blind in his or her prime, but the prospect for both me and my young family was bad enough to drive me up a tree called anxiety.

In my anxious state, I developed a nagging need to find out all I could about the various causes of adult onset deafness. This was not impelled by the ordinary clinical curiosity of a doctor. It was driven by the anxiety of a patient with insufficient knowledge. Incomplete knowledge about the causes or etiology of disorders did not panic us as doctors. We often worked with inadequate knowledge of causes, and labeled conditions of unknown cause as "idiopathic disorders," and treated the symptoms as best we could. That was not enough for me as an otherwise healthy and fully functioning psychiatrist facing deafness at the height of his clinical and academic career. As a professor on our medical school faculty, I had easy access to our professional literature and began to research and read everything I could find on the causes and treatment prospects of adult onset hearing loss.

My Growing Anxiety: Could it be an Acoustic Neuroma?

When I encountered papers on auditory nerve tumors or acoustic neuromas, as they were called, I kept going back to find more articles on them. As a surgical intern and resident, I had known that acoustic neuromas were benign intracranial tumors of the auditory nerve lying within the confines of the skull. They were benign only in the sense that they did not metastasize and spread to distant parts of the body. Nevertheless, acoustic neuromas could kill by compressing and eventually destroying vital brain tissues, which share the skull's limited inner space. Furthermore, acoustic neuromas were not that rare. What would I tell a patient like me who was hung up with a fear of becoming totally deaf, if not worse? Would I not say, "Don't just sit there. Do something. Go see a good, experienced neurologist."? So I consulted the very best neurologist I knew in Philadelphia at the time, namely Dr. Abe Ornstein at University of Pennsylvania Hospital. After Dr. Ornstein performed his neurological examination, it was his opinion that I did not have an acoustic neuroma. I should have been satisfied. What more could I want? Nothing—except x-rays. In my anxiety, I felt the need for direct, visual proof that could rule out a tumor at the base of my brain.

X-rays of the brain were not as easy to obtain back in 1972 as magnetic resonance imaging (MRI) is today. Computed tomography scans (CT scans), MRIs, and other imaging techniques today do not ordinarily require spinal taps to introduce radio-opaque materials in order to visualize the brain and detect deformities, as were required back then. Spinal taps, however, were so frequently followed by troublesome headaches that patients were cautioned to remain recumbent for an hour or more after a brain x-ray to prevent them. Afraid to temporize, and needing an answer, I felt that the downside risks of a spinal tap and brain x-rays with contrast materials were hardly as great as the consequences of missing an acoustic neuroma that might be pressed on vital brain structures within the rigid confines of my skull. So I decided to obtain a second opinion from a neurosurgeon at Temple, who agreed that brain x-rays were a reasonable procedure for me. If indeed it was an acoustic neuroma that could be surgically removed, my physical condition and general health appeared to be excellent except for some annoying prostate problems that were not infrequent in middle-aged men, and were especially common in older ones. I had paid my prostate problems little attention aside from annual check-ups with an urologist to make sure nothing was sneaking up on me from behind. So we proceeded with the x-rays.

X-Ray Results: As Much as I Could Have Wanted But Far More Than I Expected

To my great relief, the brain x-rays showed no evidence of an acoustic neuroma or other pathology. The bad news was that I developed the most severe spinal-tap headaches ever. I could not lift my head off the pillow nor get out of bed without bringing them on. My wife, Jane, was in New York for the weekend spending an overnight at her sister's and brother-in-law's apartment in New York's Greenwich Village. How many times during the weeks that followed was I to wish that I had followed Dr. Ornstein's advice for watchful waiting rather than plunging ahead as I did with the brain x-rays!

Costly Medical Misjudgments and Painful Mistakes I Made

What happened next was also the result of misjudgments of my own that taught me painful and sobering lessons. In hindsight, the first mistake was my impatience and persistence in seeking brain x-rays to rule out an acoustic neuroma. I made my next mistake in bed by over-dosing myself with liberal amounts of aspirin in attempts to relieve my spinal-tap headaches. My over-dosing with aspirin was possibly more excusable back then, since aspirin's anticoagulant effects were not so widely known. Meanwhile, whatever had triggered or resulted in my severe spinal-tap headaches had somehow aggravated my pre-existing prostate problems to the extent that at 2 a.m. the next morning, I experienced what is called acute urinary retention. If you've never heard of it, be thankful. It is a complete and torturous inability to urinate. As it happened, my wife Jane was visiting her sister and brother in-law in New York, so I was alone in the house at the time. I was able to reach the bedside phone and dial my best buddy and colleague, Sam Polsky, who lived about fifteen minutes away, and then fell back with my terrible headache and awful inability to empty my overly distended bladder.

To the Emergency Room and Urologists at Temple Hospital

Thankfully, I don't remember how Sam stuffed me into his car following his urgent call to fellow faculty friend and urologist, Dr. Lester Karafin, to meet us at the hospital. Lester provided me with an unforgettable moment of serenity by inserting an indwelling Foley catheter and prescribing a single shot of a morphine derivative, which finally relieved the spinal headache. So the next morning when I thanked Lester sincerely and profusely for having "saved my life," Lester said, "Not so fast, Mel." He then explained, "Your prostate is quite enlarged, and you are too young for a transurethral procedure. It will grow back too soon. For any lasting benefit, you will need to have a retropubic prostatectomy."

How could I argue? It was not my specialty. It was Lester's, and he was my faculty colleague and friend. The surgery was performed the next day by Dr. Karafin's colleague, Dr. Richard Newman. We had three senior faculty colleagues in the surgical urology staff at that time: Drs. Lester Karafin, Richard Newman, and Cyril Conger. Dr. Conger was their department chairman. You will meet them all, as I did during my prolonged postoperative stay.

The Operation Went Well, But Then What Happened?

Ostensibly the surgery went well, and I was feeling really fine on the fifth post-operative day when Sam Polsky dropped in to visit and chat. He updated me on the status of our several joint projects and assured me that all was under control pending my return to work. Then, a petite and lovely nurse entered pleasantly. She knew I was a medical doctor on Temple's faculty. In a cheerful, but polite and business-like fashion, she stated that it was time to remove the Foley catheter from my bladder, and she asked if Sam would mind leaving for a few minutes while she would do her quick and easy job. I told her that I would like Sam to stay, assuring her that he, too, was a doctor on our Temple faculty. This was technically

175 ❧

and actually true, but his doctor's degree was a PhD in forensic or legal medicine, and not an MD. Sam had been around medical schools and hospitals long enough to be comfortable and know that an indwelling Foley catheter was like any other urinary catheter except that it had an additional slim tube through which a few cc's of saline could be injected to inflate a small, indwelling balloon once the catheter was inserted, The balloon would then prevent the catheter from being accidentally withdrawn from the bladder. Deflating the balloon and then withdrawing the catheter through the urethra was a simple task that I had performed numerous times as a surgical intern and resident many years before.

An Unexpected, Traumatic Post-Operative Knock-Down

I've gone into this mainly to tell you how relaxed, easy, and confident I felt as a patient on my fifth postoperative day, with every favorable sign of making a good recovery from my prostate surgery. I was in no way prepared for any further drama when that ever-present matter of surgical risk made its sudden and unexpected appearance. When that petite and pretty nurse gently removed my catheter, all hell broke loose. What instantly occurred was the most alarming and unexpected sight of my own blood hemorrhaging and spurting from my lower abdominal incision.

In a bit of a shock, I tried to remain externally cool as my agile and quick-thinking nurse responded instantly and unbelievably. Grabbing a handful of four-by-four surgical sponges from her treatment tray, she literally leaped aboard my elevated hospital bed and straddled me like a bareback rider in order to press the surgical sponges tightly against my bleeding abdominal wound with the entire pressure and full weight of her perhaps ninety-pound, diminutive body. Sam immediately ran out the door to summon more help at the Nurses' Station, leaving me breathless, aghast, and momentarily un-chaperoned with that adorable young nurse.

Our emergency crew was swiftly assembled, sort of like a surgical SWAT Team, fully armed with their standard panoply of intravenous fluids, including saline solutions and plasma, as well as stat orders for blood studies and transfusions. Shortly thereafter, Dr. Kendall arrived, examined me further, and took charge. On the way out the door to write further orders at the Nurses' Station, he assured me that all would be well. And all did get well in due course, but unfortunately not before further complications that followed. I will try to avoid being overly dramatic here, and I shall stick only to the hard facts and my hard feelings about them.

Surgical Lessons Learned Painfully as a Patient: An Ode to Dr. Conger

Although the massive bleeding had been stopped, I developed a rapidly ascending infection from the urethra and bladder to my scrotal parts via the connecting pathway of the vas deferens. This further complication was also my fault since both my wife and I had turned down the frequently recommended option of a vasectomy to prevent such postoperative infections. And so, I developed vasitis and epididymytis, as well as other debilitating and painful complications that much prolonged my eventual recovery.

After my surgical wound had bled profusely into my bladder, there remained large blood clots that required evacuation. It took days and nights for the blood clots to be painfully flushed from the bladder through the urethra. This was accomplished by repeatedly injecting a large syringe full of saline into the bladder through the urethra and then withdrawing the contents, over and over, until the excreted fluids were only faintly pink, but no longer bloody. It had to be done. It was only this that would allow the bladder to contract and shrink back to its normal size.

To this day, I can still remember Dr. Conger, professor and chairman of Temple's Urology Department, feeling personally called upon and somehow responsible to flush out his fellow faculty member's painfully distended bladder at two o'clock in the morning, when a far younger, less experienced, and less patient urology resident could have been summoned for that tedious, humble, and lowly task. Indeed, such seemingly humble "scut" work was often assigned to a weary surgical intern or first year resident—but not in Dr. Conger's department. In retrospect, I painfully experienced his efforts as the menial, but self-disciplined and noble act of an unforgettable senior surgeon and a gentleman of the old school, who could have been home in bed. But that was a rare demonstration and long ago lesson in patient care that I learned during lonely nights as a doctor in pain. It was heroic post-operative work performed by a distinguished and truly dedicated surgeon.

Was My Complicated Surgical Setback Due to Too Much Simple Aspirin?

My bladder hemorrhage on the fifth post-operative day was followed by the combined consequences of blood loss, with anemia and wound contamination, as well as inflammation and edema of nearby scrotal contents and tissues. This led to marked fatigue, debilitation, and an unusually prolonged surgical recovery time. When all was said and done, what had caused things to go so wrong? The irony is that this sequel of physically costly and emotionally stressful post-operative complications was not caused by a faulty or inadequately tied ligature, but by something as inexpensive and common in almost every medicine cabinet—namely plain, over-the-counter Bayer's aspirin. In vain attempts to control my severe post-spinal tap headaches, I had overdosed myself on aspirin.

The take-home lesson for my patients and me was that almost all medications can be fatally toxic if taken in excessive doses. There were further adverse consequences beyond the physical ones that I have taken pains to describe. I was not a single player, but I had a wife on whom this entire physical setback took a toll.

Jane experienced my setback as a hard knock to herself, as well as to me. To explain her vulnerability then, I need to go back a half dozen years in our marriage.

Jane Experienced Her Own Hard Knock with "Juvenile" Diabetes at Age 34

Jane's physical and emotional setback happened some years earlier, in 1966, during a Temple-sponsored cruise of the Greek Islands. Jane and I had paired up with Max and Mary Ronis. Max, about my age, was professor and chairman of Temple's Department of Otolaryngology as his father had been before him. Jane had developed what seemed like a remarkable thirst, beyond the simple sipping of resonated wine in Greek restaurants. Max and I both noticed it, and when Jane and Mary went to the Ladies' Room, Max raised a single eyebrow and a one-word question: "Diabetes?" I, too, had wondered about that, but there was no one in her family with diabetes. Unfortunately. Max turned out to be right. Jane's uncle, Dr. Jesse Harris, had diabetes, but had kept it secret.

Jane had developed so-called "juvenile diabetes," which required insulin injections. She was particularly devastated because one of her childhood friends had been a diabetic and eventually went blind as a young woman. Further troubles ensued when Jane became convinced the contraceptive pill, which I had urged her to take prior to what I had hoped would be a romantically memorable cruise among the Greek Islands, upset her endocrine system and somehow caused her diabetes. Her gynecologist, endocrinologist, her own father, and least of all, me, whom she felt was the guilty party, tried to convince her that her theory had no actual basis in fact. Jane had been told she was a "brittle diabetic." She was very conscientious about monitoring her blood sugar and insulin dosage, and I sometimes felt terrible as I watched her struggle to control her blood sugar, at the frequent risk of insulin overdose and shock.

Chapter 17
Psychological Consequences of Serious Physical Setbacks

Wilhelm Nietzsche and Post-Operative Me

THE PHILOSOPHER, WILHELM Nietzsche, famously said, "That which does not kill us makes us stronger." He also asserted that greatness of spirit is achieved through the greatness of suffering. As for the greatness of suffering, in late August and early September of 1972, I was in free fall and was feeling helpless as my hemoglobin levels, depleted by blood loss, hovered at fifty percent of what they should have been for a man at my age. My blood was carrying about half its normal amount of oxygen to my heart, brain, and other vital organs. At that point, two weeks following my lumbar puncture, urinary obstruction, prostate surgery, and postoperative complications, I was feeling, if not close to death, depleted, in pain, and in big trouble if the treatment team could not rescue me.

Did My Surgical Setback Make Me Stronger?

What did my surgical setback mean to me? It was the first time I had experienced serious medical trouble, requiring transfusions and intensive care for a brief but crucial time. As I look back on it now, it was a mid-life harbinger of future afflictions and impairments that I would experience. I look even further back, long before I read Nietzsche's words that what does not kill us makes us stronger, to when I was a little boy, prone to hard knocks and scary scrapes. My mother used to say, "Every knock is a boost." She had never heard of Wilhelm Nietzsche, but she had the similar idea that knocks from which we recover can somehow strengthen us, or give us a "boost," as she put it. We had lots of knocks to make us stronger in the early 1930s, along with our regular boyhood games with their inevitable knockdowns, black eyes, and bruises.

The post-operative knockdown I experienced following my prostate surgery was the first time I had felt completely let down by my body. Saved in time by excellent intensive care, how little I knew at age fifty that I would live a long life that would require several more rounds with Mother Nature and Father Time before the final bell. Not many people can go for ten full rounds without knockdowns. After nine rounds or decades with Mother Nature, our arms and legs get weary and we don't hear, see, chew, digest, nor metabolize so well. Do our prior knockdowns make us stronger or help in any way? Perhaps Nietzsche was right. Serious afflictions that "did not kill me" strengthened me with the realization that we sometimes have the inner resources to recover from severe bodily tests and extended physical struggles.

When rapidly progressive hearing loss and the prospect of total deafness appeared to pose a greater potential threat, my prostate problems took a back seat. They shouldn't have, because brewing health problems should remain standing in the aisle, and not be assigned to a back seat. My prostatic hypertrophy had progressed to the point where I often needed to leave my literal seat at a good movie and go to the men's room and urinate at crucial moments in the film. This was annoying and interfered with my leisure activities some, but not my professional practice in the office nor while teaching and co-administering our Unit in Law and Psychiatry at the university. I had troubling symptoms, but was functioning well at my work.

Hard to Contemplate Further Marital Problems with a Person Becoming Deaf

Superimposed on her fears about the eventual consequences of diabetes on her own health prospects, Jane became increasingly troubled about the potential results of hearing loss in my remaining right ear. These concerns and her daily preoccupation with her blood sugar levels were projected onto the usual, normal, and tolerable issues and stresses of any decent marriage. When Jane quite frankly said to me, "Mel, if you go deaf, I can't take it," I was upset, but I could not fault her for feeling that way. And then came my unexpected, complicated, and protracted hospitalization for prostate surgery, which occurred shortly thereafter.

Jane confided in her friend, Adelaide Bry, with whom she went on to discuss her distress more openly and extensively than she had with me. Adelaide suggested that Jane should see a well-regarded psychiatrist in New York, who recommended his weekly group therapy program. Her participation in that group is why she was in New York the night when I went into acute urinary retention. We each had our own physical setbacks and illnesses that occurred in early mid-life. As a physician, I should perhaps have known better than to manage my own case, but as a patient, I was making choices that all patients need to make.

My Surgical Setback, Jane's Bad Luck, and Our Bad Timing

So, it was while Jane was in New York, staying overnight with her sister after her group therapy session, that I went into acute urinary retention after the spinal tap for my brain x-rays. That misfortune, was my fault in a way, because I was too anxiety-ridden and persistent and wanted to rule out an acoustic neuroma. So I pressed for brain x-rays, which resulted in a severe spinal-tap headache and the onset of my first major medical misadventure. I can understand in retrospect how Jane, with her own health concerns and struggle to control her insulin shots and diabetes, felt that I was needlessly complaining. I could understand that, but for a time, resented that she called Dr. English to come see me in the hospital in which I worked, where he was still chairman of the Department of Psychiatry. By then, my blood loss had been so extensive, with my hemoglobin at half of its normal amount, as to require four transfusions. After a brief look at my chart, Dr. English quickly realized that I was not in any way being a baby, and he understood my concern that Jane, as next of kin, might not be in the mood to look after me if I again became seriously ill and more dependent as I got older. That feeling of our eventual vulnerability really worked on me.

The frightening and unexpected physical setback, which I have tried to describe in some detail in prior pages, was sufficiently painful. Emotionally, however, it seemed to be a sad wakeup call for both Jane and me. We knew, from the experiences of our parents and their friends, that as life went on, the chances of my becoming seriously ill would increase. Perhaps it was due to the fact that I was ten years older than my dear wife and had recently felt the proximity of death's door, but I was left feeling that it was likely that I had experienced the way she would take care of me if and when I encountered similar physical set-backs the future. This was not the only problem, but somehow along the way, we were each taking a dimmer view of our marriage, the rose wilting, as it seems to for so many.

This dimmer view of our prospects together had led to Jane's entering group therapy in New York, where she felt increasingly confident that she would be well-advised to file for divorce. Ironically, she may or may not have been the only still-married woman in her therapy group of eight female patients. In any event, this encouraged her to file for separation and divorce. And so we proceeded with divorce with what I recall as mutual resentment, but without hatred and animosity.

Back Home

After several dismal weeks of post-surgical complications and essential hospital care, I returned to family life in our large and lovely farmhouse colonial home on our Penn Valley hilltop on Philadelphia's Main Line. It was like an almost forgotten dream. As I gratefully settled back into these familiar surroundings, Paul, our youngest, was pushing twelve. His sister, Joan, was fifteen, and David, our oldest at eighteen, was about to enter his freshman college year at the University of Rochester in New York. The three, it seemed, had suddenly grown up, albeit incompletely. Before my surgical setback, Jane and I had been about to complete our nineteenth year of marriage, with lots of effort on both sides. In the face of personal health setbacks that Jane and I had each experienced physically as individuals, and secondarily as marital partners, it was a time of emotional turmoil—not just for Jane and me, but for all of us involved.

A Time of Emotional Turmoil

After getting home, it took me several weeks to regain my physical strength, but my emotional condition was another matter. Now at age fifty, deaf in my left ear since age forty-one, I returned to my ear, nose and throat colleague at Temple, Dr. Max Ronis, who ordered a follow-up evaluation by his top audiologist, Dr. Rosenberg. Unfortunately, but sure enough, the audiograms showed further evidence of hearing loss in the my right ear. Although outwardly calm, I was thrown for a loop by the tinnitus in my good right ear. I really needed that ear. I had made my living, supported my family, and shaped my self-image, all with that good right ear for the past nine years. And it was the only one I had left. Remember that my training as a psychiatrist and analyst was essentially that of a clinically skilled, professional listener. If I could not hear, how could I listen? If I could not listen, how could I function as a psychotherapist?"

Fortunately, hearing did not decrease as rapidly in my right ear as it had in my left, which had become completely deaf in a matter of several weeks. As I write these words forty years later, I am benefited by a powerful hearing aid with which I can still hear many sounds, including the rhythmic beats of music, but not the melodies or intonation. As for speech discrimination, even with my hearing aid and an amplified telephone, my extensive hearing loss now requires me to lip-read someone whose face I can see up close, and who speaks distinctly and slowly, and in enough light. But even in my early eighties, I still heard well enough to socialize, converse, consult, and teach. However, I sorely missed the sound of music, group conversations, and children's' soft voices that had meant so much to me. At fifty, I feared not only the impact of complete hearing loss on my career, but also missing out on our extended family life with our children and their friends.

None of this turmoil showed externally when Jane and I separated pursuant to an agreement drawn up by our lawyers. Nor did it interfere with my professional work and proximity to Sam, who as our long-standing family friend counseled me in the ensuing divorce proceedings.

Back to Work

What helped my spirits was my eager return to work with Sam Polsky in our shared academic efforts at Temple. I also returned to my half-time private patients and psychiatric consultation practice, the biggest portion of which had become our work with ABC. Sam and I had two more years to complete in our five-year research project on Television Violence, Children, and Youth. Coordinating the efforts of our independent project, Drs. Bernstein, Burland, Duffy, Guy, and Hoopes, had been progressing nicely as we moved into the third year of our ongoing research studies. In addition, Al Schneider had been calling on me increasingly as ABC's Broadcast Standard consultant to review more movies, scripts, and pilot films for potential programs in the upcoming broadcast schedule. I loved all my work in both the public and private sectors of forensic psychiatry. It kept me busy, well paid, and had happily occupied, with little time for anger or brooding over my physical and marital setbacks.

Consulting in California: Serious Work in Luxurious and Pleasant Environments

It was really great for Sam and me to break away each month for a day in Manhattan, but consulting for ABC in Los Angeles and its related studios in nearby Hollywood was a special treat. I had never been to California and so close to Malibu's beach and its tempting hills nearby. It was quite another thing for two East Coast Temple University professors.

Call me sentimental. I almost cried at age fifty when I first saw the West Coast of our beautiful country while looking down at the sparkling Pacific Ocean from the high and lovely Malibu Hills. Why cry when struck by beauty? I recall thinking how sad it seemed to have arrived in southern California as a middle-aged man instead of thirty years earlier as an athletic, sun-tanned youngster with a long life ahead.

I told myself that psychiatrists are entitled to a bit of emotion too. While in Los Angeles, in my fifties, I also met my first cousin, Richard Oshman, for the first time. He was the son of my father's sister, Sarah, the only sibling of my Dad that I ever met. Richard was a lawyer, a great guy, and a devoted family man with young children. It was an emotional discovery to finally find my father's sister, a very fine Aunt Sarah, and her two sons alive and thriving in such a far-off California. As I looked back on my earliest life from the very choice, newly encountered accommodations for ABC's consultants at the Belle Air, Beverly Hills, or Century Plaza hotels, I wished I could have known her as a close aunt in my childhood.

That brings up yet another group of emotions that were there with me in those good and memorable times. I was engaged in the very serious and challenging work of studying and perhaps making socially meaningful recommendations about TV's depictions of violence, being so luxuriously ensconced by ABC's consultants with all-expenses-paid trips. This somehow was a bit much for my 1930s New England and Depression-bred sense of hard work and frugality. Why couldn't I have shared some of this unaffordable luxury with my dear parents and brother? But I fought against my pangs of guilt with a second martini at dinner, and I extended my work sessions the next day. I also dwelled often on sincere feelings of genuine gratitude. I have tried to foster that feeling whenever possible until I finally achieved, in my old age today, a sustained attitude of gratitude for blessings received, come what may.

Chapter 18
The Anatomy of An Amicable Divorce

NOT ONLY DID Jane and I refrain from saying negative things about each other to our children, but we emphasized each other's good points to them. When we subsequently and inevitably met at large parties thrown by mutual friends, the fact that Jane and I had remained openly cordial drove some of our acquaintances a bit crazy. How could two people who were divorced, they wondered, seem so "amicable" or "friendly"? In truth, we did it for our kids. Our agreed-upon policy of basic decency and respect provided enormous dividends for the balance of our lives, as well as an emotionally mature relationship to which each of us adapted happily.

In compliance with our separation agreement and the terms of the pending divorce settlement, I found the closest place to my kids where I could both reside and maintain an office for my part-time private practice. This was available at Penn Valley's nearby Oak Hill Apartments, which had a first floor that was conveniently zoned for both residential and office occupancy. It was also within easy walking distance and an even quicker bike ride for our twelve-year-old Paul. This carefully chosen location carried a message to both Jane and my kids. It said, in effect, louder than words, "I am staying nearby, close to you and your Mom. Take care of her and each other. We are not divorcing our children. I am still your dad and here for you."

Jane's Adjustment

Although the family's extended ballpark remained much the same, the ballgame itself changed somewhat. Mutual friends, Rita and Marty Eisenberg, as well as Elliot and Bernice Levin, were supportive of and sided with Jane. Elliot and Bernice were new to me. I believe that Jane had met them at the famous Barnes Museum's art lecture course given by Violette de Mazia, the long-time intimate and personal confidante of Albert C. Barnes, who became a multi-millionaire and far-sighted art collector after selling his drug company that had marketed Argyrol profitably to another company at the right time before antibiotics were available. It was a popular course for newly successful persons interested in acquiring and collecting art.

As I understood Elliot Levin's story, following his military service, he had what I thought was the amazing business foresight to anticipate the post-WWII baby boom and actually do something intelligent about it. He started a diaper cleaning company called Hushaby Laundry to service the inevitable by-product of millions of virile war veterans returning to a huge market of eager and fertile women yearning for marital love and children of their own. Elliot's company became very successful, and he and Bernice became interested in art collecting and made a few similarly minded and well-connected friends in the process.

It was through friends of Elliot that Jane met the builders of a huge new condominium development called Fairmount, where she was, for a relatively lucrative time, put in charge of sales. This helped not only in terms of earnings, but also in increased self-image as a working person in the mid-1970s real estate market. When the Fairmont condos were mostly sold off, Jane looked for other ventures. With a decade of interest in gourmet cooking and foods, Jane and a lady friend felt that the nearby shops of Narberth lacked gourmet cheese and decided to open a small shop on its small, charming Main Street, close to its suburban railroad station and liquor store, where it stands to this day.

While buying refrigeration equipment, Jane met a very nice fellow who was in the business of supplying such equipment for food shops and restaurants. His name was Marty Mellon. More important, they soon found each other to be temptingly available, mutually attractive, and divorced. And so it came to pass that Jane soon married Martin Mellon which gave her a new and rather becoming last name which Jane adopted quite comfortably, relieving me for a time of some of my Jewish post-divorce guilt. It was even more helpful to me that I liked Marty Mellon. Despite his upscale last name, he was in no way related to or connected with the very wealthy and socially lofty Mellon family. Moreover, Marty, who seemed like a well-behaved, regular guy, enjoyed a good game of bridge, a small bet, a bit of break-even gambling in Atlantic City, a pack of cigarettes a day, a martini when it was available, and a game of backgammon with my sons, David or Paul.

Jane's homemaking skills, sense of décor, good taste, and ladylike manner had great appeal for Marty, as it would for anyone, including myself. I was glad they found a new life with each other.

What About Post-Marital Me?

Between my academic and public sector pursuits in our criminal justice system, my private practice consultations with lawyers and patients, as well as our Broadcast Standards project at ABC, I had more than enough interesting and rewarding work to keep me busy, diverted, and out of trouble for the foreseeable future.

Having just failed in a marital relationship, I re-experienced my need for a mutually close, compatible, and companionable relationship. I certainly had the compatible and productive relationship with my best friend, Sam Polsky. He had been not only my professional colleague, but my closest friend and personal buddy, for the past fifteen years in working together. What more did I want than a good buddy? Much more: sex, a family, and a chance to resist mortality by continuing the blood line or DNA, as we call it today.

Sexuality and our Human Longing for Some Kind of Familial Immortality

What about the need for female companionship for which, I discovered in my youth, there was no real substitute? And here at age fifty in 1972, this need was as real for me as ever. I am talking not about sex with a passing stranger, but of physical intimacy and sexual gratification in an equal relationship with a compatible and compassionate female. If one can find moments of that kind of togetherness, it takes much of the chill out of the cold feelings of our personal and sexual isolation in the face of our pending mortality. I again mention mortal life because it is the only form of life we know. To reproduce, nurture, and raise new generations of children are the miracles that Nature bestows on each species to compensate for its mortality. Serious question: Would you rather live forever in a barren world, or in one like ours with the regenerations of new human life that can evolve creatively? We have no choice, but given our biological mortality, it is not a bad option to contemplate with gratitude.

Immortality is an invention of mankind. We must recognize that it is likely a delusional defense against the fear of death. "Be careful what you wish for," it is sometimes said. That includes longing for immortality. I believe that if our individual lives were endless or immortal, they would lack human emotion, motivation, value, and meaning. If we could look forward to endless years, we might never get around to doing anything important or creative. Death is the frame placed around the landscapes of our lives.

Jane Doe and a Few Newly Divorced Ladies

Thank God for enterprising ladies. A half a dozen of them decided to throw a party for recently divorced men nearby. Somehow I got on their list and received a phone call from a Jane Doe inviting me to a party. She sounded nice on the phone and I told her that I'd call her back. I made a few inquiries about her and was told she was a "terrific woman," divorced about a year ago from a rectal surgeon and proctologist, no less. Since I was a doctor with professional interests at the exact opposite end of our vertical anatomy, I thought that maybe a different medical specialty or personal perspective might do the trick. And so I met her and we dated, and one thing led to another, as they say.

It would have been rude and dishonest of me to turn down her unspoken invitation to sample a bit of love. She was a good lady and fine in every way, but I was far from ready to re-marry and so we broke off. About two years later, I bumped into her. She was all smiles and attractively dressed in good taste as usual. I told her how sorry I was that I had not yet been ready for a second marital commitment. She took my hand in her two gloved ones, looked me in eye, and said tenderly, "Don't worry, Mel. You taught me some new things about myself—and my body."

I felt my heart flutter for a moment. It was the nicest thing a woman ever said to me about sex, or anything else for that matter. She followed it up with the additional happy news that a year ago she had married a good man whose well-known name I quickly recognized as one of the most successful real estate operators in the Delaware Valley. All of which leads me to silver linings and happy ending stories.

A Silver Lining for my Tinnitus

Deaf for nine years in the left ear, but hearing fine with my right ear alone, the sudden sound of tinnitus hissing ominously in my right ear panicked me. I was threatened, particularly as a therapist and consultant who made his living by listening to others. Now back at work, but separated and divorced in the aftermath, what was I going to do about the ongoing threat of deafness?

I consulted other hearing specialists, who agreed with the findings and recommendations of Dr. Ronis, who referred me to his top audiologist at Temple, Dr. Phil Rosenberg. Dr. Rosenberg followed my case for a time and eventually fitted me with a hearing aid for moderate amplification of sound in my right ear. The left ear had remained beyond any hope of help. But, as had happened before in my life, serendipity and coincidence came to my rescue. Phil Rosenberg happened to be an avid sailor, and sometime sailing buddy of another audiologist named Phil, a Philip Bellefleur, PhD, who was director and headmaster of the Pennsylvania School for the Deaf in Germantown, Pennsylvania. Would I like to meet Phil Bellefleur, Dr. Rosenberg wanted to know. With Phil Rosenberg's build-up and a name like Bellefleur, my answer was, "Mais oui!" But of course!

Dr. Philip Bellefleur and The Pennsylvania School for the Deaf

Back in 1972, the Pennsylvania School for the Deaf stood on some thirty acres in Mount Airy, adjoining Germantown. The grounds contained a number of older, well-maintained buildings, some of which dated back to the late nineteenth and early twentieth century, including the Headmaster's Residence where I met Dr. Bellefleur in his den at home. This room contained a fine desk, a number of interesting objects and books, as well as a large, impressively framed, oil portrait of himself, no less. As I got to know him, Phil Bellefleur turned out to be far more impressive than his portrait. He was a friendly, open-minded, and versatile person with a wide range of interests. Not only was he a capable administrator with a special interest in deaf schools and the deaf community, but he seemed talented at almost everything he undertook from photography to sailing. He seemed equally interested in getting to know me and my special interests in forensic and child psychiatry.

As for my hearing problems and his extensive experience with cases of hearing loss, I asked what he thought of my audiograms, my clinical history, and prospects for further hearing loss. I'll never forget his answer, words to the effect that "there are all kinds of things I could tell you, but the bottom line is that I think you ought to learn sign language and prepare for deafness."

"Wow! But how?" was the gist of my slow and somewhat shocked response. He had given that some thought, too. He said, "We could use a good child psychiatrist here who is interested in hearing loss. If you could volunteer to work a few weekly hours with our children and their teachers, it would be great for our school and would help you learn about deaf kids, their families, and deafness."

And so I did just that, and it expanded and gave further direction to my career, just as my unwanted U.S. Public Health Service assignment to the maximum security federal penitentiary from 1951 to 1953 had shaped my subsequent academic and clinical career in forensic psychiatry.

Weekend Visit to the Bellefleurs' Chesapeake Home

The greatest trip I ever took was not a very privileged Mediterranean cruise on William Levitt's luxurious yacht. My very best trip did not come until four years later, in 1974. It occurred quite unexpectedly on a well-kept, twenty-nine-foot Ranger sloop that heeled nicely in a brisk puff of wind at the mouth of the Bohemia River as it flowed into the larger Elk River, heading toward Turkey Point at the head of the Chesapeake Bay. With just a bit of the windswept spray that kissed my cheek, I fell in love with my first waterborne glimpse of Maryland's Eastern Shore. My new friend, Dr. Phil Bellefleur, recognized my sailor's thrill at feeling that first puff of strong wind on a sturdy sail and graciously offered me the helm. I took the tiller with the enthusiasm of a person who long before had spent a number of boyhood days sailing small dinghies on Boston's Charles River, and much later, a few hours sailing sixteen-foot zip-class sloops along the Connecticut shore. The older sailors had said, "If you can handle the little ones and stay upright in a stiff wind, the big boats with their keel, ballast and winches are much more stable and easier to handle." But I'd never held the tiller of a thirty-foot, powerfully rigged sloop like Phil's Ranger. It was a wild ride for a time, and I was hooked. I wanted a sloop like that, a waterfront home like his, and maybe even a wife like that to share that lovely newfound shore.

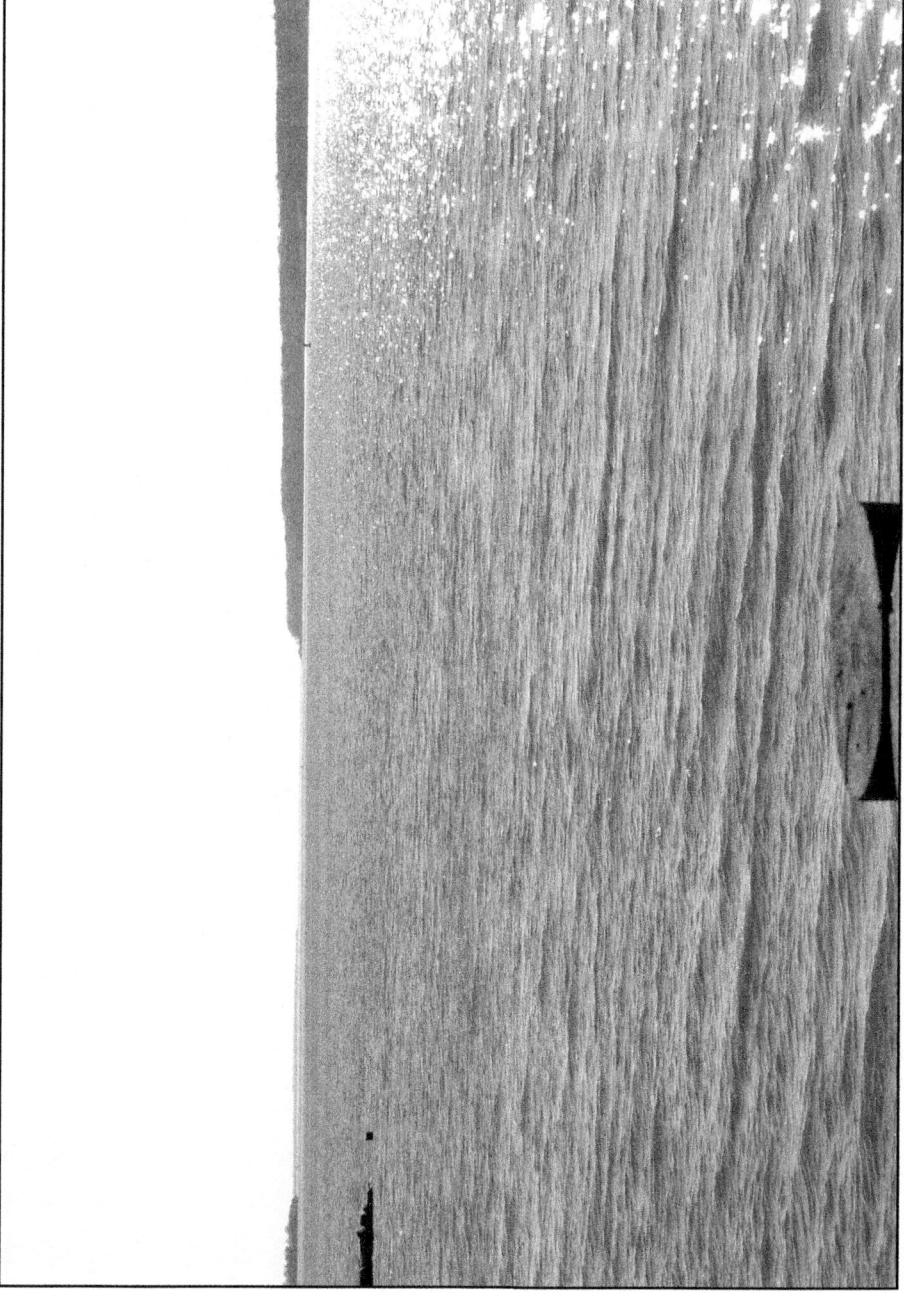

A seven-mile view from outermost piling of Author's dock (in foreground) to Turkey Point (upper right) at entrance to Upper Chesapeake Bay, with small jetty visible on left demarcating Author's son Paul's adjoining waterfront farm.

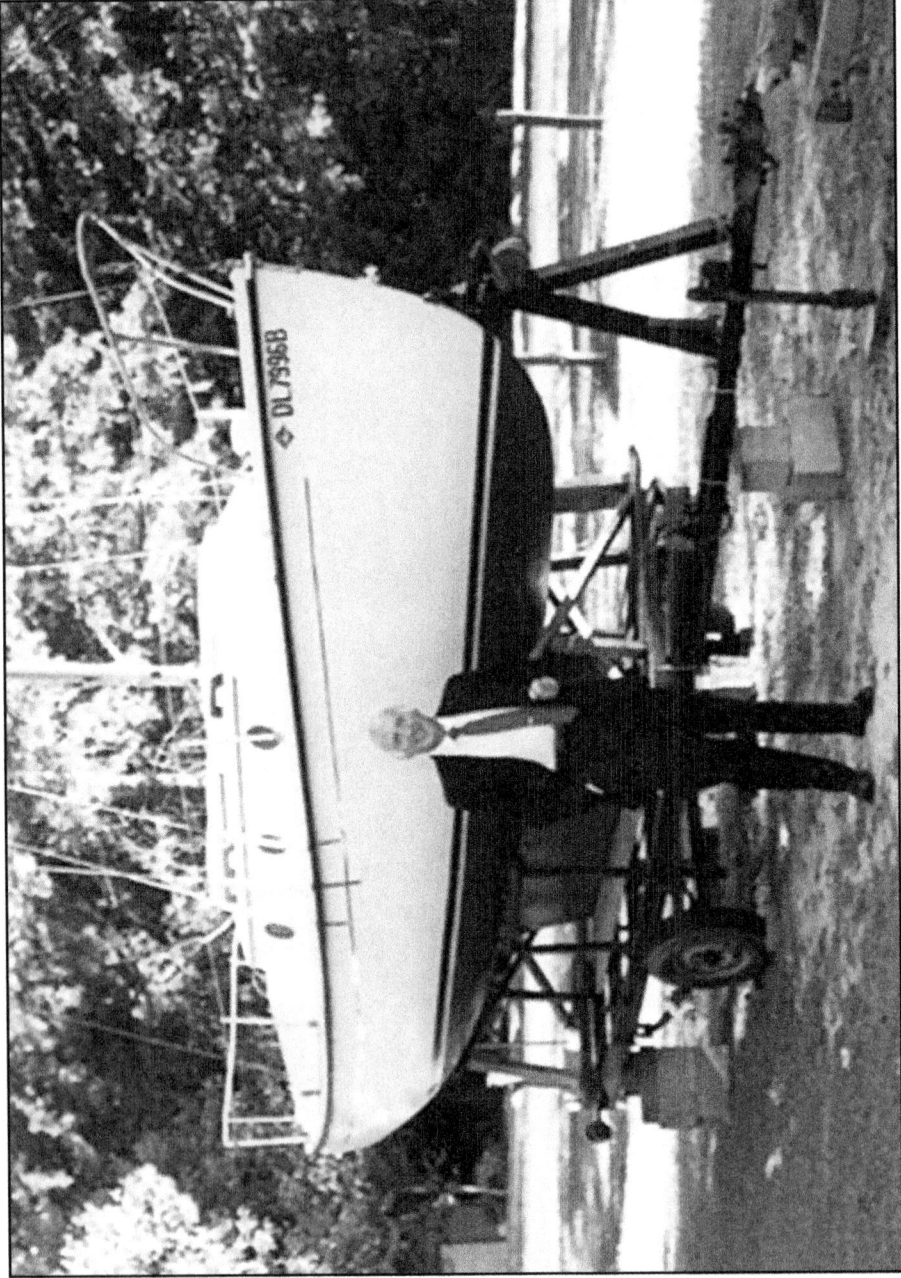

"Prime Time," long neglected on nearby neighborhood lawn, restored to pristine condition by author stopping to admire his handiwork, dressed and on way to part-time consulting at Community Mental Health Center in Delaware.

During that visit, Phil Bellefleur and his new wife, Karen, unwittingly changed the future direction, location, and geography of my life even more than their introducing me to the worlds of deaf children, their families, and their deaf community. Although Phil and Karen were ten or more years younger than I, we each had a number of things in common, including a recent divorce, and we soon became such good friends that they invited me for repeated visits to their charming weekend abode on Maryland's broad and sheltered Bohemia River. I had not realized how close to Philadelphia were nearby parts of the Maryland shore, and how unspoiled and lovely they were. And so, it was a few weekend visits to the Chesapeake home of my new friends that changed my vision of where I wanted to be.

The tradition of living on the upper Chesapeake Bay passed from the Bellefleurs through me, to my now grown children and theirs along with our family retreat. I have lived to see all of this much enhanced by son Paul's single-handed sailing skills (much better than mine ever were) and his lovely waterfront farm next door. From parents born in Europe, we have been gifted through three generations of a shared life on Maryland's Chesapeake shores.

As I look back as a widower now, with my psychoanalytic insight and my elderly hindsight, blessed with children, grandchildren and more, maybe this little piece of Maryland shore was meant to be for me. I was unconsciously conditioned for it by many things that went far back in my life, including songs my Ma had crooned to me as a little child. I still remember the words to this day. One of her favorite bedtime tunes she often sang to me when I was very little was Irving Berlin's "Russian Lullaby." As I look out at the Elk River from our waterfront family home, I still remember the words. They went like this:

"Every night you'll hear her croon a Russian lullaby
Just a little plaintive tune when baby starts to cry

Rock-a-bye my baby, somewhere there may be

A land that's free for you and me and a Russian lullaby"

This peaceful Maryland shore seemed suddenly to be an American lullaby that came true for me, for our children and theirs, and for all our dear friends, too. What will follow I do not know. We are here only for a time. Nothing is forever, except that which lives deep in our hearts.

My Loss of Sam

Sam had long maintained his busy schedule, full teaching load, and further academic duties pertaining to Temple's Unit in Law and Psychiatry. Everything had gone smoothly and swimmingly well through 1974, when catastrophe struck on August 2 of 1975, and Sam went into acute heart failure and departed from us. He had been having metabolic problems with abnormal triglyceride levels and had been seen by the top internists and cardiologists at Temple where he was a highly respected faculty colleague. He seemed to have recovered from a brief episode of heart failure earlier that summer. I remember him describing it to me as a sustained feeling of discomfort and frustration, like "being unable to breath while swimming under water," in his words. He was rescued by medication, including several digitalis-type drugs—but then it recurred, and Sam was suddenly gone. Sam Polsky was in his mid-fifties, in his prime, and much too young to die. As our faculty and students at Temple's Law and Medical schools mourned the unexpected passing of Sam at memorial services, I was devastated.

Sam Polsky's passing was not only a blow to the shared projects on which we were working, but incurred a deeply-felt sense of personal loss. Sam was not only my academic partner, but my very best and closest friend for the previous eighteen years. Like confiding brothers, we had grown to share almost everything. We were buddies. In connection with our various projects, Sam had promised me that if I would undertake monitoring and coordinating the independent project managers' work, he would assume the task of writing up the final report for ABC. I was left to do that and ended up completing a five-hundred page report for our five-year project while continuing our academic work in law and society at Temple. I discovered an interesting thing, at least for me. I did not have time to grieve, because I was so busy taking up the slack that was left by Sam's absence. This reminded me of stories I had heard that during the WWII bombing of London by the German Luftwaffe, mentally ill patients allegedly improved markedly. They got out of their beds, swept up the broken glass, and when the bombing was over and London was no longer being attacked, they regressed back to their psychoses. This reminded me that I no longer had the "luxury of grieving" because Sam's loss was like an unexpected bombshell, and I was so busy picking up the pieces.

Jane II

Following my loss of Sam, I lost my determined grip on secondary bachelorhood to a very lovely and lovable young woman who was seventeen years my junior, and too good for me in many ways, as well. She was adorable and I adored her. It takes more to make a marriage work—much more—especially with our each having children of differing ages and interests from former marriages. Her name was Jane, and my three children, who were surprised that I married a woman so young, called her Jane II, to distinguish her from their own mother named Jane. More than twenty years earlier, when Jane II was ten, I had very briefly treated her seven-year-old brother for an adjustment disorder of childhood, following the death of their father in Boston, where they grew up, and their mother's subsequent decision to move with her two children to Philadelphia and marry a well-regarded and successful lawyer, who promptly adopted the two youngsters.

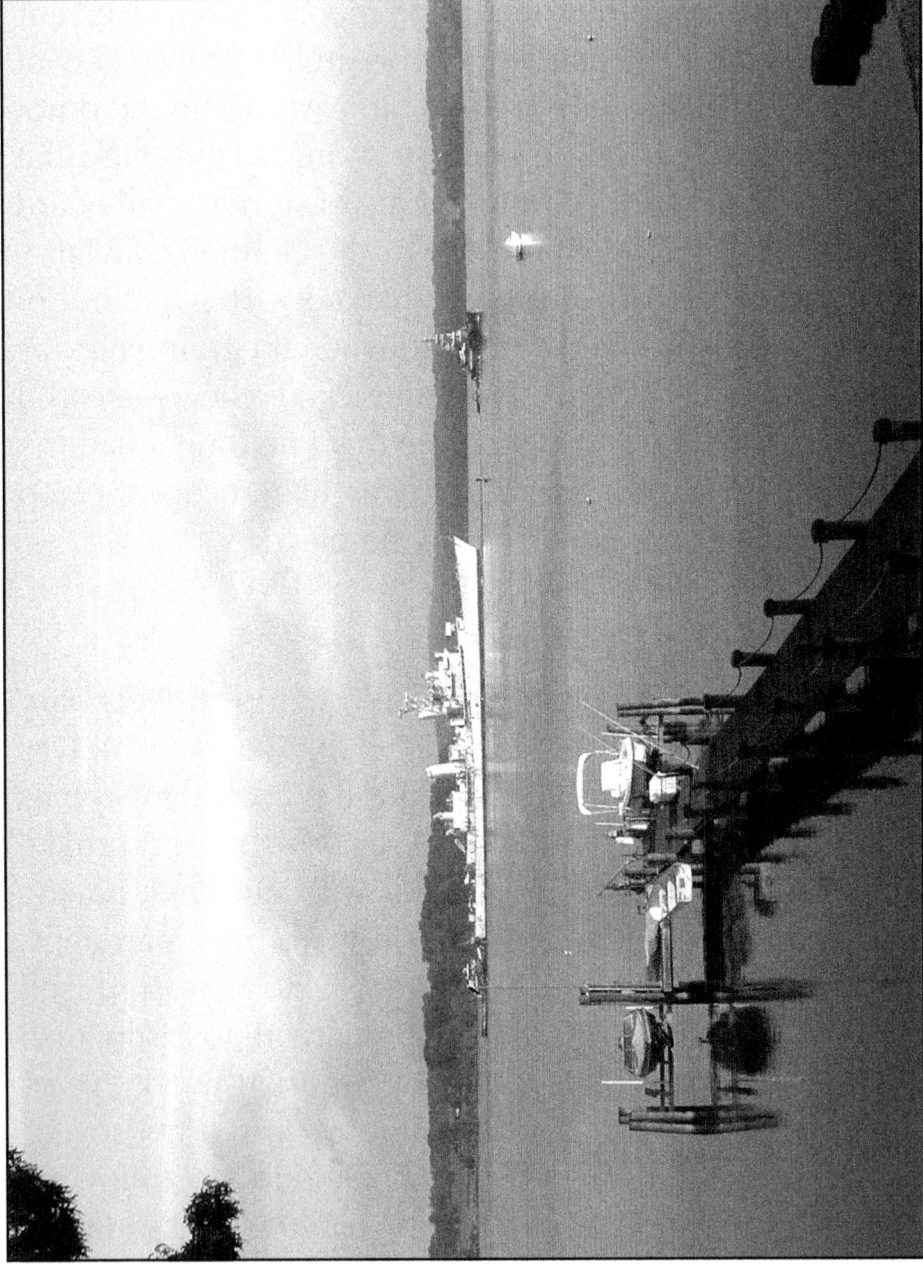

Peaceful and interesting views of Elk River traffic from Author's dock occasionally included such unusual crafts as the "Battleship New Jersey" being towed to its final resting place in Camden, NJ.

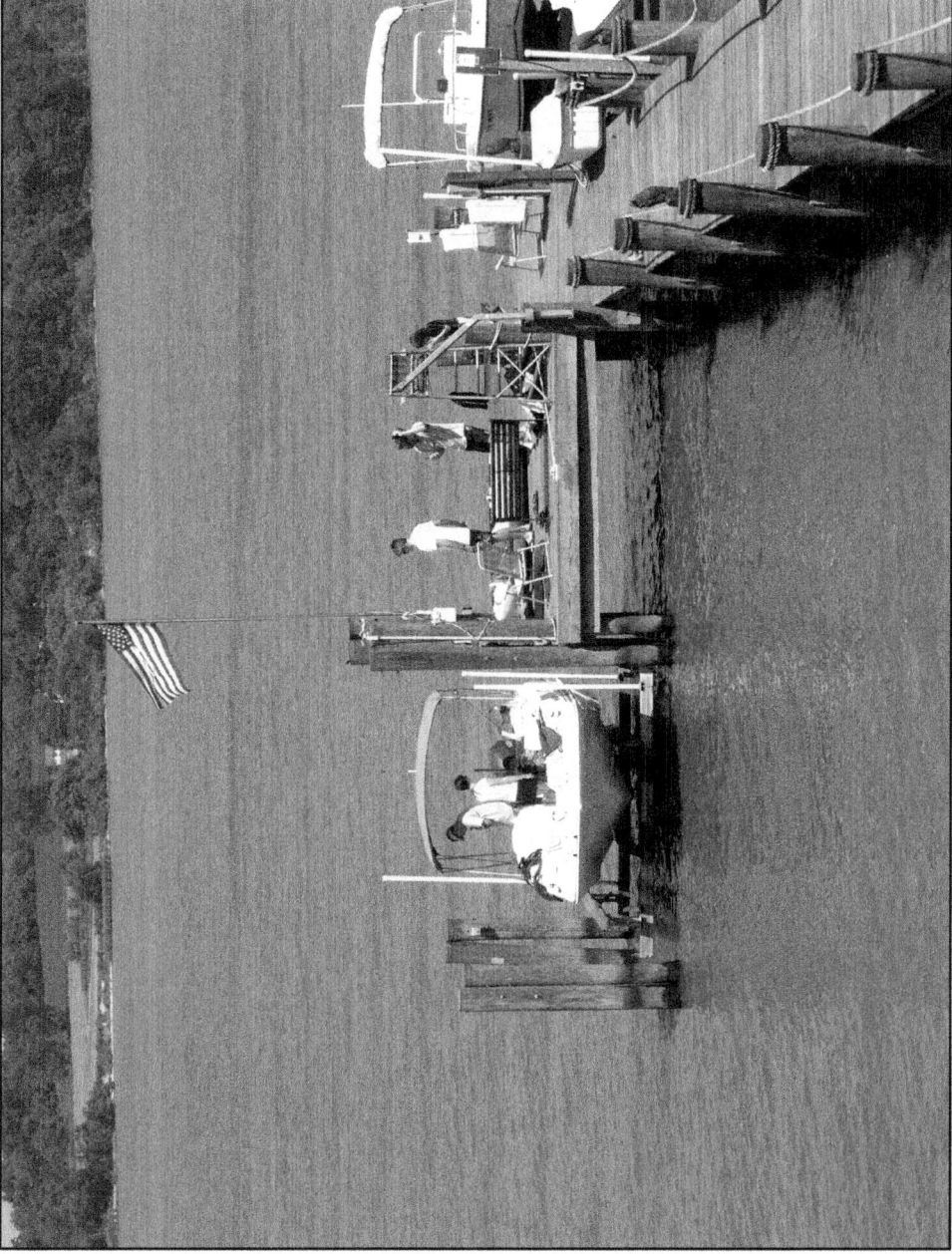

David and Paul preparing to take their kids and friends waterskiing.

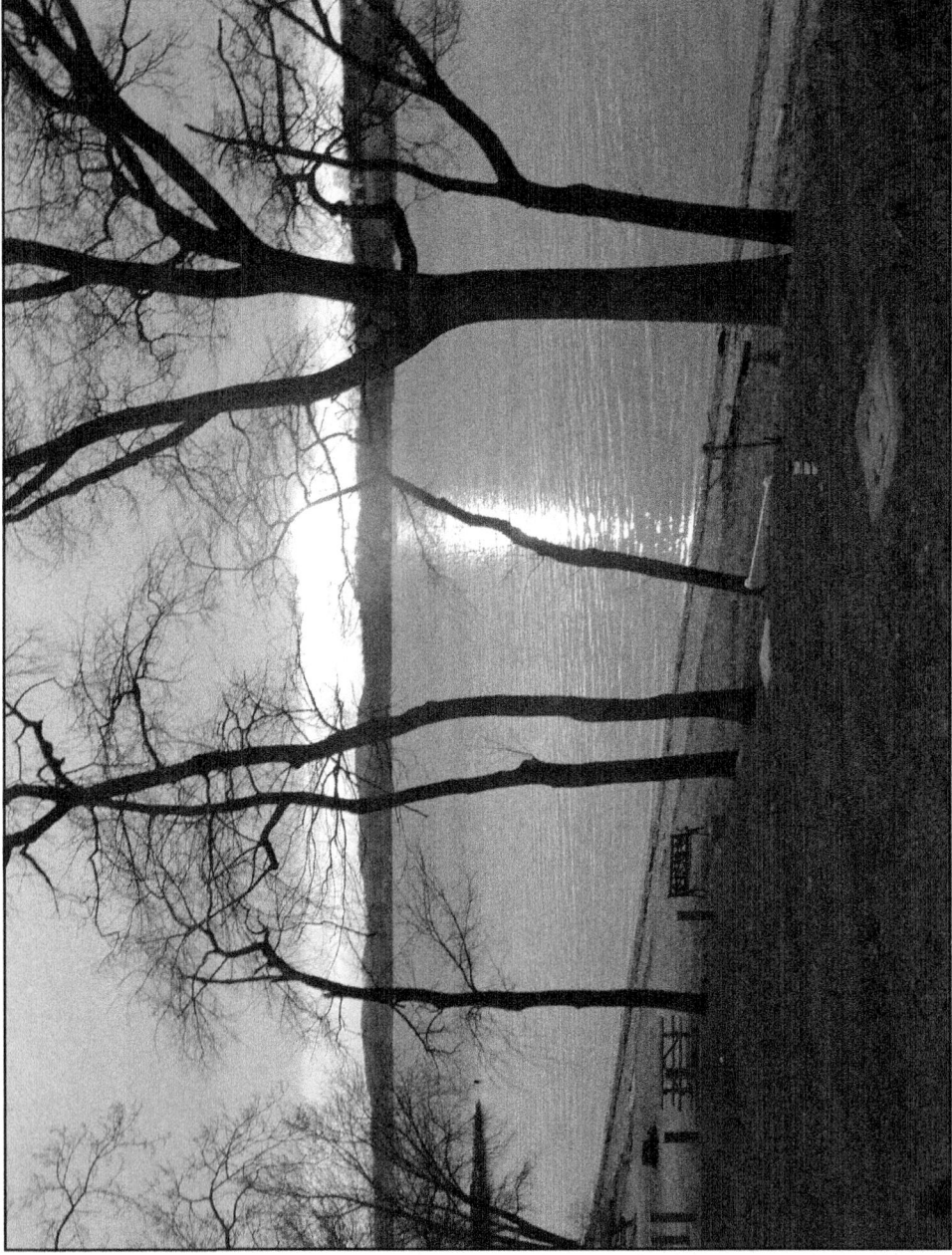

Author and neighbor's Elk River shoreline with Paul's Jetty (protruding on left) demarcating son Paul's adjoining waterfront farm.

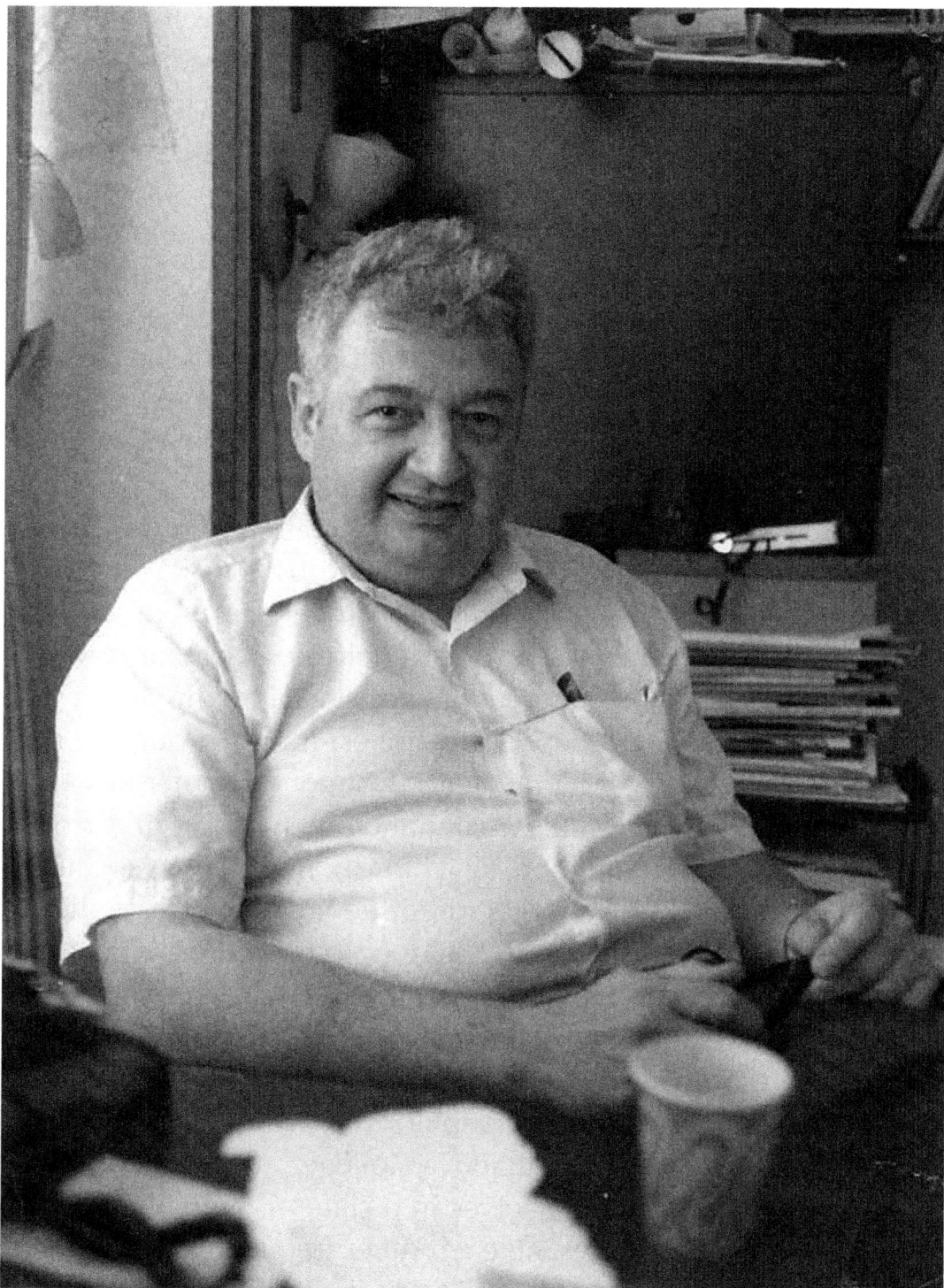

Sam Polsky, spring 1975 (photo by author).

Jane's mother was a customer of my father's jewelry shop in Boston, and so they had known each other and heard of me, which is how she happened to call me to see her little son back then. I had never treated or seen the ten-year-old sister until some twenty-five years later when, as a married woman with two sons, she phoned my office requesting an appointment for her husband, who wanted a divorce. Could I convince him to consider marital counseling, she wanted to know. With perhaps a chance, and little to lose, I felt it was worth a try. After two very reluctant joint sessions, he refused to continue but agreed to see me one more time alone, without her, during which he informed me that he was going to marry his former secretary and that it was a done deal.

"Should I tell her that?" I asked him. "She already knows. I just want us to be as decent as we can, for the boys' sake at least." I had seen far worse marital breakups. Neither of them wanted individual or further therapy, and so I felt there was no more I could do. Months later, I bumped into her at a gathering where she looked happy and well, and was all smiles. It turned out that she was living in Bala Cynwyd, practically around the corner from my home on Levering Mill Road, which I had purchased at my former wife's request to "give our son, David, a home." This was after I suggested that he take a semester off to see how badly, if at all, he wanted to continue as a pre-med student in his junior year at the University of Rochester. He left Rochester, and it subsequently took some time and doing to get him back to a Philadelphia college to finish his senior year. By then, Jane II and I had become good friends, and she was of great help in convincing Dave to finish his Bachelor's degree nearby at Villanova College.

Jane and I soon found ourselves in a state of mutually needed affection, and we began seeing each other frequently. She invited me to her home around the corner, and I invited her to join me on a visit to Phil and Karen Bellefleur. Jane II felt instantly bonded with

Karen Bellefleur, who had recently married Phil, and she much enjoyed the times we spent at the Eastern Shore.

As the relationship developed in all of its aspects, I became fond of her two nice young sons, as well as her fine parents. Jane became similarly interested in and attracted to my own three children. As our relationships intensified and the family seemed to interact well, I lost my grip on better judgment and soon found myself remarried to a woman seventeen years younger than I. It was not so much the age difference, but basically a different order of priorities. Even though we were each born of Jewish parents, it was a mixed marriage. Jane's family background placed high priorities on their synagogue, its organized community affairs, and extensive Jewish charity work. I was an ethnically Jewish person with similar moral and spiritual values, and all for charity, but essentially a more secular person little inclined toward organized religious traditions.

Stumbling Blocks

When we married, we tried our best, but my efforts unraveled as we encountered stumbling blocks in the differences between our two families' backgrounds and priorities. Ironically, the least important, but final stumble block, occurred in a Conservative Jewish temple, of all places, and involved its conservative dogma and traditional practices. It was at the time of my son David's marriage to Lauren Bronstein. In the Conservative Jewish tradition of Lauren's parents, couples got married under a "chuppah" or canopy, accompanied by their parents on both sides. A chuppah, symbolizing the Jewish home, is regarded by Orthodox and Conservative Jews as a basic ingredient of a Jewish wedding. The groom enters it first, followed by the bride and their parents or closest of kin, representing their approval in the joining of the two families.

So there we were as two sets of family members at David's

wedding to Lauren at her parents' Conservative temple. As the father of the groom, I was told by the officiating rabbi that I could not stand under the chuppah with my wife, Jane II, but only with David's mother, who could not stand up there with her new and second husband, Marty Mellon. The rabbi ruled that it must be the actual parents of the groom who stood under the chuppah, rather than either of our current spouses. The bride's parents were the "originals" and presented no such problem. It made no great difference to my son's mother. Nor did it matter to her new husband, Marty Mellon. But to my wife's parents, the sight of me standing with my ex-wife while my present wife, their daughter, was forbidden to stand by my side, was an outrageous affront, particularly to my new father-in-law, who was both an active and observant Conservative Jewish gentleman. He was a prominent Philadelphia lawyer, who did not take such insult to his adopted daughter and her mother lightly. Lacking the fabled rabbinic wisdom of a Solomon, I wondered if I should abandon my son together with his about-to-be wife and in-laws, and go sit with Jane II, my wife, and her parents. Did you catch not merely the symbolism of all that—the intense, disruptive and family disharmony of it all? Little wonder we Jews have so many troubles, I thought, while helplessly pondering the embarrassing intrusion of stubbornly adhered-to religious traditions in our complex contemporary lives.

Things had been unraveling for Jane II and me before then, but that seemed to mark the beginning of the end. My second wife and I had both hoped for the best, but we had not foreseen the problems. To be brief, I will say that our interests were different, and we parted with a mutual sense of disappointment, but as friends. Jane subsequently remarried and was living happily in a nearby suburb, from the last I heard. I dare say we each got over it, but I have regretted putting her through another failed marriage, which she did not need. But maybe we each did need it to make the next one work.

Back to Work: Professor William Traylor and Mental Health Law

Fortunately, the dean of the law school appointed Professor William Traylor to take over Sam Polsky's role in our Law and Psychiatry program. Bill, as I called him, soon became a very good friend. I had known him on the faculty, and he more than rose to the occasion. Bill, like Sam, had an excellent academic background, but quite different. Bill had been an engineering student at Purdue, as I recall, before he went on to law school. As a result, Bill seemed to me more orderly and "mathematically" organized than Sam, who had been perhaps more philosophic and wide-ranging in his approach to legal issues and teaching.

I was quick to adjust to Bill's presence and grateful for the syllabus he created each year for our new semester's work. At Bill's suggestion, we changed the name of the course from "Law and Psychiatry" to "Mental Health Law," because this was a time of substantial change of the Commonwealth of Pennsylvania's Mental Health Act, as well as those of multiple states. It was a time when reform-minded psychiatrists were teaming up with civil rights lawyers and demanding changes, if not the dismantling of gigantic state mental hospital systems, which were not adequately observing patients' rights.

Pennsylvania's much-needed Mental Health Procedures Act of 1976 clearly established patients' rights to treatment as well as to refuse treatment, as well their rights to be not unduly restrained in more than the least restrictive manner required by their behavior and circumstances. Moreover, patients were not to be regarded as dangerous unless it could be shown that they committed a harmful act against themselves or others within the past thirty days, and that the act was likely to be repeated. All these safeguards and patients' rights resulted when various courts came down with landmark decisions, which we included in Bill Traylor's fine syllabus and in our annual final exam questions for our third-year law students. The idea in the 1970s was to close down huge state mental hospitals and replace them with small, outpatient community mental health centers close to their neighborhoods. Unfortunately, the community mental health systems were never adequately funded to provide for the numbers of mentally ill persons who required responsibly monitored residential treatment. The right to refuse treatment or surreptitiously discontinue it in communities that entitle its citizens to bear arms continues to result in the tragic shootings of children and adults by mentally disturbed and emotionally distraught persons, to our recurrent sense of dismay.

Chapter 19
Life After Divorce, Remaining Amicable, Separate but Equal

How Our Dividends Continued to Grow

David Harris Heller

DAVID GRADUATED FROM the Haverford School, a very fine Philadelphia mainline school. Despite my urging that he apply to Tufts, where I had gone, one of his advisors suggested that he would be well-placed at University of Rochester. It was his adolescent privilege to follow someone else's advice, and I must admit that I again committed the sin of being a "pushy father who knows best" (with the best of intentions). Unbeknownst to me, but highly valued by David, was a hobby that he developed as the disc jockey at his college radio station at University of Rochester. Today as I write this, he is a highly-regarded news commentator with WHYY radio in the Philadelphia area. Unfortunately, my hearing loss is such that I cannot hear him, but many elderly residents of my retirement community here in Haverford want to know if I am actually the father of "the" David Heller, and they tell me that he is really wonderful at his work. That gives me joy and reassurance that he feels happy and fulfilled.

Joan Elizabeth Heller Miller

Joan married Kenneth David Miller, MD after they met as Tufts college students. Their marriage turned out to be a lifetime source of happiness, as I have watched them raise three very bright, talented, and interesting children. Joan is a two-time cancer survivor, first of leukemia at age forty and then breast cancer more recently. She has recently rewarded her potential readers with an elegant memoir called *Healing Grief: A Story of Survivorship* about these challenging experiences. She and Ken, a practicing hematologist-oncologist, offer unique and uplifting presentations to local hospitals, mental health centers, schools, and hospice organizations on issues of cancer survivorship and long-term healing.

PAUL ANDREW HELLER

Paul, the youngest, has achieved outstanding career success in the corporate world. Paul was an engineering student at Tufts and had a minor in economics. He signed on very early as an employee at Vanguard and rapidly rose to be a Managing Director. He has been the Chief Information Officer for Vanguard these past several years and is now moving over to be in charge of another aspect of their business. He is a born problem-solver who loves people, and this is reciprocated by the many friends he has. He is an avid sailor, and I take pride in having introduced him to that hobby when I first showed him the ropes and the points of sail, and which way the wind blows, so to speak. Today he is a much better sailor than I ever was and enjoys navigating his twenty-three-foot "Com-Pac" sloop, which is ideal for the Chesapeake, with many shallow inlets to explore.

MY GRANDCHILDREN

My daughter, Joan, and her husband, Ken, provided me with the greatest gift of my first granddaughter, Cara. While obtaining her Master's and PhD degrees in Clinical Psychology at Gallaudet University, Cara acquired a specially trained service dog certified by Canine Companions for Independence (CCI). She wrote an excellent PhD thesis on service dogs for deaf individuals, and she continues to volunteer her services to CCI as President of CCI's Maryland, Virginia, and D.C. chapters.

Julie, Cara's younger sister, completed her Master's Degree in Social Work at University of California Berkeley, with an emphasis on gerontology. Julie has recent part-time employment as an adjunct instructor and service-learning coordinator at Northeastern University where she co-teaches and guides groups of Northeastern University students on various cross-cultural teaching tours of European, Asian, and African countries. Extremely capable and energetic, she works as a Research Associate at the Massachusetts Institute of Technology AgeLab in her other part-time job. She will be beginning her PhD in Social Work this coming year.

Last but not least of the Miller children is Jeremy who graduated with top grades, high honors, and a Phi Beta Kappa key from University of Massachusetts Amherst. He will be entering Johns Hopkins Medical School, where he will train to become a fourth generation physician, starting with his great-grandfather, Dr. Benedict Harris, myself as his grandfather, and his own father, all of whom have had clinical academic careers as practicing physicians. So I anticipate and pray that he, too, will emerge as a strong, resourceful, and successful teacher and clinician in his forthcoming medical career.

My youngest son, Paul, and his wife, Laurie, brought me my grandchild John. As I write these words now, this tall, handsome and strong grandson is getting back on his feet after a traumatic car accident, recovering with all of the help that his very capable and supportive parents can supply for their only child.

David and Lauren brought me two grandsons, Cody and Jake. Like my own father and brother, Cody, at age twenty-three, is a capable craftsmen and skilled jeweler. He has a remarkable talent for producing unique pieces of silver and gold as free-form creations, embedded with semi-precious stones, for which he has created an online internet business and a professional website from which he makes a living.

Jake is a bright, athletic, and agile young man who is a sophomore at Temple University, where he seems to be interested in ecology and environmental studies. In my view, he is just beginning his undergraduate life, and he testing his strong young wings with which he seems capable of doing many good things.

I Was Determined to Remain Single—But It Was Not to Be

As for me, after two failed marriages, I was determined to remain single, but unable to live a life of religious, let alone secular abstinence, I dated a number of women over a course of many years, and developed extended relationships with a couple of them. Divorced and separated people encounter each other with multiple needs, some of which are conscious and many of which are not. I usually had good conscious reasons and intentions with the women I met between my first two marriages. So wanting to avoid becoming passing ships that meet in the night, one enters into ongoing affairs, which not only become intimate, but meaningful in different ways to each party, as I discovered. The basic problem with a love affair is that if it is really gratifying, one or the other partner wants to turn it into a commitment called marriage. I had been determined to remain single. My best intentions to remain single began to waver somewhat with several truly lovely and sincere women with whom I found myself increasingly involved. And yet I dreaded undertaking what I really knew deep down were the true responsibilities of a marriage: a commitment "until death do us part."

MIDDLE AGED LESSONS LEARNED IN BETWEEN MARRIAGES

Following my marriage to Jane II, I was all the more determined to resist a third such commitment and marriage, as I sampled the illusion of free love between consenting adults. I did not relish the bachelor's life, as I learned belatedly and very sadly that ongoing, consensual sexual affairs between adults who were legally free to marry were by no means totally free. They worked freely only for a time. If I were free to marry a person in a mutually gratifying relationship, and claimed to love that person, how could I justify a lesser relationship? If sex and the relationship were really that great for both, then why not convert it into the maturely trusting and full commitment of marriage, with or without prenuptial agreements? If things were really not that great, why continue it? How could one be sure things might not improve if less than great, or that great relationships and situations existed only in the movies? Monogamy, in contrast to monotheism, seemed much more difficult, restricting, and demanding to practice. Then, when I expected never to marry again, I met someone very different, and things changed.

Chapter 20
Shopping for a Crockpot, Ending Up with a Wife

I WAS SIXTY years old, and I had taken to having a sandwich or something very light for lunch, and then visiting a couple of local thrift shops on the Main Line. I thought it would be good if I could learn to cook a bit, and maybe even set up a meal at the beginning of the day with a crock pot, which seemed to be popular then. One day as I was going by the Jefferson Hospital Thrift Shop, called Penny Wise, I spied such a crock pot in the window, went in, and was approached by a charming lady who wanted to know if she could help me. She volunteered that she had many crock pot recipes. This turned out to be so. Her name was Irmgard Foulkrod, the widow of John J. Foulkrod III, who came from a prominent Main Line family, formerly from the Germantown section of Philadelphia, where there is a Foulkrod Street.

This sweet lady took an interest in me and told her fellow volunteers at the Jefferson Hospital Thrift Shop that she was determined to get to know me. Indeed, she invited me on a chartered bus trip to New York sponsored by the Philadelphia Country Club, of which she was a member, courtesy of her widow's rights for the previous seven years since her husband had died. The trip was to a Vatican art exhibit at New York's Metropolitan Museum of Art, and it was a great day. I reciprocated by inviting her to dinner the following week at her favorite restaurant in Gladwynne.

She expressed further interest in me and since I had seen her home in Gladwynne, she wanted to see where I was living in a small cottage in nearby Penn Valley, which I used mainly to see private patients while continuing with my academic and clinical responsibilities at Temple's Schools of Law and Medicine. When she saw my neat little cottage, she pronounced it "charming," but insisted that I allow her to plant a few decorative flowers and a bush. She offered that gardening was something she did with pleasure. It turned out that she was in charge of the annual plant sale for the Gladwynne Library and had raised considerable funds because of her volunteer work. To make a long story short, I soon realized that she was a very unusual, reliable, and mature person, particularly when I learned of her background, which was truly remarkable, I felt.

Not Exactly a Nun's Story, but Close Enough

Irmgard had been born and raised in Bad-Aachen, Germany, Charlemagne's ancient capital on the German border with Belgium and Holland. Irmgard's father, Heinrich Bellingrad, was of Swiss-German background, and was a highly-intelligent, successful businessman, who was head of Dunn and Bradstreet for Western Germany. Irmgard was the older of his two daughters who, like her father, was raised Lutheran, whereas her younger sister, Katie, like her mother, was raised Catholic. When Irmgard was eighteen, girls her age in Nazi Germany were being sent to Hitler Youth camps to mingle and perhaps bear more children quickly for their Fuhrer.

Irmgard's father took a dim view of this prospect, and he smuggled her out of Germany under the assumed last name of Boulanger to a colleague of his in Belgium. Sworn to secrecy and to not be in touch with her parents until after the war, it had been arranged for her to enter a student nursing hospital program under the auspices of the Ursuline nuns. There in Belgium, she spent the war years as a student nurse taking care of not only Wehrmacht soldiers, but Allied soldiers and others who dropped from the sky. She saw much heavy duty warfare, and even the nuns' hospital was subject to bombing and errant German rockets.

As the war turned against the Germans, highly-placed Nazis were pretending to be soldiers and got themselves admitted to the nuns' hospital to avoid arrest and prosecution as war criminals. Meanwhile, on Eisenhower's staff was a young attorney from Philadelphia named John J. Foulkrod III. He was Eisenhower's officer tasked with ferreting out highly-placed Nazis, who were posing as patients in hospitals and other places of refuge. One day, he arrived at the Ursuline nuns' hospital in his Jeep with his enlisted driver, armed with an automatic weapon, and knocked on the door asking to meet the Mother Superior. In his politest manner, he asked if anyone there spoke English. Mother Superior said yes, and brought forth student nurse Irmgard Boulanger. Captain Foulkrod asked if she would translate for him. This brave and determined young woman looked him in the eye and said, "Yes, but only if you give me penicillin for my patients." And so he did, and she did. This led to a swift relationship. Captain Foulkrod was single, and he took a liking to her.

After several weeks of working together, he returned to the hospital in dismay after learning it had been bombed. His translator was nowhere to be found. He had enough political and practical clout to commandeer a bulldozer. "Where was she last seen?" he demanded. They said she was last seen coming out of the delivery room with a newborn infant in each arm. Putting two and two together, with his commandeered bulldozer, he rescued her from the bombed stairwell where she had been buried for seventy-two hours with a newborn under each arm and not a drop of milk for them nor water for her. She also had shrapnel wounds on her lower back and buttocks. To make a long story short, all three of them survived, and Irmgard was doubly grateful to JJ Foulkrod III, who was increasingly interested in her welfare.

In due course, he went to his boss, General Eisenhower, and confessed that he was in love with an "enemy alien." He told Ike the story of her bombing and survival. The general said, "Don't worry, I'm going to Washington next week on some urgent business." In due course, as Irmgard understood it, Congress passed the first "enemy-fiancée" act in contrast to "war-bride" act. After the war terminated, Irmgard was placed on a four-engine Constellation, together with her little Springer Spaniel and several cartons of Pall-Malls, with which Foulkrod had supplied her to ease her way through various European stops.

Irmgard's American Story and Her Children

Upon her marriage to Foulkrod, Irmgard was informed by her newly met mother-in-law that the Foulkrod women did not work as nurses or in any other capacity, but did volunteer work instead. Irmgard was dutiful and fell into this new routine with all of her capable ability to adjust. In due course, she gave birth to JJ Foulkrod IV, who became a big strapping youngster, and a son of whom any man could be proud. Irmgard had not only done her duty, but repeated it with a follow-up act, which presented Jack Foulkrod with the apple of his eye, a beautiful daughter also named Irmgard. The young Irmgard did not find this to be a popular American name, and in her early school years, had it changed to Bonnie. She grew up to be as lovely a daughter as any parent would wish. In due course, Bonnie married one David Rees from Pittsburg. David Rees went on to Temple Medical School in Philadelphia, where quite by coincidence, I had lectured to his class on several occasions about medical-legal issues they might soon encounter as physicians. When I came into the picture, Bonnie and Dave Rees had young children. Bonnie worked as a substitute teacher when her children grew older, while her husband's career in orthopedic surgery flourished at Reading Hospital.

When Irmgard expressed curiosity about my rural weekend home on the Elk River in Maryland, which I had purchased in

January 1977, I brought her down to see it. She exclaimed, "It's beautiful! It's nicer than the Rhine." "You bet," I said, never having seen the Rhine. To make a long story short, once again, we began living not exactly in sin, but frequently sampling it. Over a period of time, she wondered if she could stay in Maryland to "plant a few flowers and tidy things up," she said. I returned to work during the week at Temple and my small office practice in Penn Valley. Far more than tidying up, she planted azalea gardens and transformed what had been a nice place into a real home.

As for her son, John, he had gone into the Air Force as an enlisted airman and was assigned to be the Chaplain's assistant. In the course of that work, he became increasingly interested in religion and through David Rees, I believe, met Cinda Hess, whose father was a Methodist bishop in the Ohio conference. In due course, Irmgard's son, John Foulkrod, and Cinda each became ordained ministers, and when I met young Reverend John Foulkrod, he was the pastor of a very substantial congregation in Ohio. That is true, but not exactly so, because when I first met him, he was sitting relaxed in a chair next to my hospital bed, in which I was recovering from major chest surgery, a lobectomy for lung cancer, at age sixty-seven. I awoke to see a large, heavy-set fellow, who sat there calmly, quite motionless, and seeming almost like a Buddha, exuding a sense of peace and well-being. In my condition, I was more than grateful to have a supportive clergyman of almost any denomination in my hospital corner, and family at that point.

In a rather short time, Irmgard and I took to each other's children and grandchildren as if they were born to us. Together, we collected six grandchildren from my issue and seven from hers for a total of thirteen—and still counting, in terms of great-grandchildren. The third time around, it seemed that I hit the jackpot. I think my unexpected Irmgard was the best wife that I could possibly have found, but I didn't realize it until I found her crying one day in the bathroom when I returned to Maryland from Philadelphia. Wanting to know what the trouble was after we had been living together in visible sin in front of our children and other prime folks, she said, "I'm crying because I want to be a Mrs." I suddenly knew how right she was for me—and, why not?

And so I married for the third time. Under the circumstances, and all things being considered, I felt and still do that she was meant to be for me. We truly loved each other and our shared children and grandchildren. For the time we were together, Irmgard was a strong woman both in body and will for me. She shared my concerns, as I shared hers. Together, she helped me to build a beautiful home on the Eastern Chesapeake Shore, where our children learned sailing, the fun of crabbing, swimming, boating, and waterskiing, among other hobbies and friends we shared.

Our Loss of Irmgard, But Not Her Family

Sadly, around 2004, Irmgard developed a pulmonary condition and then atrial fibrillation. One of her greatest pleasures had been to invite her German family of cousins and her only niece, the daughter of her sister, Katie, to enjoy our Elk River home and surroundings. Irmgard's niece was named (guess what) Irmgard, and was married to a very nice young man named Uwe Bennink. Uwe was a very bright guy, who was well-placed with the German state or federal police system where he was in charge of teaching newly-recruited personnel and familiarizing them with essential computer skills, as well as other necessities of their occupations. My wife's sister, Katie Ault, lived in Holland, close enough to frequently visit her grandchildren, a beautiful little Alina and her brother, Fabian, who were approximately eight and five when I first laid eyes on them. Irmgard had a lovely family.

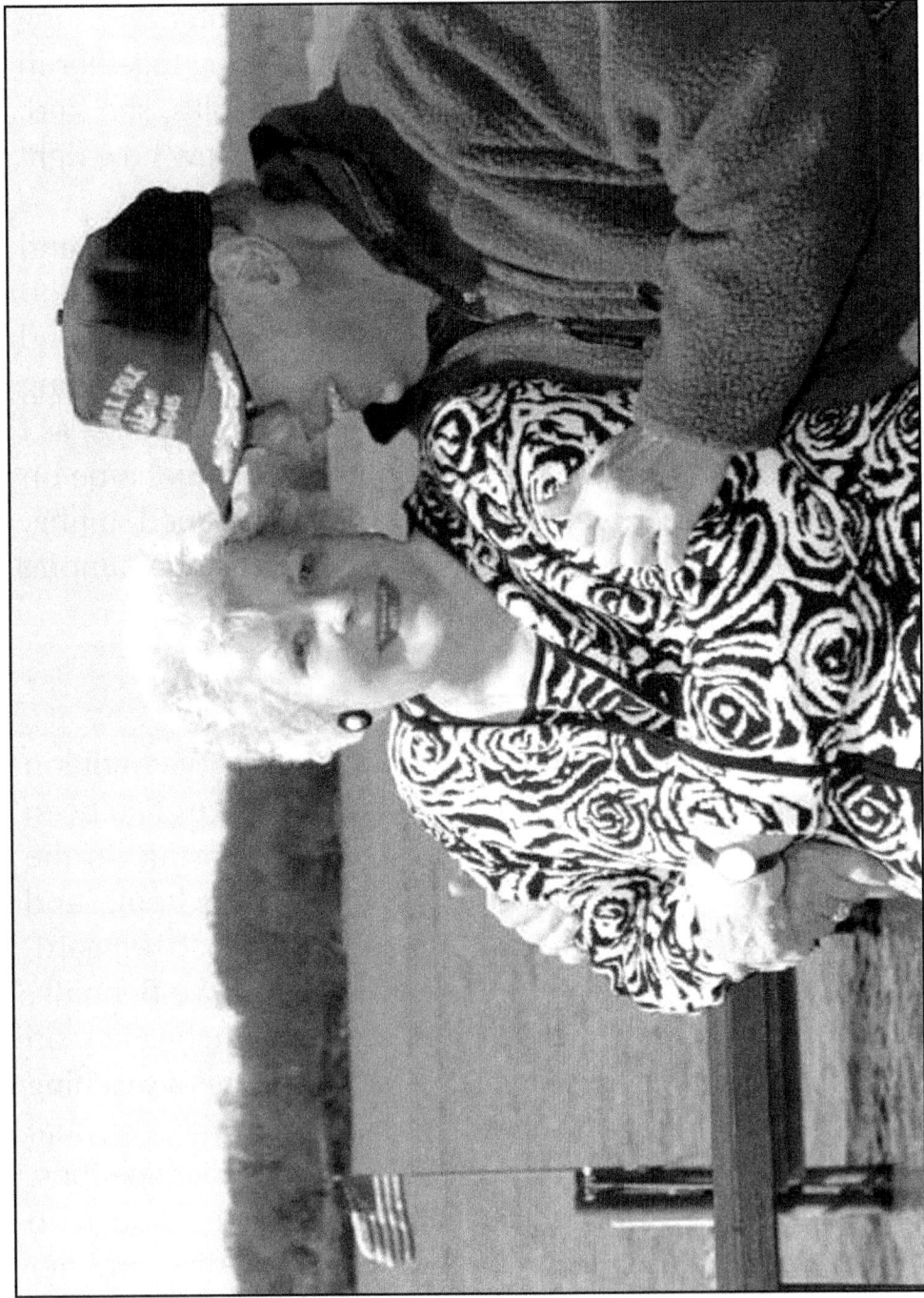

Author with recently married wife, Irmgard Foulkrod Heller, pushing into their early seventies together, knowing how lucky they were to have found each other.

Now years later, as I write these words, the home at the Chesapeake Bay is hallowed by our departed Irmgard's ashes scattered and sown among her living gardens of recurrently blooming azaleas. Her daughter Bonnie and husband Dave's children are grown up with children of their own. Their daughter, Elizabeth Rees, won the Latin prize at her graduation from Wyomissing High School in suburban Redding. She went to Duke, and then work in Washington, D.C. for a federal agency in which she could not openly discuss the nature of her work. In due course, she met a Marine captain named Anthony Giardino. Anthony was no ordinary Marine, but a graduate of Annapolis, to which he had obtained entry by virtue of the fact that his father and uncles had all served in Vietnam. Elizabeth and Anthony got married in a lovely ceremony at the U.S. Naval Academy's Chapel under the drawn swords of his chosen classmates. Irmgard, dressed in a long rose-colored gown for the occasion, was enormously proud to be part of this ceremony, as I was equally proud and grateful to be included as the happy couple's step-grandfather.

Chapter 21
Middle Age Brought Me Added Perspectives of Pa and Ma

IF WE ARE blessed with parents who live long enough for our paths to cross and continue for many years thereafter, we can sometimes be gifted in our middle age by new pictures of them that revise, augment, and tell us things we had not known about or seen in our parents before. I have two such experiences to share with you. The first is a story about my father as told to me by my cousin, Sam, years after my dad had died. The story was subsequently confirmed by my brother, Saul. Both Sam and Saul had worked for many years together with my Dad in his jewelry shop. I had departed from Boston long before, to pursue my further medical career in Philadelphia where my Boston cousins, Sam and Shirley Geffin, caught up with me at a wedding in Philadelphia. Sam and I had been close as youngsters in Boston, but had not been in touch for a long time. Accordingly, it was so good to see him, and the following story he told me about my dad, his Uncle Herbert, affected me so deeply that I wrote it up when I got home, and later typed it into my computer as a personal essay. What I wrote back then was the following:

Herbert and the Archbishop's Cross (My dad as told to me by Cousin Sam Geffin)

I realized that I had seen too little of Cousin Sam and the others following my departure from Boston some twenty years earlier. We now stood, glasses in hand, savoring the occasion and surveying the growing crowd of noisy guests in the formal ballroom. Soon Sam and I found some chatting space off to the side. It was a fortunate spot, a bit away from the main crowd, yet only a few steps from the sumptuous bar which had been laid out for the bar mitzvah festivities for the son of Sam's wife's cousin. To make the event more special, the bar mitzvah boy's father was now a prominent Philadelphia rabbi, whom I had seen perhaps once or twice since he himself had been a teenager at Sam and Shirley's wedding in Boston long before. So there I was with Cousin Sam, extending from the bar, as extended family should on such occasions, and talking of old times. As mentioned, I had seen Sam only rarely, and not since his Uncle Herbert, my father, had died a few years before.

When he was a young man just out of the service, cousin Sam had apprenticed himself to my father who was a master jeweler in Boston, and a demanding taskmaster with unyielding opinions and principles. But his Uncle Herbert, who could generally be depended upon to blow up in brief intermittent squalls of temper, was also a forgiving and loving man. It was Uncle Herbert's essential warmth which made things emotionally tolerable, if not always tranquil, for his small crew working together in the close quarters of a small shop over the years.

When Uncle Herbert, the Boss, was out on a call, his crew found frequent respite from the boredom of routine jobs and the tension of delicate ones by indulging in rugged verbal games which featured recurrent familiarities and uninvited insults which passed as comradely humor. No one's weakness was immune from being outrageously lampooned, nor safe from an eventual carefully crafted retort.

So Sam, like his Uncle Herbert and other memorable characters in that and similar small shops, spent the better part of a working lifetime toiling over other people's precious stones and settings at the jeweler's bench. With the margin for error so small and costly, the only defense was the development of that experienced, discerning and critical skill known as the jeweler's eye with which they regarded not only their work, but from time to time, each other, their customers and colleagues, as I said. While good-natured, these appraisals were often exquisitely accurate, detailed, and sometimes quite hilarious.

And so we recalled that the rabbi had been such a likable youngster when I first met him at Sam and Shirley's wedding so many years before in Boston where we had all grown up, more together than not. We were proud that he was now the prominent and respected rabbi of such a large Philadelphia congregation.

Perhaps it was our unspoken but certain knowledge of the kinds of philosophical questions that Uncle Herbert would sooner or later have put to the rabbi if given half the chance, even at his son's bar mitzvah, that made Sam break our moment of silence to remind me of the story about my father and The Archbishop.

"What Archbishop?"

"You mean you never heard about your father and the Archbishop? I can't believe it. I better get us each a refill. Here, let me have your glass." I watched Cousin Sam go off, already smiling and relishing the story that he was about to reveal.

Sam was a short, but very coordinated fellow, sort of like Mickey Rooney. I watched him with his small bald spot, which he seemed to share with my Dad and me, as he skillfully maneuvered himself to the front of the bar. Soon he returned without spilling a drop, and with an invitation to sit down together off by ourselves. "This story is too good to be interrupted," he explained.

It all began at A. Stowell & Co., that fine Boston jewelry establishment that had seemed to call on Uncle Herbert for their most demanding jobs, if not the most profitable ones. Although he had neither the appearance nor the pedigree of even a salesperson at Stowell's, my father was regarded by Stowell's management as just about the finest precious metal worker in all of Boston. And

224

there were a few really good persons at the bench in those days, or "mechanics," as they called themselves. But let me tell the story as I heard it from Cousin Sam.

"So the boss at Stowell's phoned and asked if Uncle Herbert had time to walk over and look at a job—something very unusual, and confidential, he acknowledged. And so I remember how your father eventually comes back with a small cardboard box, like a shoe box, in a brown paper bag. And Carney Filino whispers to me that maybe Stowell's sent him back with a little lunch for all the shop, loud enough for your father to hear, and he tells Carney not to be fresh.

"'Come in here,' he says, and I'll show you something special. So he opens the box: And then inside the box, he unwraps several layers of tissues, inside of which is cradled in a very soft polishing cloth, a gold cross, maybe five inches one way and three the other. I had never seen anything like it. Very rare, like in a museum, maybe. Beautifully worked, with strands of rope woven out of very thinly drawn gold, and set with many cabochon rubies and emeralds, and old-cut diamonds too. Renaissance, they thought.

"It belonged to Archbishop Cushing. Stowell's said he brought it in himself last week. They had called to say he was coming, of course. And Uncle Herbert was told how he arrived there with his limousine with his chauffeur and the Monsignor, and a couple of motorcycle cops as escorts. Out gets Archbishop Cushing, and after suitable greetings, he is quickly ushered into Stowell's private office. Then the Archbishop takes out the cross, along with a small piece of wood maybe four or so inches long." Sam paused to savor his drink along with his story of Herbert and the cross, as I did too. And then he continued.

"The wood was said by some to be from the original Cross, and the Archbishop believed that this might indeed be so. It was very old, but not smooth or finished in any way—just a very old small piece of wood that had been secretly preserved and handled with great care over the centuries. Now the gold cross was made of wood too, Uncle Herbert had explained, but the outside was completely covered with gold, perhaps one-sixteenth inch thick, or a bit less in places. What the Archbishop wanted to know was if Stowell's had, or knew a special person who might be able and willing to carefully make a little cupboard in the cross, after cutting away just enough of the outside gold so that it could be fastened and hinged as a door, about one by four inches. It should be properly made so that it could be closed to conceal, or opened to reveal the special piece of wood.

"'Herbie, do you think you can do it? Stowell's asks Uncle Herbert. Uncle Herbert says he'd need to study it carefully and would let them know. So straight into the safe it went, and several times during the next week, Uncle Herbert would take it out after the shop was closed and there was no one around except me. And he would stare it at for maybe ten minutes, scribble some note on a piece of paper and put it and the cross back in the safe without saying a word.

"The upshot was that Uncle Herbert, never one to shrink from a professional challenge, even one posed posthumously by some master jeweler of the Renaissance, decided to take the job. But it would take time, he said. What he would need to do is figure the best way to cut through without damaging the thin metal layer entwined with woven strands of gold and set with gems. Who knew what lay underneath? Where and how to dig in would be not unlike finding an approach, a path to ascend some forgotten, unscaled, sheer mountain wall. So, Uncle Herbert told Stowell's that he'd have to study the piece further, and keep going back to it until a way to proceed would be revealed. And Stowell's told the Archbishop that the job was very delicate and required further study. And the Archbishop told Stowell's that he was in no hurry, but that great care needed to be taken with the ancient cross.

"Get the picture?" asked Sam. And there the matter rested, until

Uncle Herbert felt ready to proceed. He announced that he would need to carefully make a series of small holes, by slowly turning the piece by hand on a small lathe. That the shop had no such lathe posed no problem. Ira Ohanian had just the right watchmaker's lathe in his nearby shop, and old-timers like Uncle Herbert and Ira felt honored when a fellow craftsman needed to borrow the use of some special tool or other. Perhaps the borrowed use of an infrequently used piece of equipment justified its original expense, or the space it continued to take in a busy shop crowded by various, out-dated and invariably bulky pieces of heavy machinery rarely used, but sentimentally retained. Such apparent relics of the industrial age stood in a corner like some sacred cow, and generally could not be retired until its owner was ready to do likewise.

Anyway, one evening after the help had left, and undisturbed by the daily distractions of a busy shop, Uncle Herbert left the shop with a plain brown paper bag under his arm. He had told Ira that he had something unusual he wanted to try on Ira's lathe, but Ira was in no way prepared when Uncle Herbert pulled that cross out of the bag and laid upon the bench.

Ira, a usually very good-natured, agreeable and calm person, became agitated when Uncle Herbert explained what he proposed to do with this delicate and quite remarkable cross that belonged to the Archbishop himself. Uncle Herbert became the very model of calm and measured reassurance when he explained to Ira exactly how and why he would proceed with the careful exploratory "surgery," making only the smallest holes through which they could see the underlying condition of the piece—and only that for now.

Uncle Herbert could, after all, be persuasive and even charming when he wanted to be, and Ira had great respect for his skills as a jeweler. What finally calmed Ira a bit was Uncle Herbert's reassurance that he would use Ira's lathe mainly to steady the cross which he would turn only by hand, very slowly and carefully.

And so they proceeded by hand. And after a time it became clear that the work was moving slowly indeed. Not too slowly for Ira who kept reassuring his old friend that they had all the time in the world, but too slowly for Uncle Herbert, who was getting a bit tired, and observed that the night was getting later and later.

And so he turned on the power, reassuring Ira that he was "only going to touch" the cross on the now spinning lathe "just to make a start in the metal."

"Careful, Herbie."

"Don't worry, Ira."

So, you can guess what happened next. Somehow the cross got snagged on its gold ropes or something, and went spinning across the room. Herbert, the machine, and time itself stood motionless. There lay the cross in a far corner of the floor, twisted and bent. And there lay also numerous broken cabochon rubies scattered all over. The silence was broken only by the sounds of uneven breathing.

The first words were Ira's. They began as whispered low moans, intruding themselves softly, almost inaudibly, but persistently until they burst forth in a calamitous crescendo.

"Oh, my God! Oh, Oh, Oh...My God...Oh, my God."

"Shhh!"

Finally Uncle Herbert, regaining just enough command, opined, "Ira, the first thing we need is a drink."

Not having any better ideas, Ira quickly produced a bottle reserved for special occasions, as well as the medicinal benefits of a couple of shots in quiet contemplation of life and its vicissitudes.

After a time, Uncle Herbert asked Ira for a dust pan and brush. And then on his knees, as though positioned in penitence, Uncle Herbert began his punishment by scouring and sweeping the dark shop floor for torn strands of metal and scattered gems. He was soon joined by Ira who, though innocent, kept saying, "It's my fault, Herbie. I should have stopped you."

"No, no, Ira. It is all my fault, my impatience. You had nothing to do with it."

"But what are you going to do, Herbie?"

"I'll do what I have to do. I'll fix it, no matter what"

And so, the two old men in their sixties swept long into the night. Cousin Sam went on to describe how many additional nights for the next six months, Uncle Herbert had worked alone in his shop, often sleeping for just a few hours before morning, on a folding cot he kept there for that time.

It seems for a time that the Archbishop's cross became my father's to bear. He sent to Brussels for matching rubies and emeralds. And he went on and carved out the cupboard, and created the hinged gold door that the Archbishop had envisioned. He skillfully repaired not only those damages that might show, but he remedied as well those that were invisible, for they constituted the test of his integrity even more than his skill.

Uncle Herbert could be a very stubborn man. He would complete the job that Stowell's had undertaken for the Archbishop no matter what it took. He matched and recreated the strands of gold and wove them into the ropes. And he replaced and paid for all of the broken or missing gems out of pocket, and went quite broke doing so.

And one day a few months later, he told Stowell's that job was done, and that afternoon, bearing the Archbishop's cross in a brown paper bag, Uncle Herbert brought the completed job back to their elegant store. They were very pleased and much impressed with Herbert's work, and told him so.

Then Herbert told them the story about the disaster with the lathe, and at first they couldn't believe it, for there was no evidence of repairs. But when Herbert drew their attention away from the cupboard and gold door he had created, and directed their expert appraisers' eyes to newly woven strands of ropes and the replaced emeralds and cabochon rubies, they were stunned at how seamless the work appeared.

It took only moments for Stowell's to conclude that they would tell the Archbishop merely how difficult the job had been, indeed beyond expectation. But this particular customer had cares enough, with no need to concern himself with the technical details of the trade.

Although I had never known of that story, nor had my father ever mentioned it to me, I immediately recognized that it was true. There was no way that Cousin Sam nor anyone else could have known that at the time of those events which Sam related, my father had come to me. He wanted to know if I had any money. I told him that I had saved about two thousand dollars from my military pay, and he wanted to know if he could borrow it to make payroll. Of course, I gave it to him.

I hardly thought about the money in later years when I had paid the mortgage and succeeded sufficiently not to be concerned about that forgotten matter. My brother, Saul, who had been there then, and who took over the shop when Dad died, had known, but had never told me the story. Subsequently, when I had written up this story as our Cousin Sam recalled it, I sent it to my brother Saul, who confirmed it, and described the cross to me in further detail.

Cousin Sam's eyes glistened and were moist as he finished the story. It was a belated Bar Mitzvah gift, with dividends indeed from Sam's Uncle Herbert, my departed Dad, to all of us.

Now, years later, as I type this story onto my computer from its earlier paper manuscript, I wonder briefly if our dad ever considered raising his price for that difficult job and his arduous labors. Knowing him, I doubt it. In his business dealings, Herbert was as proud of his word as he was of his work. A philosophical man, if not a religious observer, maybe a part of him felt he had been done a favor in being put through some kind of inner, but very real comprehensive and final exam of himself. Perhaps he took payment and satisfaction in knowing that he passed it with high honors.

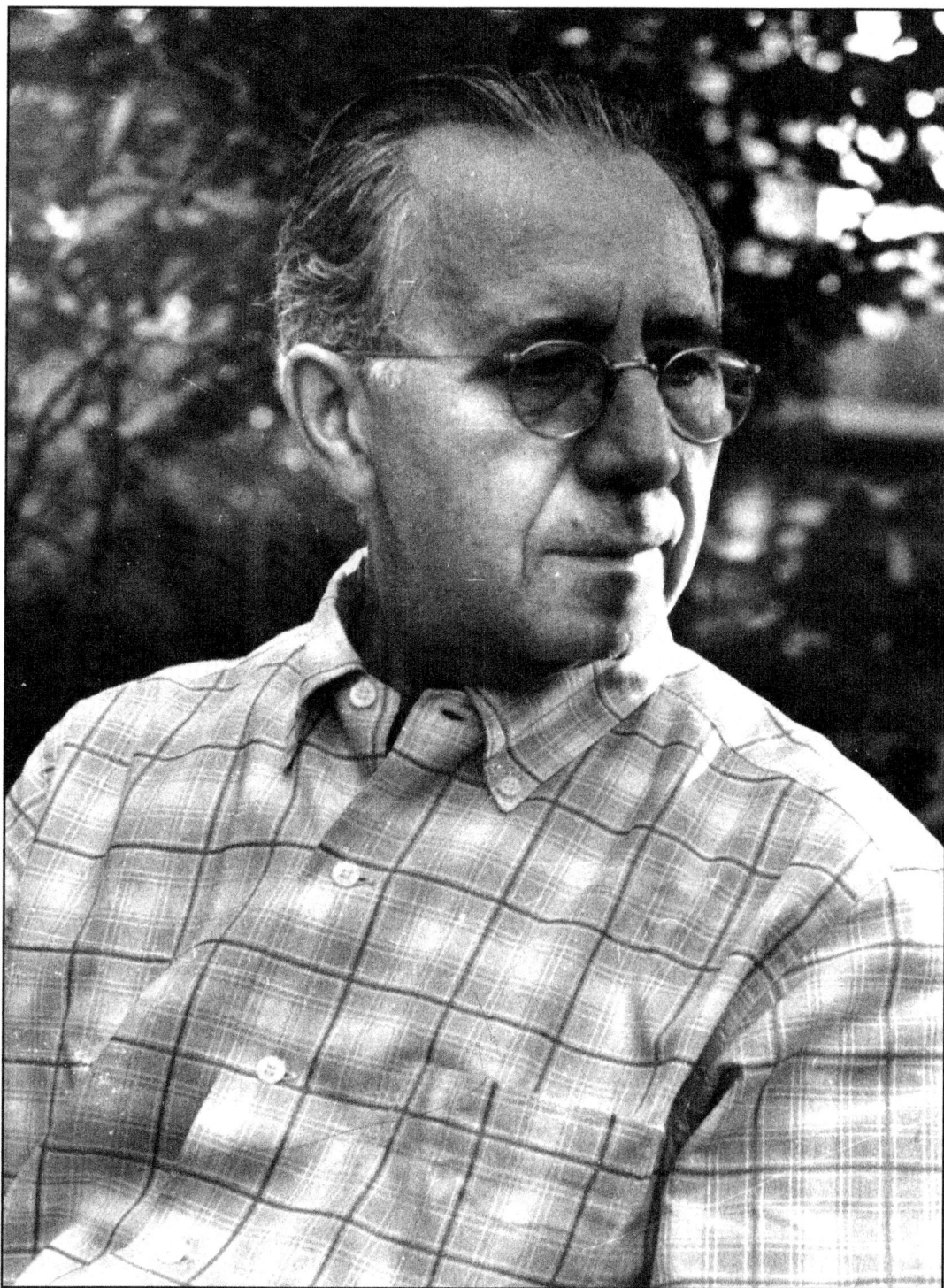

My dad, age 64, circa 1958 (photo by author).

Don't hang up the phone. I have an equally powerful story that gave me a second view of our widowed Ma and her ability to create a new life for herself and us when the good Lord presented her with that opportunity.

A Year After Dad Died, Our Ma Found a New Life

When our Dad died on May 30, 1966 at the age of seventy-three, our Ma was bereft and left alone. My brother, Saul, then in his early fifties, conscientious, capable and concerned as always, called her daily. Saul had inherited and taken over our father's jewelry shop, as well as the cumbersome legalities of handling Dad's personal estate, very modest as it was. What about his widow, our Ma? My wonderful older brother, Saul, and sister-in-law, Ellen, came up with the ingenious idea of creating a job for Frieda, our Ma, at Herbert Heller & Co., the small but busy shop in the Jeweler's Building in downtown Boston. The Jeweler's Building had a number of floors housing many wholesale businesses and manufacturing shops in Boston's fine jewelry trade. Our Ma could easily do the trusted and important errands of picking up and delivering orders and pieces of work that required reliable transfer between various shops and businesses. She would not need to leave the building and would be welcomed and safe among the various artisans and tradespeople who had known her deceased husband, Herbert.

So, it came to pass that while in the building's elevator to deliver a work order to a familiar shop on another floor, our Ma was greeted by Louis Chalpin, a recent widower and fellow jeweler who had known our dad as well as my brother, Saul. Mr. Chalpin and our Ma regarded each other briefly, until the elevator arrived at her floor. But, after bumping into each other several more times over the next few days and chatting, Louis invited Frieda for tea in a little shop next door, and soon thereafter for dinner. Satisfied that he was a gentleman and a good person, Frieda reciprocated by inviting Louis for a home-cooked meal. She was a good cook with lots of old-country recipes. So, you can guess what happened. They fell in love.

Down in Philadelphia in 1968, I had not yet heard a word about any Louis Chalpin, but my brother Saul in Boston had sensed that something was brewing between Mr. Chalpin and our Ma. And so she phoned me one evening and asked if I could call her back since she had a lot to tell me. As I could afford an extended long-distance call better than she could, I was intrigued and wondering what was up. I said, "Sure, Ma. I'll call you right back." She picked up the phone immediately and said, "I have something to tell you." She launched at once into the story about how she and Louis kept bumping into each other in the elevator, and that they soon discovered that they had a lot in common besides their need for a new special friend.

It was a remarkable coincidence, she felt—as though it were somehow "beshert" (a Yiddish word for pre-ordained or meant to be), in that each was a recent widow and widower, and each had two sons, one of whom lived nearby in Boston while the other son lived in Philadelphia. That was coincidence enough, but when they discovered that both their younger sons were not only physicians, but psychiatrists and analysts, that seemed too much of a coincidence, especially since neither Frieda nor Louis knew quite what a psychoanalyst was. But that was not why she called.

She then took a deep breath and said, "Melvin, he wants to marry me, and I really love him." She then went on to describe that he was a thoughtful, good-hearted, loving, and affectionate man, with clean habits. I was stunned, and why not? It was as though I had been suddenly hit, not by a brick, but by a dozen roses. "Wonderful, Ma! If you've been together and known each other for two years, and it feels right, it makes me very happy to know that another man loves you, and that you love him in return. "

And so I called my older, wiser brother, Saul, in Boston and asked if this Chalpin fellow was for real. "Yes, he's a very nice guy, Mel. But why do they need to get married?" Where starry-eyed me saw dozens of roses, my brother, with both feet on the ground, knew that roses have thorns. "What if he gets sick?" he asked. I responded to his concern too impatiently, saying "For Crissakes, Saul, what if *she* gets sick?" (I would have reason to remember that reply in years to come when my Irmgard died.) And so, Louis moved into Ma's apartment on Washington Street in Brookline, Massachusetts. They married in a civil ceremony in Boston when Ma was seventy-six.

Our Ma's New Life With Dear Louis Chalpin

They were truly sweet and dear with each other. And why not? Although she complained that it was now getting wrinkled, our Ma still had a pretty face to which she applied little or no makeup. She had nice skin and a solid chunky build that never got fat, but felt softly feminine or "zaftig," as such bodies were affectionately termed prior to the subsequent Twiggy look in fashion magazines. Louis also made a nice appearance, and I always felt they were an attractive couple.

The next thing I heard after they were happily married and getting along fine for about a year was that Louis alarmed his bride by wanting to take her on a honeymoon. It was not the honeymoon that alarmed her; she was all in favor of domestic love and romance. It was where he wanted to take her. Louis yearned to show his wife the region of Russia where he had been born and grew up, and he wanted to see who and what remained. When our Ma telephoned me about Louis's honeymoon plans, she seemed halfway between being petrified at the prospect of setting foot on Russian soil on the one hand, and wanting very much, on the other hand, to please her husband's desires that she accompany him.

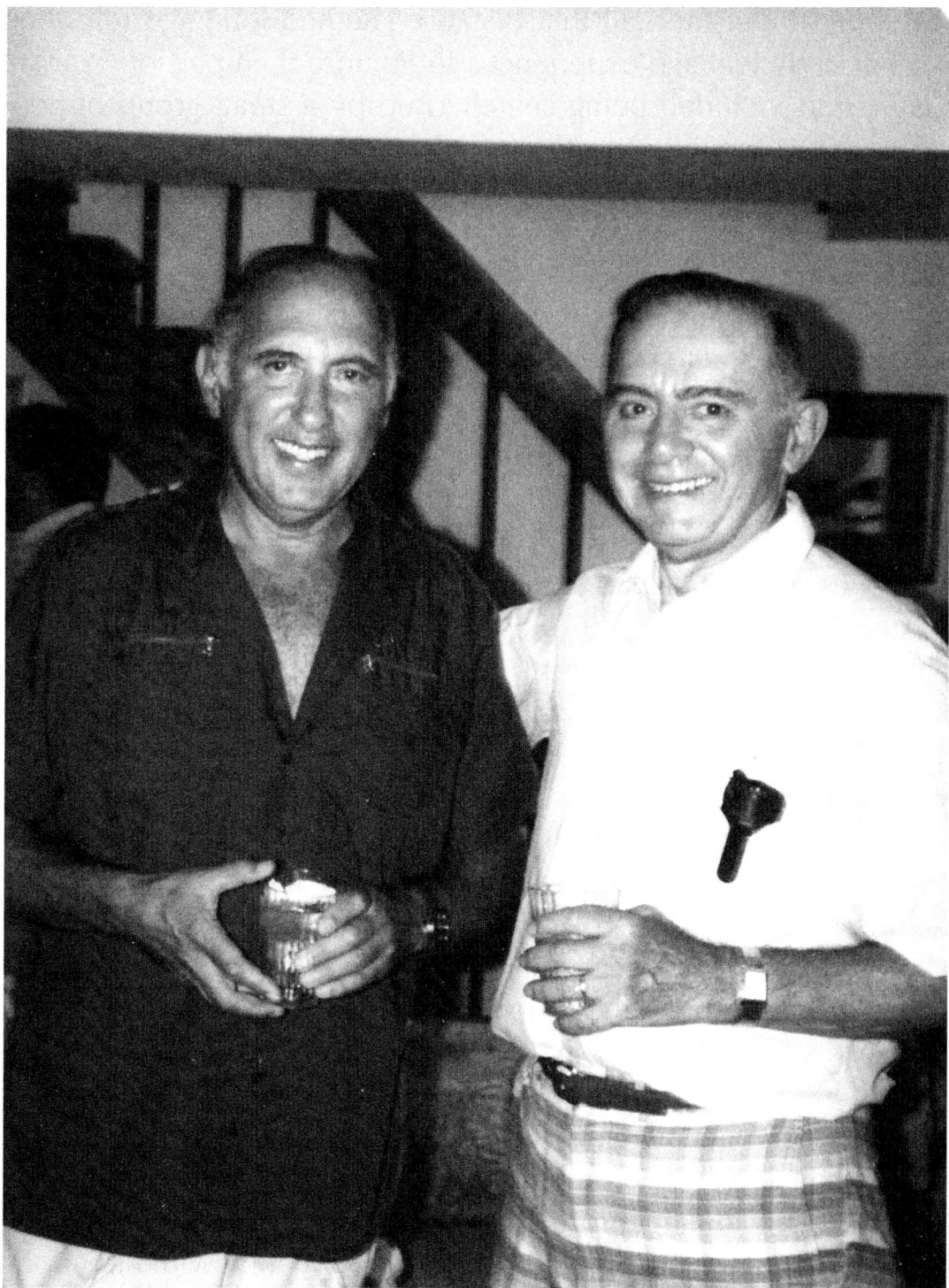

Author age 59, and brother Saul age 65, on Saul's rare summertime visits to our Chesapeake shore home, but together as always.

I could understand all that because she had long ago told me that her early teenage experiences in Poland, then part of Czarist Russia, had included being snatched up by a small group of her adolescent companions in the town square, and then grabbed by her waist-length hair and thrown over a saddle in the middle of a shouting troop of Cossacks, who tossed her into the local jail. About fourteen or fifteen years old at the time, she had never gotten over the emotional trauma of captivity and the humiliating knowledge that her father had to somehow raise funds to bribe the chief guard to get her released.

Ma's Fears of Foreign Travel and an Unexpected Visit With Dad's Lost Sister

Louis understood his wife's fear, but calmly reassured her that neither Cossacks nor the Soviet's secret police posed any danger to American tourists in the presence of our alert U.S. embassy. I felt it was in Ma's best interests to abandon her longstanding fears of Russia and replace them with the current and rational concerns about their honeymoon wishes and the practical travel needs of two elder adults abroad. As I think back on it now, I recall that I had associated "Galloping Cossacks" and "Coastal Raiding Vikings" as earlier versions our modern day terrorists. They now include recurrent waves of suicide bombers and mass murderers who cowardly strike at schools, public buses, cafes, and crowded market places to blow their innocent victims to pieces while they themselves feel assured of having earned a place in Paradise, and the added bonus of a few weeks of high-profile publicity in their sub-culture's mass media. And so, in comparison to my small current concerns about the isolated, intermittent, but frightening risks that can strike unfortunate travelers abroad, I sided with Louis and urged our Ma to venture forth confidently with her good husband and American passports to Odessa. But sure enough, our Ma had not been entirely wrong in her apprehensions.

They were not in Russia more than a few days when a couple of soft-stepping, secret police types approached Louis and said in English, "You speak a very good Russian." Without batting an eyelash or feeling openly threatened, Louis replied truthfully by saying with a pleasant smile and Russian accent, "That is because I had a very good teacher." Indeed he had. Being born and raised there, Russian was his native language, which, unlike his equally fluent English, he spoke without any trace of a foreign accent. Perhaps because he was old, relatively short, stocky, relaxed, and casually friendly, speaking so much like one of their own elder parents or other folks at home, they left him alone with his dear American wife, who smiled politely, but spoke no Russian—and to mother's relief, they never showed up again.

Our Ma related that she was much impressed with her husband's cool and confident manner when questioned. I agreed that his personality was such that he neither took nor gave offense. Ma told me that, no longer feeling spied upon, she relaxed and enjoyed the sights as well as a number of authentic Russian tea rooms where Louis continued to practice his very good Russian and think about the next prudent steps he might take in finding evidence of any surviving relatives of his in Odessa, or our mother's in Poland. Sadly, he found none of his, but they unexpectedly discovered one of my father's older sisters, who had quite miraculously and resourcefully escaped eastward from a rapidly occupied and Nazified Lithuania into Soviet Russia's equally frightening and dangerous territory.

Somehow Louis, years later, made contact with someone from Kaunas (Kovno) where my father grew up. Our Ma's very cool, inauspicious-looking and multi-lingual Louis succeeded in tracing and eventually contacting an older sister of my father's, who, under an assumed name, had been a medical doctor during Stalin's formerly dangerous and conspiracy-minded rule, which apparently had left her still shaken and secretive. Having admitted to Ma and Louis her hidden identity as a Jew, our father's very frightened and elderly sister was anxious to get rid of both of these American strangers, and begged them to leave and have no more to do with her.

Ghost Stories of the Twentieth Century

I cannot vouch for the authenticity or further details of this very sad story. It obviously shocked my dear Ma and Louis, and I thought they would have told it, not only to me, but to my brother, Saul, but he and I never discussed it. What was there actually to discuss? In comparison to keeping up with each other, our kids, and more immediate concerns during our infrequent visits with each other in subsequent years, Ma's story about our Dad's lost sister surviving mysteriously in Russia was not high on our agendas. Similarly, I never told it to my kids until many years later, and so I have lived with it as a ghost story, a chilling fragment of the Holocaust, which sits like a silent cat that occasionally haunts surviving Jews, Germans, and ethnic others of our dwindling WWII generation even today in places far away and long removed from Nazi Germany.

And so, Ma's deep fears of Cossacks were passed on to me in the form of equally deep regrets that none of my dad's siblings survived Hitler's European Holocaust except for one elder sister, who apparently wished forever to be unnamed and forgotten as such. That seemed kind of horrible, and I can only hope that this unknown, hidden, and lost Jewish-Lithuanian aunt of mine had somehow, somewhere in the vast Eurasian land mass of Russia made a life and legacy for herself, with children, as I have been able and free to do, and write about in these many pages.

My widowed mother's marriage to Louis Chalpin enriched her life in many ways, and mine as well in bringing me for a time two middle-aged step-brothers, Louis's sons, Bill and George. The younger brother, George, lived in Boston and I met him only a few times. However, the older brother, Bill, lived with his wife, Irena, and their two lovely daughters quite nearby in Berwyn, one of Philadelphia's Main Line suburbs. Bill Chalpin was a well-regarded chemical engineer at Sunoco and a very pleasant fellow. In our fifties, we got to see a good deal of each other when Bill usually beat me at tennis.

In retrospect and most important for me, I think that my mother's late life marriage to Louis set for me an optimistic example of what new love can sometimes bring to senior citizens, even in their elderly years. As you have read in these pages, I followed my mother's example by sharing some twenty years of my life with Irmgard Foulkrod. Irmgard was a wonderful wife whom I married in 1988 when I was a young sixty-six and she was an even younger sixty-four. We did not quite match my mother's and Louis's daring leap into marriage when she was seventy-six, but their example inspired me to try to do likewise for as long and well as we could.

Chapter 22
When a Doctor's Parents Die

My Son or Daughter, the Doctor

AMONG MY UNSPOKEN fantasies was the idea that I might, as a doctor, be in a position to spare my parents some of the distress, pain, and nagging worries of their illnesses and impairments as they aged. If we live long enough, we are likely to be inflicted with arthritis, arteriosclerosis, cardiovascular disorders, skin cancers, and worse. Geriatric impairments, like wear and tear on old machines or appliances, seem inevitable if we live long enough. Pursuing medical care, like shopping for expensive jewelry, can be pretty much a blind article for most people even today, despite such online resources as PubMed, Medscape, Google, and Wikipedia, especially in the face of blatant commercial advertising to the public by pharmaceutical companies and competitive heath care providers, including some of the biggest university-affiliated medical centers.

If one can afford the best care, come to America where medical care is not only a complex, business-managed affair, but a huge government-regulated commercial industry, both for better and worse. Choosing the right doctor at the right time in the right place can be difficult for anyone, even for a physician who requires special surgery or other treatment for a complex condition that may not be that frequently encountered. Under such conditions or at any time of need, it is good to be able to ask someone you can trust, who is in the know or knows someone who really is. Believe me, I've been in that position myself and knew who to ask where the best places and people were likely to be found.

As one's parents age, it is nice for them to have someone in the profession to guide and introduce them to experts in the appropriate surgical or medical specialties involved. It is not that our elder patients and parents want something wholesale, but they feel no longer at the top of their game and feel instead a need for a real family doctor whom they can trust to guide them when medical decisions must soon be made. Who better than their son or daughter, the doctor? How did I feel about all that as a doctor and a son when my parents died? The short answer is "'like everyone else, only more so." Why talk about this kind of thing here in my memoirs? What more significant moments should we recall and ponder in our lifetimes? Let me write first of when my father passed away.

When My Dear Dad Died

I've written much about my Dad in these pages, but here is a bit more about him. My father died unexpectedly and rather abruptly in Boston on a Monday, May 30, 1966, at the age of seventy-four, as officially recorded. I mention Monday because on Sunday afternoon, May 29th, I was fortunately free on the side lawn of our suburban home in Philadelphia, having just finished putting together a large, brand new, jungle gym for our four-year-old son, Paul, when my wife came bursting out of the house and pulled me quietly aside. She said, "Mel, we just got a phone call from Boston telling us that your father has some kind of serious cardiac emergency, and they are preparing him as soon as possible for major surgery today at the Beth Israel Hospital...Don't call Saul and Ellen back. They are on their way to the hospital right now." A beautiful Sunday of relaxation at home had turned suddenly into a highly pressured and awful day of alarm.

"Oh my God," was all I could say in the next breath. Then, as I got my head together, I quickly added, "Let me wash up and change my clothes. While I do that, please call the airport and get me on the first flight to Boston. Then please pack me a small overnight bag, and I'm out of here. Once I'm gone, please call the hospital to let my father, and the doctor who is in charge of his case up there, know that his son from Philadephia is on the way." Jane, a cardiologist's daughter, was good at these kinds of things and was not rattled.

Arriving at the Boston airport, I took a cab and went directly to the hospital, where I was expected and was told to go directly to the operating room where my dad's surgery was already in progress. Familiar with the Beth Israel Hospital, where I had completed my own surgical internship some fifteen years earlier—an era that suddenly seemed like yesterday to the rushing, but puffing and less fit, forty-five-year-old man I seemed suddenly to have become. Arriving at the O.R. door, I peered through the small glass window into the room and gently knocked. One of the masked surgeons looked up. Apparently recognizing me as the patient's son, he signaled the nurse to bring me in. She quickly provided me with a surgical gown, cap, and mask while telling me that my father had been in ongoing surgery during the past hour for a large aneurism of the thoracic aorta.

That didn't sound very good. I had never witnessed, let alone assisted at, such an operation during my internship or subsequent surgical residency at Yale and its affiliated nearby VA Hospital in Newington, but I knew immediately that a thoracic aneurism was a dangerously weakened and distended, or ballooned-out, section of the body's largest blood vessel. Blood leaves the heart through the thoracic aorta under considerable pressure. Quickly processing if not yet digesting this ominous news, I nodded to the two masked surgeons who hovered over their patient's surgically draped wound, and quickly placed myself immediately next to my dear father's anesthetized and intubated head. Urgently but gently leaning over, and paying attention only to him, I said words I'll never forget.

"Hi Dad. It's me, Mel. I'm here with you. Can you hear me?"

Of course, even if he could hear me, I quickly realized that he couldn't answer me with that tracheal tube stuck in his throat and distending his vocal cords. So I reached down and squeezed his hand and said again, "Hi Dad. It's me, Mel. I'm here."

To this day, I believe that I felt him squeeze back with the firm grip of a man whose hand had been strengthened by years of work at the jeweler's bench. I could not swear to it back then, but I can still recall his hand squeezing mine to this day. But only silence followed in the Operating Room until I heard a strangely familiar voice that I couldn't quite identify say, "Hello, Mel. Welcome back. Sorry we meet again like this."

I looked up in disbelief. Could it be the same Dr. Eddie Frank, my former chief resident and surgical instructor at the Beth Israel, who stood alongside me fifteen years earlier when I did my very first appendectomy, and as I made the initial incision whispered, "Gently, Mel. Gently like a bride."?

Yes, it was Dr. Ed Frank, a fine general surgeon who was assisting his older brother, Howard Frank, a thoracic surgeon who had answered the call in response to my father's emergency. My father never woke from this major emergency surgery. Nor did I ever hear his words again until I began faithfully recording some of them in these pages. But the thoughts still trouble me. The attempted surgical repair to the thoracic aneurism could not be completed as planned, and they brought him, with surgical forceps and clamps still in place, back to his room where he never regained consciousness. He died sometime after midnight on Monday, the 30th of May. So much for living another day. Sunday had been a very long day. My dad was dead. Little Paul had a new jungle gym he would not remember and had lost a grandfather he hardly knew and would not remember. And I was devastated and remember it all to this day.

I write these pages as an old man who just turned ninety-three. Looking back, could I, or anyone, have saved my Dad if I had been living in Boston in 1966? Aortic aneurisms, even large ones, can lurk for months and years without causing any symptoms at all, until they burst and present themselves as life-threatening emergencies. To this day, most aortic aneurisms are picked up accidentally on such widely-used imaging techniques as CT scans and MRIs ordered to diagnose or investigate other conditions. Fifty years ago in 1966, we did not have the routine use of today's imaging techniques. Most important, thoracic surgery was still in its relative infancy. Today, the surgical treatment of aortic aneurisms is a highly sophisticated procedure performed by experienced cardiac teams of surgeons and physicians from a number of related medical specialties. At top cardiovascular institutions such as the Cleveland Clinic, as many as one thousand aortic aneurism repairs are performed on selected cases each year with good long-term results. My poor Dad, and Drs. Howard and Ed Frank, didn't have a chance with a large thoracic aneurism under emergency circumstances. The Massachusetts General Hospital had a few more thoracic surgeons in 1966 than the Beth Israel's good Dr. Howard Frank, working alone with his brother Edward, a very capable general surgeon but without specialized thoracic training. If I had been there, and had it been possible to get my Dad quickly over to Massachusetts General, I probably would have suggested that. But it might have made no difference. Even if my seventy-four-year-old father had survived the difficult surgery, he would have faced weeks and months of discomfort and debilitation in further post-operative care.

Our younger son, Paul, was present when his dear mother, my first wife Jane, recently died following a massive pulmonary embolism from a blood clot in a fractured leg that had been immobilized in a cast. Sad and doleful as some of our assembled family was in remembering her, at the end, our steady Paul lifted his glass and said with a sigh of resignation, "At least it was quick." I remembered thinking that very same thought as I was flying back to Philadelphia fifty years before, after his grandfather died.

When My Mother Died

I must confess that I have been sometimes afflicted with nagging feelings of remorse or guilt when I think about the circumstances of my mother's death. It is not uncommon when our parents die that we think we should have done more for them while they were alive. It was not that so much that bothered me. It was my feeling that somehow I should have done more for her at the very end, when she was facing death. Too much was in my hands and up to me. It wasn't as though I could have called in a priest or rabbi and left it up to him or her. There were medical decisions that needed to be made and she trusted me, her "son, the doctor," for guidance in making them.

Unlike my Dad who, with his long history of peptic stomach ulcers, had little faith in doctors and their old "Sippy diets" of milk and cream, my mother thought that doctors knew something, if not everything, and kept me informed about her medical condition. Although she was not a complainer or hypochondriac in any way, she sought my personal opinion about each of her aches and pains. She also showed me her medical reports, and so I knew about her aortic valve stenosis or narrowing, moderate hypertension, and cardiac condition. Although I was not a general practitioner, and hardly a cardiologist, I had read up on aortic valve stenosis as I did on most illnesses when I encountered them in close family or friends, and particularly in myself. Some thirty or more years ago, aortic valve replacement was not the everyday occurrence that it is now, even with selected elderly patients, at top cardiac surgery centers. And so, cardiologists practiced "watchful waiting" and treated them with standard medications, as required.

Ma Came to See Her Son, the Doctor

Toward the tenth year of their marriage, as Louis and Ma advanced into their upper eighties, travel was no longer easy for them, but they came to visit me anyway. The latent agenda and purpose was to see what their son, the doctor, and his faculty-connected medical friends had to say about her worsening heart valve problem. I turned to Dr. Norman Lerner, a close friend who was a top internist and medical professor at Temple, and asked him to examine her. Dr. Lerner was known as a so-called "doctor's doctor"—one that we went to when we ourselves had a troublesome medical problem that required consultation.

I also had a further relationship with him because Norm Lerner was not only an excellent physician, but also a capable pianist with whom I had practiced violin-piano sonatas on occasion. I learned that Norman was not only a better physician than I was, but also a more persistent and disciplined musician than I had been in my post-medical school years. In short, I admired and trusted Norm Lerner as a personal friend when he examined my mother as gently as though she had been his own. He ordered electrocardiograms, a chest film, and basic lab studies as I awaited his verdict.

"Not so good," he said to me.

"What's to be done? Do we have any decent options?" I asked.

"Let me talk to a couple of our cardiologists and heart surgeons," he replied.

He came back with the news that they all advised against surgery. They would not put this eighty-six-year-old woman through major surgery in her condition.

"So what do you want to do, Ma?" I asked her.

"I'd like to like live a little longer if I could," she replied.

It was well after midnight when I discussed this calmly with her dear husband, Louis. He sighed. We had been at the hospital all day. It was even more tiring for him, an old man, than for me. I suggested that we get some sleep. He agreed. In the morning, she was gone, quietly they told me, in her sleep, just like that. I cried that night like a child, because when her time came, there was nothing I could do for her. Sometimes it is hard to be "my son, the doctor."

Aging and the Passing of Generations

I was sixty-six and hardly a youngster when my mother died. I found myself thinking of many things when both my parents were gone. Up to then, I had found it strange, even after my own children were born, that I continued to feel sometimes more like a son than a parent. While my own parents were alive, they somehow reawakened the enduring and unspoken childhood bond that, when all was said and done, sometimes reminded me I was still their kid. Of course, I was both a father and a son, but it was only after both my parents died, and I became an "orphan" so to speak, that I realized I had been assigned a new and more difficult role to fulfill than "my son, the doctor" had been for me in my parents' elder years.

I have since lived long enough to become, for a further time as the parenting cycle continues, a psychological father-figure or patriarch for my grown children's families. That role, too, would become a changing and diminishing one as I went from ripening on the private vine of our own home, to aging with our fellow geriatric residents in a rather elegant retirement facility for variously impaired elderly folk in Haverford, Pennsylvania. It was here that I began the work of writing these memoirs between periods of rest and recovery from the seemingly inevitable medical challenges of our geriatric journeys.

Chapter 23
Forensic Psychiatry, the FCC, and Sex on Network TV

AFTER CONSULTING WITH us at least monthly for five or more years, as described in previous chapters, and following Sam Polsky's early death in 1975, ABC kept me on as Al Schneider's known and trusted Broadcast Standards and Practices consultant. In the ensuing years, I was called upon regularly to view and write my professional opinion on new scripts, rough-cuts, films, and series under consideration for broadcast in ABC's new season of competitive entertainment programming. In addition, increasingly successful made-for-theater movies were being assessed for purchase of their re-broadcast rights as TV entertainment fare with requisite BS&P cuts and edits. Big stakes were involved as writers, producers, and network programmers were eager to introduce more controversial, but hopefully meaningful and significant adult themes, including serious sexual issues, into network entertainment programming. Sexual issues and themes had always been more controversial and taboo than violence for network affiliates in the bible belt and Midwest. But meanwhile, the movies were "growing up a bit" in terms of portraying sexual, social, and other adult controversial issues that were kept in the closet or swept under the plush carpet of network TV. The Constitution protected the rights of adult consumers to read books of their choice or purchase tickets to view what they wished. The networks depended on revenue from sponsors and advertisers for their very lucrative, but mandatory, government license to broadcast.

It Was Not Just Violence, But Sex and Other Broadcast Standards Matters at ABC

During the 1970s and early 1980s, sexual issues were particularly troublesome for some of ABC's network affiliate stations in the South and Midwest. So, Al Schneider, a corporate vice president, was called upon by ABC's top brass to come up with a rational and balanced set of guidelines for depicting sexual content on network TV. This was no small matter in the major networks' ongoing competition to attract the largest numbers of viewers as a market for commercial TV's sponsors and advertisers.

Accordingly, as my consultation contract with ABC was renewed for the next thirty years, our alert, competent, and experienced BS&P editors asked my opinion about sexual portrayals of everything under the sun, the moon, or the bed sheets, it seemed. A handbook for making such decisions and outlining the network's policy in doing so seemed highly desirable. Always the thoughtful attorney and network executive, Al Schneider reached out to academic experts and found Philip Sarrel, MD and Lorna Sarrel, MSW at Yale to serve as his special consultants on Broadcast Standards issues regarding sexual matters. I had never known the Sarrels, having completed my psychiatric training at Yale long before they arrived there, but I had heard good things about them.

An Unexpected Request from ABC

I was a bit surprised one day in 1980 when Alan Wurtzel, a young psychologist and capable statistician, came to see me with a message that Al Schneider wanted me to write a monograph on ABC's guidelines for the depictions of sexuality and sexual content in entertainment TV. It was a big and time-consuming job that I thought Schneider would have assigned to Dr. Philip and Lorna Sarrel, and so I was somewhat taken aback. It was because Schneider was tied up during my scheduled consultation visit to ABC in New York that young Dr. Alan Wurtzel, a recently hired research psychologist, came to me with Schneider's urgent message and request. Schneider was sorry he couldn't meet with me, but had allegedly specified that my monograph or booklet should be "non-controversial, understandable, non-technical, and readable by our Broadcast Standards editors, as well as the general public."

"Wow!" I thought. First, there was no way to write a non-controversial or bland booklet about sex that was worth reading, especially if it dealt with feelings and community standards. That was because sex itself was not bland and shouldn't be. When I asked for specifics, I recall quite well what was wanted. "Just give us, in your own words, in forty double-spaced pages, the rationale, the psychological reasons which you can put down on paper on the subject of sexual editing." The hope was also expressed that the work would be succinct, interesting, and informative. Grateful for all these suggestions, I went out the door with my head spinning slightly. Before I could get away, however, my young network colleague, Alan Wurtzel, gave me the following small-craft advisory: "Remember, no value judgments."

The First Sexual Rule in Broadcast Standards Editing

I was paralyzed at the typewriter for an entire week while I was condensing two file-drawers of materials I had previously sequestered in anticipation of a lengthy book on the same subject. Then, like an apple falling on my head, came my discovery of the First Sexual Rule in Broadcast Standards Editing. It went like this:

There is no way to avoid value judgments in responsible sexual behavior, nor in its responsible depiction on television. Once the connection was made between sexual intercourse and its potential consequences, value judgments were inevitable and essential, if sometimes belated. That was what this booklet was about—value judgments. Not yours or mine in particular, but the reasons or rationale for making both sexual decisions and editing judgments concerning the depiction of sexual content on network television.

The Work of Broadcast Standards Editors

Our Broadcast Standards editors were trained to review and advise at every stage of program development from initial concept to finished product, in a hopefully cooperative relationship with the writers, producers, and the programming community. But sometimes, it became adversarial, as sex itself can sometimes seem. Our West Coast editors, under the competent leadership of Tom Kersey, a former fighter pilot who was not cowed by verbal adversity or heated argument, persistently considered matters pertaining to audience demographics, sensitivities, contemporary tastes, and the balanced presentation of responsible viewpoints and values. Our Broadcast Standards editors required an open set of clear reasons, which were free from hidden agendas and secret policies. As a psychoanalyst and child psychiatrist, I emphasized some of the early origins of sexual attitudes and the sensuous side of infant care in our making of broadcast standards.

The Sensuous Side of Infant Care

I indicated that the nurturing of infants and care of the young involve both instinctive and learned experiences that are reciprocal and intimate. Infant care features such daily sensuous behaviors as rocking, nude nuzzling and bathing, stroking, kissing, sucking (any finger will do), and in the human offspring, the frequent exposure, anointing, patting dry and powdering of tender genital parts. You thought infants just ate and slept? Babies are neither stone cherubs nor rubber dolls. They come complete, with many needs and nerve endings. I felt that if an editor wanted to know about sex and sexuality, they needed to understand the dimensions and dynamics of our pre-genital childhood experiences, and I spelled these out for them.

Comforting and loving infant care is sensuous, I explained. It is as natural and essential for infant development as mother's milk. Tender intimacy, however, does not come in a bottle. It is instinctual and expresses the mammalian heritage of infant care, adapted to human need. I indicated that the sensuous experiences of infancy contribute profoundly to our earliest patterns of personal and interpersonal development through behavioral modeling, imitation, and social learning. These experiences mold our basic attitudes toward sensual intimacy and interpersonal adaptation from that time on. Such early pre-verbal, intimate experiences express a parent's sensuous attitudes by deeds, rather than words. Human sexuality begins with these first crucial imprints.

Similarly, as any parent knows, there is more—much more—that must be accomplished in preparing a child, if not for high society, at least for kindergarten. There is a social side to child care. After learning to eat with a spoon, to sleep through the night, and a few basics about who's who, and what's whose at home, the next social milestone is toilet training. This milestone is very big because it is usually accompanied by the introduction of that essential ingredient of group living or civilization—the sense of shame. It is perhaps a shame that shame is so important for the development of a sense of a conscience or superego. Aside from our brain size and finger dexterity, shame is the main thing that distinguishes us from other mammals. Persons who are substantially immune to shame are deficient in superego development, as well as unreliable, untrustworthy, and sometimes dangerous. Only animals and infants lack it completely. Each civilized generation teaches shame to its children along with the alphabet.

The Development of a Sense of Shame

The development of a sense of shame is so essential a milestone in individual and human history that it marks the end of childhood innocence in each of us, and the banishment of our lot from the Garden of Eden. This remarkable biblical event records the eating of the forbidden fruit of knowledge after Eve's temptation (by no less a phallic symbol than the snake), as well as the earliest origins of sexual shame, guilt and modesty, including the invention of the first bikini—the fig leaf. Coming quite early in each person's life, as it does in Genesis, we are, thereafter, each marked by shame and guilt.

I described for our Broadcast Standards editors whom I felt should know these things, that with some early sex instructions and the further development of shame, life changed radically for each infant, as it did for mankind after The Fall. Parental indulgence, I explained, was increasingly replaced by discipline and responsibility. The self-centered, sensuous pleasures of infancy were curbed by the carrot of encouragement, and the stick of shame, weighted (as shame always is) by the further threat of deprivation, ostracism, or other punishment. You don't remember? For those readers who need reminding, the sexual instructions at this age were quite specific, standard, and familiar: "Pull your dress down. Pull your pants up. Don't run around like that. Don't let me catch you peeking again. That is private. You are bad. Go to your room. Don't say those words. Those are bad, dirty words. Nice children don't say those words. Shame on you!" Now that I came to this stage of the child's sexual and social development, our Broadcast Standards editors, like these young children themselves, were ready to look at sex and television in the home.

A Note on the TV Depiction of Nudity at Home

As for the depiction of sexuality and nudity at home, a powerful, self-conscious preference for privacy distinguishes human intercourse from animal copulation. Lovers generally do not want to be observed in their act, except by each other. With children running about, some parents cannot always count on each other's undivided sexual attention and may find themselves making love to a cocked ear instead of the passionate person they married. Parental privacy can be a precious commodity, not just for intercourse, but for plain, uninterrupted conversation. It is easy to see why many parents get edgy. Once we understand the pains to which most parents go in order to keep their own sexual behavior from being observed or even heard by their children, it is not hard to understand how much parents would resent seeing the very same acts being depicted by others on TV in front of the very same children at home.

What about nudity itself? Well, there is total, partial, frontal, silhouetted, dimly lit, tribal, infant, and burlesques of nudity, to mention only some that are encountered in Broadcast Standards review. Any adult with really big problems over infant nudity is unfit to change a diaper, and not much help around a house full of babies. Children frequently see their little brothers and sisters naked, and no one, including network television, should make a big deal out of it. Tribal nudity, a la "National Geographic" is invariably covered by at least a small frontal apron. This, too, is no problem if that is the way the tribal people normally go about, and their nudity is not unduly ogled, or otherwise exaggerated for the audience by the camera. It is not the editor's role to distort otherwise sensitive depictions of authentic tribal life by adding sarongs or other imagined trappings of decency. The reasonable depiction of nudity in art and sculpture does not require Broadcast Standards editing, as well. "Reasonable" means portraying the entire work as the artist depicted it, and not focusing the camera unduly on the sexual parts alone. The nudity of art requires neither emphasis nor exclusion. Such nudity is entirely appropriate when not presented as a peep show.

You get the point. And so it went in numerous consultations on sexual content that I pursued with our West Coast BS&P editors in Los Angeles, as well as with our East Coast editors and Al Schneider in New York. We learned much together in applying our Broadcast Standards rationale and guidelines to the actual script portions, filmed rough-cuts, and practical programming materials and broadcasting issues encountered by our editors back then. Similar work goes on to this day. Sex itself has not changed that much, if at all, since then, but network television has with the growing advent of cable TV, along with our shifting attitudes toward controversial sexual practices and the social consequences or morality of out-of-wedlock reproductive activity. Despite all that, I felt that the rationale in my monograph entitled *Sexuality, Television, and Broadcast Standards*, published by ABC in 1984, still applied in 1992, when I retired from my TV consultation work at ABC.

As for mammalian sex itself, this is not a book or chapter on the sex lives of mice, men, and women. Human sex is a developmentally personal and sub-culturally shaped instinctual drive, or "biological hunger," if you will. How do I view it as a child and forensic psychiatrist and elder psychoanalyst today? Writing now as an old man in the second month of my ninety-forth year, what kind of sex life might I wish for my beloved, creatively playful, studious, hardworking, and grown-up grandchildren? Would I wish upon them a constipated lifetime of recurrent sexual frustration and prolonged abstinence? Or a life of responsible, mutually gratifying, and fulfilling fornication within mutually committed and meaningful interpersonal relationships? That is more easily said than accomplished when it comes to momentary or sustained human urges, as well as the swift passage of time which waits for no man or woman. Despite our best laid plans, experiences, and transient human accomplishments, Father Time and Mother Nature will have their way with us in episodes of mortal combat and physical impairment, especially as we age. Geriatric medicine and surgery could be a spectator sport like boxing, wrestling, or speedway auto racing if we weren't afraid to watch the suffering results of Nature's bodily combat with us, and its unfair use of choke holds in massive heart attacks, strokes, and inoperable metastatic cancer. I have had none of these, but I have gone a full ten rounds with many cruel knockdowns, with no cold complete knockouts for good thus far. What was it that Nietzsche said about "that which does not kill us makes us stronger"? Let us think about that as we look in on my medical and horizontal surgical battles with Mother Nature.

Chapter 24
My Knocks and Boosts in Going Ten Rounds with Mother Nature

MY VERY PERSONAL career in surgery started long ago and way back with an abrupt circumcision before I knew what it was all about. That, I am told, was followed some ten months thereafter by an unrelated mastoid operation behind the left ear. Since I remember neither of those operations, I shall spare us those details. But I do remember relishing a welcome dish of ice cream following my tonsillectomy a few years later. With that bit of pediatric surgery and ancient history, I am eager to address some of the subsequent, more major surgeries without which I might not be alive and functioning today. I've already described Round One of my lengthy tussles with Mother Nature in Chapter 16 of this volume, entitled "Round One: Tinnitus and Anxiety About Hearing Loss." That was back in 1963. Recovering from that one, and living long thereafter, I encountered a number of further knockdowns in my fight to the finish against Mother Nature's unpopular, but all-time, world-reigning champion, "Two-Fisted Mortality." Round Two follows.

Round Two, 1989: Chest Surgery for Lung Cancer

Let me set the stage. I was sixty-six and Irmgard was sixty-four when we got married in 1988 in nearby Elkton, Maryland. Elkton had been widely known for a time as The East Coast Capital of Quick Marriages. We weren't sneaking off, but we wanted to be married quietly and officially. I promptly added Irmgard to my medical insurance policy and retirement benefits plan. In connection with the medical insurance form, I suggested that she should have a mammogram, which she never had before. She agreed, providing that I would take the time to get a routine chest film.

I had been a moderate smoker, but Irmgard, who had lost her first husband to throat cancer, insisted that as a wedding present to both of us that I give up that "filthy habit" once and for all. Thankfully, her mammogram was fine, but my chest film showed a distinct lesion in the lower lobe of my left lung. Treatment? Remove the lobe, if not the entre lung, followed by prayer and lots of luck. I must have had good luck because I am still here thirty-five years later to tell the story. But I didn't know I would be spared, and I was initially devastated by the diagnosis of lung cancer—bronchioalveolar carcinoma, to be exact. It is currently called an adenocarcinoma, and although distinctly malignant, is now regarded as not the very worst type most likely to quickly metastasize and spread.

But before I knew all that, I had some bad luck, too. I was taken from the postoperative recovery room to my private room to more fully awaken, but with still groggy awareness of extensive bodily edema indicative of an adverse cardiac event. The cardiologist who had apparently been called to see me on an emergency basis in the operating room was now being assailed quietly, but very forthrightly by Irmgard, who had been awaiting my return. I still recall her voice and some of her words to the effect that, "A couple of hours ago, I sent you my strong, very healthy husband with only a small spot on his lung. Look at him now. What have you done with him? What went wrong? I need to know."

Not used to this kind of outspoken performance, the cardiologist mumbled something about the likelihood of a transient heart attack in former smokers. "Is he going to get better?" my new wife asked. "'We certainly hope so, and expect so. He is getting diuretics and other medication for that, but right now he is a cancer patient."

As I watched our cardiology colleague beat a hasty retreat, I was still getting out of my anesthesia and could hardly believe my ears. Then I noticed on the other side of my room was a very large and solid young stranger, who seemed well over two hundred and fifty pounds, meditating peacefully in the room's most comfortable and relaxing chair. I knew immediately who he was. It was Irmgard's son, John J. Foulkrod, the Methodist minister from Ohio. I had met his younger sister, Bonnie, and her husband, Dr. Dave Rees, from nearby Reading, Pennsylvania, but the Reverend from Ohio had been too busy with his church and young family to make the trip until now. Looking over to me with a smile and in his deep pastoral voice and tone, he said, "Hi, Mel. I'm John. I've just been praying for you, and I'll bet you a double scoop of ice cream that you're going to get better very soon." Realizing that his ministry prevented him from wagering anything much stronger, like a double Scotch on the rocks, I loved him immediately.

The cardiologist's suggestion that I had experienced, as a sixty-seven-year-old man a not-unheard-of, ordinary heart attack during major chest surgery was not the complete story. One of the doctors there who knew me personally from around our hospital later confided that the firmly tightened, mechanical rib-spreader had suddenly sprung loose and struck my heart, causing a sudden cardiac dysrhythmia. This, in turn, had caused a flurry of action, including an emergency call to the cardiologist, who had not fully explained to Irmgard exactly what had happened. Of course I was there, but being deeply anaesthetized, had no idea of what was going on. I was not a litigious person and certainly would not want to sue my own university hospital or colleagues. Besides, and more important, my heart had settled down to a steady rhythm known as Right Bundle Branch Block (RBBB). It has been with me ever since, but has caused no problems. Still gratefully alive and doing so well for so many years after my lung cancer surgery, why should I be a "sore winner"?

Following an initially scary, painful, and disabling setback, I got well fairly quickly. With Irmgard's fine post-hospital care and skill in managing our home together, and regaining strength, I experienced no pain except occasionally at the costochondral junctions where bone adjoins cartilage at the ribs. I could live with that, as well as with some diminished vital capacity or breathing power reflective of the fact that my remaining four lung lobes could not always do the work of the original five when called upon to do so. I declined the recommended and proffered chemotherapy. Instead, I proceeded to oversee the building of additional decks and a long dock, with its electric boat lifts extending one hundred feet out into the Elk River, where it still stands after all these years. Irmgard, likewise, planted our shore home with her gardens. We extended our own lives and those of our families for another generation of mutual care and affection between a man, his wife, and their shared loved ones. It was dear Irmgard who had made this happen for us. I felt well and looked forward to a more healthy future.

About the only good thing I can say about the nagging post-operative fears of recurrence or metastases that many cancer patients endure is that these anxieties distracted me for a time from further concerns about additional hearing loss. Between 1989 and 2001, all went well except for a relatively easy gallbladder excision with the then newer technology called laparoscopic cholecystectomy. This was performed with visual and flexible surgical equipment inserted through several small incisions that allowed adequate abdominal access. This innovative procedure was in marked contrast to the long ago gallbladder surgeries at which I had assisted in my surgical internship and residency by patiently holding retractors or eagerly inserting a few final sutures in closing the abdomen. Actually doing gallbladder surgery was reserved for our senior and chief residents. So the new technology was continued medical education for me as both a patient and a former surgical trainee. Aside from this gallbladder event, I had no significant physical problems. Again healthy at age seventy-nine, I was in no way prepared to understand what was about to happen next.

Round Three, 1992: Coping With Progressive, Adult-Onset Hearing Loss

Although none of these rounds with Mother Nature was fun, I learned hard lessons in what it was like to be a patient, and a good deal about pathology and surgical procedures from the horizontal perspective of a patient. What taught me the most about what it means to be a patient, however, was neither as dramatic nor life-threatening as my lung cancer nor a second experience with cancer, of the stomach, at age seventy-nine, with its continued potential for recurrence. Instead, what has clobbered me the most, and has provided me with a deep and recurrent sense of what it feels like to be a patient, has been my experience with progressive hearing loss. Deafness might seem like an unlikely, if not ironic script, especially for a psychiatrist. Perhaps not as bad a soap-opera as that of a surgeon going blind, but bad enough. In any event, back then when it first happened, I had little idea and less choice about the matter.

My hearing loss did not descend on me like the suddenly threatening dark cloud of cancer. Instead, it slowly but increasingly separated me from things I loved or needed—like music, casual conversations, or spoken directions about how to get back on the highway when people took the wrong exits, not to mention being unable to participate at large professional meetings or continuing medical educational lectures. Missed even more were the intimate and tender whisperings of love in the dark because the simple expedient of turning on the light to lipread would quickly break the spell. Picture it for a moment, if you will…

As I previously described in Chapter 16 of this book, it all began in 1963 with a feeling of fullness and a soft hissing sound in my left ear. When the feeling persisted, I consulted a well-regarded otolaryngologist, who was a neighbor. After a brief examination he told me that I had fluid in the inner ear—cause or etiology unknown. He thought it could be viral, perhaps too much exposure to loud noise, or maybe a toxin. "Not much to do about it," he added. "We'll just watch it. Your right ear is fine." Audiology tests thereafter were consistent with "severe to profound sensorineural hearing loss," or so-called nerve deafness, in the left ear. No treatment was available and the left ear was beyond any help that a hearing aid could provide.

I could still hear a pin drop with my right ear and so I went back to my work and to my busy life, grateful that my right ear was perfectly fine—until one day when the other shoe suddenly dropped, nine years later. I was shocked not by a loud noise or bang but by a soft, quiet, and hissing sound far more frightening to my ear. It was the long familiar tinnitus of my deaf left ear that was now hissing ominously like a snake in my good right ear. That threw me for a loop. I really needed that good right ear with which I had made my living and supported my family. Hearing had been essential in the further shaping of my identity and self-image during the past nine years of being both a teacher and a therapist. My training as a psychiatrist and analyst was essentially that of a clinically skilled, professional listener. If I could not hear, how could I listen? If I could not listen, how could I function as a psychotherapist?

The acute anxiety I felt made me want to run. I remember bursting out of my chair and literally running over to the Ear, Nose, and Throat Department. There, I was told that my friend from whom I sought a consultation would be doing surgery for the next several hours. Even though he wasn't there, the brief dash to his office seemed somehow to have helped.

I now sensed in my right ear that same feeling of fullness I'd had in my left ear nine years earlier. I began walking in circles while ruminating over my symptoms and speculating aimlessly about their origin. Worst of all, I worried about how much time I might or might not have left to hear. In short, I was walking in the shoes of a patient. However, in the office of my doctor, Max Ronis, an unexpected calm came over me. I remember he alternated between calling me "Mel" and "Doctor," perhaps because of his own anxiety about knowing me first as a friend and colleague, and now as a somewhat panicked patient. We psychiatrists notice things like that. Max, remaining professional, told me the audiogram he had ordered confirmed that my left ear indeed appeared finished, "kaput." It also showed, unfortunately, a substantial decibel loss and a diminution of word discrimination in my right ear. Of course, I took this bad news very seriously, but I continued to feel strangely calm. At least, I was getting some answers.

Max then confirmed my own hunch that there was little or nothing much further he could recommend medically, surgically, or diagnostically. There was no doubt that it was sensorineural hearing loss, so-called nerve deafness, profound in the left ear, and currently moderate to severe in the right. Adding that we should obtain follow-up audiograms at regular intervals, Max concluded with the encouraging news that I would probably benefit from a properly fitted, more powerful hearing aid.

Referred to the audiology department for further tests and measurements, I began to gain confidence that perhaps I could carry on and function in my work with a hearing aid. For two days, I was in suspense, awaiting the ear molds required to try a powerful hearing aid. They fit nicely, and after three long minutes, but in only three short words, *I could hear* more than well enough to converse again! I believed with sudden confidence that the little amplifier behind my right ear might indeed be, if not a cure, then a practical, reliable, and effective solution to what I had, the day before, feared might soon be followed by the end of my hearing days. "How long would my hearing last?" I asked Max. Of course, he did not know, nor did several well-known experts in other cities to whom he subsequently referred me.

Although I had stumbled badly into it by virtue of my own substantial hearing loss in middle age, and would continue to develop a special professional interest in hearing loss issues, the world of the deaf was not my world, as I explored it back then. My interests, priorities and family, as well as my work and career, were all deeply and irretrievably embedded in the world of the spoken word and in our written language. For whatever time I might be able to hear with the blessing of my new hearing aid, I needed to live in my own hearing world. Let me add quickly that the left ear mold was soon laid to rest in the back of a desk drawer, for no hearing aid then, or since, was able to restore useful sound to that cosmetically balancing, but non-functioning appendage.

Incidentally, but prophetically, the head of our nearby Pennsylvania School for the Deaf, Dr. Philip Bellefleur, who had became a close friend, looked at me one day back then and sincerely advised me to prepare myself "to go deaf," in his words. "You're probably right," I thought to myself as I wandered off. "Yeah, Phil, you're probably right, but just how does a fifty-year old guy with a family and kids to send to college do that?" Those words would come back to haunt me in later years, but I was much too involved back then with the pressing obligations of my immediate world to prepare for an unknown future in a deaf world.

So, I plugged in my trusty new hearing aid, packed a couple of spare batteries, and threw myself back into work in less than a week. For those who asked about my hearing aid, I said that I had experienced a sudden hearing loss that likely was due to a virus, and it probably was. Spins aside, I tried never to pretend to hear what patients or colleagues said if I hadn't heard it, nor was I ever reluctant to ask them to please repeat their words—and not quite so fast—if I hadn't caught them the first time. That was an important and early rule I made for myself, and one that I invariably followed back then with everyone. Hearing-impaired patients, adult in so many other ways, are frequently too shy or embarrassed to ask you to repeat what they missed. It is sometimes important to remind discouraged patients that it takes a certain attitude—a certain dignity and a patient regard for impatient others—to get the most out of their hearing aids as well as their increasingly strained relationships with others. By some good grace or favor of destiny, and for no medically explainable reason, my right ear did not follow the same rapid downhill course that my left one had. I continued instead to be able to converse quite normally, and conduct my business affairs on an amplified telephone.

If anything was different, I seemed more conscious of the privilege of being able to work, and so I worked harder and better than ever. I continued to see both private and clinic patients, to teach our residents and students, to obtain and co-administer university contracts, to supply and supervise psychiatric evaluations of defendants for our state courts, to conduct meetings, and to design and consult on research projects. Despite substantial hearing loss, I was functioning, and began to hope that I would no longer be walking in a patient's shoes, but in my own shoes, as a doctor. In retrospect, I really had been granted only an extension—a gift of extra time to go on with my work and responsibilities. How long could my luck last? Nine years, precisely.

Later when I experienced a further episode of hearing loss, I ran back to Max, and sure enough, the audiogram showed another distinct dip. Most disconcerting was that my word discrimination ability had also dropped substantially. We were puzzled by what could bring on hearing loss in episodes like mine, spaced apart with maddening and confounding regularity by nine years. They can occur with Meniere's Disease, but Meniere's includes problems with balance, dizzy spells, or vertigo, none of which I ever had. So we quickly dismissed that as a possibility. Max and I both had been practicing long enough to know that some things in medicine are just puzzling, like "FUOs," or fevers of unknown origin. In medicine, we have a name for conditions whose cause we cannot discern. We call them "idiopathic" rather than "idiotic," and we let it go at that. So, was I simply running out of time?

Retiring From Temple

The year after my lung cancer diagnosis and surgery, I turned sixty-eight—a polite, traditional, and for me quite convenient time for a graceful retirement from the faculty positions which I had held for more than thirty years at both Temple University's Schools of Law and Medicine. What to do next? I really didn't have to work immediately, or ever, if I wanted to live with the concept of New England frugality with which I was raised. In fact, I could easily have gone fishing, and pursued my numerous hobbies instead of my profession. Our youngsters were grown, and the mortgage was paid.

Somehow, however, by working as hard as I could, and for as long as I could, in the hearing world, I had perhaps through plain luck, come to a place where I had a reasonable number of choices to continue to function as an increasingly deaf doctor. And are not such choices, and the freedom to make them, what the good life is all about, I wondered? As a practicing physician, I had really loved my profession, and felt that I was finally beginning to know something about the mystifying, fascinating, and frequently humbling specialty of psychiatry. I had earned my credentials in both adult and child psychiatry, and I had learned some valuable things about mental and emotional illness in the process, I thought.

Why let all that go to waste on the golf course or fishing and sailing on the river? While I could still enjoy some of that, I could also throw myself into learning more about deafness and hearing loss, I reasoned.

So that is what we did for the next several years. I say "we" because, though it was not one of her life's greatest joys, my wife became the proactive partner of an increasingly deaf spouse. Communication can be a recurrent problem in the best of marriages when we fail to listen adequately to the words, needs, and messages of the other. But when a deafened spouse cannot hear a simple request, or misinterprets and resents an innocent comment, married life can congeal into a mutually resentful and punitive stand-off in which each spouse may feel alone and even abandoned. This, I had found, was a risk, especially for older people who need their partners to face life's challenges when their children are gone, and their health may be failing. Thankfully, I did not learn these painful lessons in my own home, but in my long experience of working with couples, and in my increasing work with deaf and hearing-impaired people following my so-called "retirement."

Although she was also fluent in other languages, my wife and I studied sign language and finger-spelling together. Indeed, we were still at it when we got to it relatively late in our lives with the stiffened fingers and set life-patterns that are a part of older age. We had easily learned the names of many things, but becoming really fluent in American Sign Language (ASL) was as difficult for us as it would be for any old immigrant couple coming to learn a new language and speak it properly in a new country with a different alphabet. We kept sliding back into the language we spoke in our own hearing land. Sign language drew attention to itself, and especially when out among strangers, my wife and I were loathe to bring added attention to ourselves as a gesticulating couple. Still, we tried hard. We bought books and cassettes to practice signing, found a local sign language teacher, and made several trips to the premiere university for the deaf, Gallaudet in Washington D.C., where we spent a number of interesting and pleasant days.

As for my professional options, there is little shortage of work for an otherwise healthy but deaf doctor who knows his or her stuff, and keeps up with the literature. Consulting regularly at a nearby school for the deaf, I soon achieved a kind of parity in signing with pre-school and kindergarten children, since our sign-language skills were equally elementary. In a sense, we were children learning new words together, and when we made mistakes, it was mutually enjoyed fun. As a mainstream child psychiatrist, I previously had little meaningful exposure to the psychological, emotional, and educational challenges experienced by deaf children. The great majority of hearing-impaired children are born into hearing families and to perplexed parents who need enlightened guidance and help with long-term planning. Such counseling has been a rare commodity for both deaf children and their parents, as well as for most patients with adult-onset hearing loss, I was to discover.

In less common cases, when an otherwise healthy deaf infant is born to deaf-mute parents, the child is perceived and greeted as a special gift. It is the biological continuity and affirmation of the deaf couple's own kind, and their sub-cultural legacy. Such proud and productive deaf folk see themselves and their children as perhaps different, but in no way handicapped.

The happy work with hearing-impaired pre-schoolers did not last very long. Because I was signing only a few hours each week, it seemed that the little ones rapidly outgrew me with their increasing fluency in signing. Also, I was no longer energetic and limber enough at the kind of play-therapy that pediatric psychotherapists sometimes need to use with little children. In understanding and relating to such little patients with their need for emotional props and toys, one must often join with them at their own level, which is frequently right down on the floor. I soberly concluded that hearing loss was not my only problem. I was getting too old to pursue a successful career as a pediatric play-therapist with deaf children, while learning to sign with the other hand.

In retrospect, my loss of Sam Polsky through his early death was also an aggravating factor in my hearing loss back then. I did not realize that among the many things for which I missed him was a special kind of hearing. How is that? Have you ever noticed how often spouses, close friends, colleagues, and business partners, add to and augment what each other hear? Even casual friends, wanting to know what news they may have missed, greet each other with "Hi. What's up? What's cooking today? What have you heard?" We hear through our own ears, and those of our closest friends. Sam was my closest friend and we heard twice as much together as either of us could hear by ourselves. That's the way it is with close partners and friends who needed to keep few, if any, secrets from each other. Despite increased hearing loss and the loss of my best friend, my academic life in forensic psychiatry at Temple continued with Professor William Taylor, who very capably took over Sam's duties. A number of years later, I was to discover that there was still a professional life "after deaf."

After retiring from Temple at age sixty-eight, my psychiatric career continued with my private cases and ongoing consultation work at ABC for a time. I also began to do some consultation work at the Sterck School for the Deaf in Newark, Delaware. As I recall, it was somehow through that connection that I met a licensed psychiatric social worker, who had successfully raised her own deaf and blind daughter, who was by then a junior in college. The remarkable mother, intimately familiar with sign language, had been treating a substantial caseload of mentally ill, deaf adults as their counselor and therapist at a community mental health center in Wilmington. I was then recruited to work part-time with her as a Community

Mental Health Clinic psychiatrist in the assessment and treatment of their special population of mentally-ill, deaf patients for whom there were so few treatment facilities elsewhere. This work enabled me to gain further experience with sign language and the deaf sub-culture, as well as some of the extra communication problems that deaf persons encounter in medical and mental health facilities.

These were also interesting times, because the tides were changing rapidly in community mental health, as well as in psychiatry generally. In the last decade, and in the early years of our new, current century, the practice of psychiatry continued to shift its emphasis away from talk therapy toward psychopharmacology, and the so-called neurosciences. The writing of prescriptions and emphasis on drug therapy became a major therapeutic function of a new generation of public sector psychiatrists, aided and abetted by the pharmaceutical companies and third-party payers.

Clinical psychologists and licensed social workers were easier to find, and readily available at substantially lower salaries than physicians. Who really needed expensive psychiatrists in community mental health clinics, except perhaps to write prescriptions? This was then a decade made to order for any increasingly deaf psychiatrist like me, with a great many years of clinical experience, and a fresh supply of prescription pads. I had, prior to that, been selectively writing prescriptions for psychotropic medications when we had a relatively limited psychopharmacological armamentarium and choice of effective drugs—until things really took off with the advent of Prozac, it seems.

For a number of ensuing years, I wrote prescriptions for our deaf patients, as well as some of my hearing ones. But I had my reservations. Psychiatric time in community mental health clinics was scheduled essentially for prescription writing and periodic case evaluations. Although I was turning eighty, and still seeing a few private patients whom I could hear close up at a maximal distance of two to three feet, fishing and sailing were beginning to look more attractive than prescribing routine psychiatric drugs or their latest variants. I was seeing "cases" rather than treating patients. Psychiatric times were changing along with my post-retirement hearing ability.

Hearing impairment has been for me a long walk in a patient's shoes. Was coping with progressive deafness in the same league as surviving cancer, which also occupied me for a time? For me, the answer is not yet clear-cut. You see, I got over my cancer, and eventually came to terms with my worries about potential recurrence and death. But I don't think I have yet come to terms with my adult-onset hearing loss. Hearing loss can really get to you over time, especially if you were not born that way and did not grow up in the deaf sub-culture.

Like a number of persons with profound hearing loss, I can "hear" you fine, up close and one-on-one if you are looking at me in reasonably good light, and if your newspaper, moustache, soup spoon, or hand is not hiding your lips. Those are a lot of "ifs." But I am no longer in denial, and no longer pretending I can hear. For the many who cling to denial of their hearing loss, the final, undeniable, frustrating, and maddening inability to understand phone conversations is our last stand, our auditory Waterloo. When the phone rings, and you cannot discern the stranger's name and figure out that it is not a man's voice, but your own wife who is calling, you know you have a problem. People are functionally deaf when, for example, their word-discrimination is no longer sufficient to understand spoken language over the telephone. My hearing affliction has included a long journey through that awkward stage of hearing loss.

What have I learned as a doctor in becoming "legally" deaf, so to speak? Many things, not the least of which is what it is really like to be a patient with a chronic, incurable, and personally diminishing impairment. But even more important, perhaps, I have also learned something about our human resolve and resilience, and our considerable potential for coping with very humbling affliction that distances us from the mainstream, and diminishes our prospects for spontaneous relationships with others.

Between 1989 and 2001, aside from learning to deal with hearing loss, I had no significant physical problems except for a relatively easy gallbladder excision. So in 2001, again healthy at age seventy-nine, I was in no way prepared to understand what was about to happen next.

Round Four, 2001: Partial Gastrectomy for a Stomach Sarcoma

Round Four for me started out with what seemed like an upset stomach and bad bellyache, which was a rare event for me. I thought that maybe if I could have a good BM, all might be well, but no luck. Nothing happened. No stomach rumbles, not even a sound. It seemed unusual. I began to get concerned and speculated that something else might be going on. The last thing I remember before waking up on the bathroom floor was wondering why it was that it is sometimes so hard for humans to have a normal bowel movement when elegant horses of either sex could simply lift their tails and defecate quite openly with aplomb, if not admirable savoir faire, in mixed company while standing up. I must have been getting a bit delirious before passing out.

I had apparently fainted in the bathroom and was quite surprised to see both dear Irmgard and Dave Rowan, my neighbor and frequent boating buddy, staring down at me sprawled on the bathroom floor with my pants down. "No pictures, please," was my first thought. Obviously dazed, I asked what happened. Irmgard was speechless, but Dave said, "Mel, you fainted while you were on the john, and we've called an ambulance. It should be here any minute now."

I was in no condition to argue.

The ambulance took me to Elkton's Union Hospital where Dr. Henry Farkas, my good medical friend and Emergency Room doctor, quickly assessed the situation, and thought I might encounter more than our local hospital could handle back then. After gently advising me that he thought I'd be better off at Christiana Hospital in nearby Newark, Delaware, he phoned ahead and ordered the ambulance to take me there forthwith. Receiving a swift and thorough workup, I underwent surgery the next day by Drs. Smale and Kahn, who encountered what the pathologists had diagnosed as a Gastrointestinal Stromal Tumor (GIST). I had never heard of it. Neither had most doctors and surgeons. It was not a new disease. We had previously called these malignant tumors leiomyosarcomas, but new immunohistology techniques had identified them as coming not from mutated smooth muscle cells, but from connective tissue or stromal cells in the lining of the gastrointestinal tract.

Dr. Smale was a pleasant, but no nonsense middle-aged man with a good head of hair styled in a military or butch cut. He came right to the point and said, "Dr. Heller, the first thing you need to know is that it was malignant, and we had to take out a portion of your stomach to which it was attached. And the second thing is that the tumor had ruptured and bled, sending little pieces into the abdominal cavity to seed it with potential metastases. Dr. Kahn and I flushed out the entire abdominal cavity thoroughly. We think we got it all, but we cannot be sure. And by the way, we had to remove your spleen because in was in the way."

Then Dr. Smale examined my drains and dressing and said. "Everything looks fine. How do you feel?"

"Pretty good under the circumstances", I replied.

"Are you in any pain? Can I get you something?"

"A new spleen would be nice."

That got me a wry smile and a gentle pat on the head from Dr. Smale, who knew I was grateful that he had tried his best.

I was shook up by the surgical pathology report. Its findings indicated that I was at high risk for recurrence of my sarcoma. However, my super son-in-law, Dr. Ken Miller, a very capable and fine oncologist, quickly took hold and guided me personally, and literally by the arm, to Memorial Sloan Kettering Hospital in New York City, where he introduced me to Dr. Ronald De Matteo, who was conducting a clinical trial on the new drug called Gleevec. I qualified for the trial, and because GIST is a sneaky and unpredictable sarcoma, I remained on the drug for ten years despite its side effects. I studied what I could find out about my sarcoma and joined an online GIST support group, where I learned a good deal more from my fellow patients and their caregivers. In 2003, I obtained a consultation with Dr. Margaret von Mehren, a nationally known GIST expert at Philadelphia's Fox Chase Cancer Center. Guided by her follow-up counsel, I have remained free of manifest recurrence of my sarcoma to date. But what seemed like a simple upset stomach ended up as a problem that still concerns me to this day.

If you are curious about sarcomas, they are not my medical specialty, but here are a few words about that term. Sarcomas are simply one of the two large designated groups of cancers. Sarcomas arise from so-called mesenchymal stem cells in the middle layers of normal embryonic tissues. These mesenchymal cells are those that give rise to our normal muscle, bone, fat. cartilage, tendons, blood and other tissue. When damaged or genetically mutated, these cells can grow wildly on their own to form a group of malignancies or cancers called sarcomas. Members of the other large group of cancers are called carcinomas. Carcinomas originate from embryonic epithelial cells, which form skin and glandular tissues. With that brief explanation, let us proceed to an entirely unexpected and brief knockdown that almost proved fatal.

Round Five, 2001: Episode of Gross Hematuria

My GIST sarcoma surgery healed well and on November 7, 2001 Irmgard and I were heading back to Dr. Smale's office for what we hoped would be a routine postoperative check-up. It was my tenth postoperative day, and I was feeling pretty good, but not yet up to par. Irmgard was driving, and we had gone only about four miles from our driveway, almost to Route 213, when I looked down at my pants and saw that I was having a hemorrhage. It was not from my abdominal sarcoma wound, which had healed nicely. I knew immediately that it was a large bleed from my enlarged prostate gland, because I had had a couple of them several years before, and had been taking Proscar until Drs. Smale and Shah discontinued it prior to their surgery. So I told Irmgard to drive us to Union Hospital in Elkton, which was only about fifteen minutes away.

There we discovered that my busy and capable young urologist was away (on his honeymoon, if you would believe). The ER technician had great difficulty inserting a Foley catheter into my bladder. He did not realize that he had inserted the catheter only as far as the prostatic portion of the urethra where he had pushed its firm tip into the prostate itself, which then continued to bleed all night. My hemoglobin dropped to dangerous levels requiring blood transfusions and a 3 a.m. phone call to Irmgard to come up because they were not sure I was going to make it. By this time, I was sedated and pretty much out of it. Obviously, I lived or I wouldn't be writing these words today. I was saved by a very fine urologist, Dr. Ronald Tutrone, who drove up in the early morning from close to Baltimore, I was told. Dr. Tutrone promptly removed the catheter, inserted a cystoscope, flushed out the bladder's blood clot with saline, and stopped the bleeding.

The problem had been due to the preoperative discontinuation of Proscar at the time of my GIST surgery ten days earlier, and not getting back on that medication promptly thereafter. Such seemingly simple slip-ups and errors should not happen in hospitals, but they still can even with today's increased safeguards.

In comparison to my major surgeries for two separate cancers of the lung and stomach, this all-night urological bleed and seemingly easy procedure might seem like a minor event. But had it not been for Dr. Tutrone's alacrity and skill many years ago, I would not be here to tell the story. The emergency cystoscopic procedure that finally controlled the bleeding was duly recorded in Dr. Tutrone's operative report of November 8, 2001. I shudder to think, had I died, whether or not my hospital death would have been investigated. Such things happen, and whether or not we are deaf (as we all may be under anesthesia), we need someone close, strong, nearby and informed to watch over us at any age, and particularly in our senior and elder years.

I still fear that my inevitable departure might yet be triggered by my troublesome prostate, in the form of a bleed or an acute urinary retention, which I have yet to forget after being almost knocked out cold during Round One way back in 1972. Dr. Tutrone and subsequent urologists did advise me to make sure that any future catheterization should be done by a urologist. At age ninety-three, I don't know how much I can be sure of as a hearing-impaired patient in a hospital's emergency ward or operating room. In 2005, however, I was facing surgery once again.

Round Six, 2005: Spinal Stenosis and Peripheral Neuropathy

Narrowing or stenosis of the spinal column by such common causes as ruptured discs, old vertebral fractures, or bony spurs can cause serious sensory and motor impairments as well as severe back, buttock and leg pain. Any or all of those symptoms may be diagnosed as spinal stenosis. In 1975, I had a ruptured inter-vertebral disc problem and was seeing a neurosurgeon, who had operated on my tennis-playing colleague, Dr. Ted Cohen, who indignantly insisted that he had done nothing more to bring on his affliction than simply to bend over to pick up a small dish or cup that had fallen to the floor. I, on the other hand, had played a good deal of late-middle-aged volleyball, and had been lifting and moving some moderate-sized, but heavy boulders for my dear wife's new rock garden on the grassy upgrade from the sandy beach along our Elk River waterfront home on Maryland's Eastern Shore.

So I was thinking about all those things and ruptured discs when I began to feel less strength in springing up from a low chair, or on climbing a steep set of stairs without pulling myself with my arms upward along the banister. When I actually fell backward onto the sidewalk while ascending three steps to enter a building at my granddaughter's graduation from college, I knew that something was wrong. I consulted my internist, who ordered an MRI of the lumbar spinal vertebrae, which showed a ruptured disc and spinal stenosis. Further consultation with a neurologist for peripheral nerve testing led to a definite diagnosis of peripheral neuropathy. With the distinct findings of both spinal stenosis and peripheral neuropathy, I needed to study the matter further and obtain more consultations. Once again, I was walking in my patients' shoes, as I previously had when my prospects for total deafness had seemed so imminent and threatening.

What was I to do now? I consulted two additional, highly qualified neurosurgeons, Dr. Paul Marcotte at the Pennsylvania Hospital and Dr. Yakov Koyfman, an experienced neurosurgeon of European origin at Christiana Hospital in nearby Newark, Delaware. After carefully studying my records, MRIs, and neurological findings, Dr. Koyfman stated, "Dr. Heller, I do not think you have much to gain from neurosurgery at this time." On the other hand, Dr. Marcotte, who made a similar study of my records, recommended surgery, but said that it might be complicated and difficult because of a "subluxation" or partial displacement of one of the vertebra's surfaces against its neighboring vertebra. That sounded anything but reassuring, and gave me further pause.

The next thing I must mention is that just as cancers come in two types, carcinomas a sarcomas, surgeries are of two types: elective and non-elective, including emergency surgeries where there is little or no choice but to operate. Enthusiastic surgeons and especially eager patients need to know not only when to operate, but also the equally important ability to judge whether or not to operate at all. This can be particular important in cases of elective surgery for acute or chronic back pain, as I discovered in my sixth prolonged adventure of walking as a doctor in a patient's shoes

The next step I needed was to consult with my trusted step-son-in-law, Dr. David Rees, married to Irmgard's daughter, Bonnie. David was and is a very capable and experienced orthopedic surgeon who, after reviewing my records, wrote back to me that with his own spinal stenosis patients he regarded surgery "as the last therapeutic modality" after trying all other means. He advised pain medications and physiotherapy first. On the other hand, my capable cardiologist, Dr. Chris Bowen, who had been following me for a slowly progressive stenosis of the aortic valve, warned me quite sternly that if I did not have the operation right now, I would lose the future use of my legs. What is the ordinarily intelligent patient to do? Although I was a doctor, in this instance I was primarily a well-informed patient. That was the very point. The informed patient has, and should have, the last word, the final say. After contemplating further details about my neuropathy, and considering some other development that were then emerging, I declined the spinal surgery option for a number of reasons. Among these were my changing circumstances and situation at home.

It Was Not Just Me; My Wife Was Ailing Too

It was not just my back that was hurting. The woman at my side, my wife and side-kick, was hurting much more. My spouse got suddenly knocked down, too. It started when Irmgard developed an uncommon, but not entirely rare pulmonary condition from a microbe called mycobacterium avium intracellulare. Neither of us had ever heard of it before. We consulted a pulmonologist, who explained that her cough and fatigue were due to a non-contagious form of bacteria commonly found in the ground, and that it affected small numbers of usually older women who enjoyed gardening and bird feeding. Irmgard seemed equally fond of both hobbies, as did I.

Although she continued to see the pulmonologist and consulted with other specialists, her quiet cough and sense of fatigue failed to respond to treatment. She then developed atrial fibrillation (Afib), an irregular heartbeat that was of far greater concern to me than my own back problems. The reason for my worry was that atrial fibrillation can lead to a pooling of blood in an upper heart chamber called the atrium, where pieces of clot, called emboli, can break off and enter the blood stream to reach the brain and cause major and fatal strokes. Unfortunately, that is what happened to my wife. Irmgard suffered a major stoke from which she never recovered, and which eventually caused her death on December 7, 2005. That infamous date became my personal Pearl Harbor Day.

I have related how in 1989, I lost a lobe of my left lung from cancer, and in 2001, how I lost my spleen and a portion of my stomach to another cancer. None of all that was as painful as losing a spouse, a whole person who had been such a devoted, heart-warming and beloved part of my life.

For a while after I lost Irmgard, I tried to hang in by myself down at our rural shore home, with hopes that perhaps I might find a middle-aged or older ex-service man and his wife to move in, rent-free, to look after me and our lovely waterfront property. No such luck. My aching back, balance problems, and unsteady gait got worse. Hard as I tried to prevent it, both Irmgard's gardens and her ailing husband slowly went to seed. Finally, I knew I needed to find an all-purpose retirement facility. My capable kids helped to find such a place, called the Quadrangle, in Haverford, Pennsylvania, and moved me in on October 31, 2006, I remember the exact date because it was Halloween, and some of the staff wore holiday costumes over their regular clothes. At age eighty-four, I was not in good shape and did not expect to live much longer, but I am still here at ninety-three, in much worse shape, but still able to think, recall, type, and share the story of a long, fully lived, fortunate and privileged life. God willing, I hope to live a bit longer.

A Place Called the Quadrangle

The Quadrangle is a full-care retirement facility with a well-staffed clinic, as well as ample provisions for assisted living and long-term nursing care. For the past eight years, I've been living alone in so-called independent living status, while busying myself with these memoirs, assorted doctors' appointments, and thankfully, my nearby offspring.

The Quadrangle is a luxurious place. It was built on the former Lloyds estate. No, not the famous Lloyds of London, but right here in the U.S. before the days of present taxes. The estate's spacious and well-kept Manor House and several hundred, well-tended acres on which stand many additional new buildings, attest to its former opulence. If you need a private, full service retirement facility with a decent staff, and a cluster of nice, elderly, generally well-educated people, who are fairly well-fixed, but too impaired or tired of trying to make it in their own homes, you will find few, if any such retirement places nearby that are any better. I have a nice apartment, with a second bath and bedroom for my offspring or grown grandchildren to visit and stay overnight if they wish. It is all the home I can handle physically. I walk very slowly and carefully now with a four-wheeled walker called a rollator. I now move about with caution because I already fractured my right femur. That required a total hip replacement, which was no fun, but it now works pretty well. Presently, I have only one original hip left, hopefully with many miles to go without falling again.

With those limitations (and there are more), I am trying to finish these memoirs before they finish me. That thought is something special, but also sobering. There can't be much time left since time flies fast and comes crashing down regularly on my aging cohort here at the Quadrangle. That is because our overall average age here is now above eighty years. Who's next?

Individuals I have known and shared remembered time with seem to be dying almost every day, and sometimes in clusters of two or three. Their passing is noted and set forth tastefully for a few days on a handsome table decked with flowers near our frequently used elevators, where we cannot miss noticing their passing. I call it the Falling Leaves Table.

So I have been thinking that I wouldn't be here today were it not for my lengthy career in surgery—horizontally that is, as a patient. You thought I had left surgery in 1950 to pursue a long career in psychiatry? Well, to be truthful, I've had an even longer and more exciting career in surgery than in psychiatry, especially in the last twenty years. As a matter of fact, I wouldn't be alive today if I had not returned to surgery often enough.

Round Seven, 2009: Surgical Aortic Valve Replacement (SAVR)

After moving into the Quadrangle, I did pretty well for the next three years. But a couple of years before the ongoing spinal stenosis issues had emerged, my Maryland cardiologist, Dr. Chris Bowen, had informed me, back in 2003, that I had aortic valve stenosis. So I was not surprised to see the valve become increasingly constricted in subsequent echocardiograms and follow up studies. Aortic valve stenosis is not uncommon in eighty-year-old persons.. It was what had caused my mother's death at age eight-seven. So my question inevitably came down to when, where, and how I would proceed to have my aortic valve replaced. My primary care doctor referred me to a fine cardiologist named Timothy Shapiro, who took over from Dr. Chris Bowen when I moved from Maryland back to Philadephia less than a year following Irmgard's death. The first thing I asked Dr. Shapiro was, "Who does the most and the best aortic valve surgery in this country?" Without batting an eyelash, Dr. Shapiro, who had trained at Yale and Penn but not in Cleveland, responded with two words: "Cleveland Clinic." Little did I know that those two words would figure prominently in my final decision about where and how I would have my aortic valve replaced.

Shopping and Researching for Elective Heart Surgery

The first cardiac surgeon that Dr. Tim Shapiro sent me to was Dr. Scott Goldman at Lankenau Hospital in Philadelphia. Dr. Goldman was one of the top-rated cardiac surgeons in the area. On review of my records and further exam, Dr. Goldman said he would be glad to do my surgery forthwith. He had a fine reputation, but I needed to think further about Dr. Shapiro's immediate and candid assessment of Cleveland Clinic as the best place when I first met him. This was not an ordinary appendectomy on a healthy twenty-year-old, for example. This was to be open heart surgery on an old man with a large, recent, and complicated cancer operation, and in poor shape with a relatively new anti-cancer drug that caused edema and substantial anemia, among its untoward side effects with me. Without chest pain, shortness of breath, or other cardiac symptoms, I had wanted to save the forthcoming summer for some family-shared vacation and birthday times. There was no rush in undergoing elective surgery, and so Dr. Goldman said he'd be glad to see me if I chose to return in September. My son Paul, who finger-spelled and was glad to accompany his hearing-impaired father at such potentially crucial meetings as key medical consultations, was much impressed with Dr. Goldman.

However, Dr. Shapiro had additionally suggested that I might look into a new alternative that, if successful, did not require opening the thoracic cavity. The new procedure was called a Transcatheter Aortic Valve Implant (TAVI) and was undergoing trial at the Hospital of the University of Pennsylvania (HUP). Also referred to as the Percutaneuous Aortic Valve Implant (PAVI), the operation consisted of inserting an ingeniously rolled up, artificial aortic valve into the heart via the femoral artery. This new, potentially ingenious approach would avoid the risks of stopping the hearts of very elderly persons, as they would be when undergoing standard aortic valve replacement surgery. So, I met with Dr. Bavaria, a top cardiac surgeon at HUP who was in charge of the Transcatheter Trial. After examining my numerous medical records, Dr. Bavaria felt that I would be at very high risk if I underwent standard surgical aortic valve replacement, and urged me to see whether I could qualify for the Transcatheter trial at HUP. I did that, and was about to complete their extensive "Trial Inclusion Workup" when my views began to change.

The Patent's Role and Responsibility in Providing Informed Consent

If you've ever undergone even a mildly unusual procedure at a clinic or hospital, you were required to sign previously prepared legal papers called Informed Consent documents. Not only as a forensic psychiatrist who had co-taught this subject to third year law students for some thirty years, but now as an elderly patient, I took this responsibility very seriously for my own good as an informed, high-risk patient. While going through Dr. Bavaria's intake process, I had been studying everything I could find about aortic valve replacements on old persons like myself. It helped to be a doctor, but you don't need to be one to learn about elective medical and surgical procedures. In true emergencies, it matters less because we have little choice even if we are still conscious and know what's going on. But in non-emergencies, you should try to understand what you are being asked to consent to. Don't sign the consent papers as blindly as most persons do, with or without a silent prayer.

Absent an emergency, and with the help or your library, and espciallly a computer with search engines like Google, Medscape and numerous others these days, literate persons can learn to make informed judgments about their medical and surgical options, and to have more enlightened and self-empowered discussions with their physicians. If your doctor dismisses or evades your questions, find another, if possible. Sometimes, no matter what you are able or unable to do to help yourself, coincidence and luck are often ongoing factors in one's medical affairs. Let me tell you how those factors influenced and determined my final decision about the two alternatives for undergoing aortic heart valve replacement in 2009.

Some Added Luck While Researching my Surgical Options as a Patient

By what turned to be a very fortunate coincidence, Mark Mendel, a very bright and close friend of my son, Paul, since their early teenage days, was visiting him for a weekend at our conveniently shared Elk River homes in Maryland, and I joined them for a friendly fatherly chat. What has that to do with us and our discussion of aortic valves? Well, I had forgotten that young Mark Mendel, whom I hadn't seen for a number of years, had obtained his PhD at University of Pennsylvania in Bioengineering. And when the talk eventually turned to my forthcoming aortic valve replacement, Mark who is not a physician, turned out to have had much more contact than I would have imagined with the bioprosthetic science of aortic valve replacement. This, to my surprise, was based on Mark's prior experience in working closely with a fellow bioengineer, Ivan Vesely, PhD, who for some ten years had ran the Cardiac Valve Research Lab at the Cleveland Clinic, no less.

Just before that I had been trying to study as much as I could find about my own surgical prospects as an elderly patient in need of a surgical atrial valve replacement (SAVR). Several recent reports and items added further light on the subject and made me a bit more circumspect, if not leery, about the risks versus benefits or trade-offs of between Transcatheter Valve Replacements in contrast to SAVR.

I read through informative articles on aortic valve replacement procedures by highly qualified experts. Based on their enlightening discussion, and on my further perusal of the subject not as an expert, but as a prospective valve replacement patient, the following seemed evident to me. First, complications and adverse results from the newer "Transcatheter Aortic Valve Implant" (TAVI) were fewer than with the standard SAVR only in the first postoperative year. On the other hand, the pre-existing, standard SAVR would be more reliable throughout the second and subsequent years after the surgery. What really grabbed my attention, however, were the statistics of adverse outcomes for TAVI the first thirty postoperative days.

Adverse Outcomes for Transcatheter Aortic Valve Implants

As I pondered the figures, it seemed that some of the risks and serious complications of the newer TAVI procedures were very sobering, to put it mildly. For example, if my age cohort of octogenarians underwent the allegedly safer transcatheter procedure, one out of every ten of us would be dead within thirty days, and if still alive after that, one out of every four of us would need a cardiac pacemaker with good batteries for the remainder of our lives.

On the other hand, if the open-chest SAVR patients got through the first year, their future prospects for the next five years were substantially better than those who had their new aortic valves ingeniously snaked through the skin and the large femoral artery to reach the heart and replace the valve. Although such procedures were an amazing development, if I were to undergo the risks of a transcatheter aortic valve replacement, I would be looking for more than the one-year advantage it allegedly provided in the first year. Moreover, the experienced cardiac surgeons at the Cleveland Clinic that Dr. Shapiro had told me did the best and the most aortic valve replacements did not embrace the transcatheter procedures. That tipped the balance for me in favor of the SAVR. So when Mark Mendel recommended the Cleveland Clinic-trained Dr. Michael Banbury, now the chief cardiac surgeon at the nearby Christiana Hospital in Newark, Delaware, I hastened to make an appointment to see him, with my son, Paul, on September 26, 2009.

Dr. Michael Banbury

The rest was easy. Dr. Banbury was not much older than Paul, barely fifty, if that, and at the top of his game. I asked him how his results compared with those of the Cleveland Clinic. He replied more confidently than modesty with, "Just about as good and in some ways a bit better." I didn't need Paul to finger-spell that. Dr. Banbury spoke loud and clear. He had examined all my records, which I had sent to him ahead of time, and when I asked him whether he thought I was a suitable candidate for aortic valve surgery, he replied without hesitation: "Yes." I liked him and Mark Mendel's confidence in him. So my next question was, "Dr. Banbury, would you do my surgery?" He replied, "I'd be honored." So, on October

10, 2009, after further workup, Dr. Banbury implanted in my chest a new aortic valve made of bovine tissue. The new valve has been doing its job very well these almost five years since.

I cannot deny that open heart surgery and replacing an aortic valve was quite a hard knock that required recovery time and a cardiac rehab routine. But the concomitant boost was a big one. It came in knowing that I was still lucky as a patient that could think his way through a difficult and carefully considered decision. That the decision turned out to be right was quite a boost. Cardiac surgery was far from my specialty. But one does not need to be a doctor to make carefully considered decisions about surgery, plumbing, roof replacement, or aortic valve replacement. Just investigate and study the matter by reading reliable and reputable sources, seeking second opinions, and sharing what you are learning and thinking about with your doctor. Try it.

Round Eight, 2010: Total Hip Replacement

Only a few months after my cardiac surgery and cardiac rehab sessions, I was feeling much recovered and stronger. My son, Paul, and I were heading down to our Elk River Shore home in Maryland. He picked me up at the Quadrangle, and we were starting down the long carpeted corridor to load ourselves and my overnight baggage into Paul's car. Hurrying along with my heavy overnight bag in one hand, and leaning on my wobbly cane with the other, I underestimated both my age and my spinal stenosis balance problem. Down I went on the soft carpet. I landed on my hip, somewhat athletically, I thought, as I had fallen many dozens of times during my college football days seventy years earlier. Shaking off Paul's concern as he helped me to my feet, I assured him that it was "nothing, just a bruise."

I thought that the hip was merely bruised even when its mild discomfort continued while we did a bit of boating the next day, and even when the pain seemed no better as we headed back to Pennsylvania the day after that. My Quadrangle Clinic doctor ordered hip x-rays to be taken at the nearby Bryn Mawr Hospital, but they showed no evidence of fracture. When the pain worsened the following day, we repeated the x-ray studies and, sure enough, they now showed a linear facture across the upper, right-angled neck of the thigh bone (femur). So they kept me at the hospital, where I was soon seen by a tall, young, bright, and very cheerful orthopedic surgeon named Eric A. Levicoff, MD, of whom I had never heard, but who seemed okay. After walking with a broken femur for three days, I was in no mood to go shopping for referrals for the total hip replacement surgery that he advised. He did it the next day, and it turned out fine. I've been grateful for my artificial hip joint hardware these past five years.

Except for the surgical wound, which healed quickly, hip replacement was not an easy postoperative experience. It was a hard knockdown that required both physical and occupational therapy to learn how to use a "pick-stick" instead of kneeling or bending down to pick things up from the floor, and how to maneuver oneself to insert one foot and then the other into their proper segment of our trousers—daily abilities we ordinarily take for granted, along with tying our shoelaces. The new hip joint seems to be working adequately except that I cannot flex my thigh far enough for me to reach and trim my toenails, which can sometimes be a substantial matter in geriatric podiatry, and life in general.

I'm not trying to make light of this orthopedic achievement, but I've had bigger things to worry about during the past five years since my right hip was done. So why am I telling you this particular story among the successive knocks and boosts encountered in my geriatric surgical adventures?

First, because prior to operating on me, Dr. Levicoff had discontinued the Gleevec therapy for my cancer that the nationally known sarcoma expert, Dr. von Mehren, had prescribed to control it because she felt that my surgical pathology report indicated that I was at "very high risk for the cancer's recurrence." Discontinuing Gleevec is fairly routine prior to most major surgeries, so there was nothing unusual in Dr. Levicoff's decision. Nevertheless, discontinuing Gleevec was anxiety-inducing. GIST sarcomas can be so unpredictable as to become a source of ongoing anxiety for many people who encounter each other in our online sarcoma support groups. The secondary emotional effects of cancer on patients, their families, and caregivers is a huge and widely experienced human story unto itself.

Next, through my broken hip story, I wish to alert you to the high incidence of avoidable knockdowns and serious falls among geriatric folk, with their weakened neuromuscular systems and thinned calcium-deficient bones (as in osteoporosis, and osteopenia). Needless knockdowns happen to elderly people ignoring or denying their geriatric diminutions of energy, strength, endurance, and almost everything else. Our large cohort of fellow octogenarians fall weakly and weekly, if not daily here at the Quadrangle. We develop mostly bruises, but also fractures. Some of these are more than simple cracks, and may require weeks of immobilization in a cast. With circulation problems, blood clots may form and break off, causing pulmonary embolisms and sudden death. That fatal sequence following a lower leg fracture took the life of my children's' mother, Jane, here at the Quadrangle not long ago.

So, where was the gain or boost from the hard knock of hip replacement surgery? I have since developed wise caution and great care in moving about in my apartment, or wherever I go on foot. "Be careful" is now my watchful mantra. I feel that caring voice inside me like an attentive inner companion. I realize that there is no fool like an old fool, as I now move about very carefully, aided by my trusty, four-wheeled rollator.

Round Nine, 2010: Endoscopic Retrograde Cholangio Pancreatography (ERCP)

Ten months after the hip replacement, I underwent a two-hour Endoscopic Retrograde Cholangiopancreatography (ERCP) to remove two gallstones and some "sludge" in the left hepatic duct. This endoscopic surgery is performed by specially trained gastroenterologists. The procedure allows the gastroenterologist to access organs within the abdomen by passing a tube through the esophagus into the stomach while the patient is under general anesthesia. Thereafter, the gastroenterologist is able to pass thinner, more flexible tubes from the stomach into the duodenum, which is the next section of the gastrointestinal (GI) tract. The duodenum contains the openings of the bile ducts from the liver into the GI tract. By manipulating the flexible tubes (called catheters), the operator can maneuver the thin tube into the liver's hepatic duct. I've gone into this brief anatomic discourse to explain how ingenious is this surgical method, which enabled the operator to find two bile stones and some "sludge" that were dangerously obstructing my hepatic duct and causing inflammation, sepsis, and recurrent fever.

The alternative would have required major open abdominal surgery and cutting into the liver, a much larger procedure. I did not, however, get away scot-free. The two very capable gastroenterologists and an anesthetist working as a team encountered great difficulty in getting the endoscope through the upper level of the esophagus on three attempts. I was told afterward of this difficulty, which explained to me why I was having trouble swallowing large pills. Not to get into further details, I subsequently developed dysphagia, a problem about which I had heard and knew very little before encountering it. I have experienced increasing difficulty in swallowing, to the point of choking on food and aspirating it. That led to several episodes of aspiration pneumonia, requiring hospitalization for septicemia and bacteria in the blood stream. This was like getting hit by a bus.

Challenged by Dysphagia and Aspiration Pneumonia

Next I was referred to swallowing disorder therapists, who visualized my swallowing during a test and concluded that I needed a feeding tube in order to get enough nutrition. This understandably dismayed me. An ENT (ear, nose and throat) doctor strongly advised me to have a feeding tube. My dear son-in-law, Dr. Ken Miller, an oncologist, said, "Dad, it's easy." "Easy on whom?" I wondered. Asking both Ken and the ENT specialist, "Who would help me clean it?" I concluded that I'd rather choke to death on a delicious hamburger than end my days with a feeding tube. Dr. Toan Nguyen, my gastroenterologist at Bryn Mawr Hospital, who was much experienced with feeding tubes, supported my view and preference to work with a speech and swallowing therapist.

I worked with two very capable physiotherapists for dysphagia and swallowing disorders. They taught me to thicken my foods and drinks, to take small sips and small bites, and then to swallow only with my chin down and pressed against my chest. Carefully practiced by a formerly occasional glutton, I think it was much better than a feeding tube would have been. However, to avoid talking while I ate, which brought on spasms of gagging, choking and aspirating food, I now eat mostly by myself. I have missed the casual lunch and dinner conversations, but in this way, by eating in solitude, I have succeeded in swallowing enough food and drink to maintain my weight and energy level. As time went on, I can now drink small sips and handle a tasty glass of wine, or beer, slowly and happily with my sons, and feel those small blessings most thankfully in my throat on a hot summer's day.

I've gone into this, hopefully in not too boring detail, for a special reason. My swallowing disorder that followed the ERCP in Round Nine, along with my progressive hearing loss, described in Round Three, combined to disable and knock me down far more completely and permanently than my two major surgeries for cancer and the aortic heart valve replacement. That was because the dysphagia and adult deafness combined to isolate me. I could no longer hear ordinary social conversation, even in small groups. I could no longer dine regularly or casually with people, and eat and drink sufficiently without choking and aspirating. Mother said "Every knock is a boost" so often that it became the title of these memoirs. "If the knockdown doesn't kill you, if you can just only crawl away and manage to survive, it will one day make you a stronger person," she insisted.

Where could I eventually find, or even imagine, any kind of "boost" from my combined hearing loss and swallowing disorder? I wondered about those setbacks for a long time. And then it came to me. I remembered that some people actually took voluntary vows of silence. Vows of silence are common in a number of religious orders and faiths. My involuntary and lasting experience with silence boosted me into periods of solitary reflection and introspection. These not only disciplined me, but enlightened me about myself and people with whom I had formerly been able to chat gaily and daily without caring or wondering what our easy conversations were all about.

Despite the above limitations in easy chatting, I have remained the same sociable person that I always was, and have maintained meaningful relationships with members of our Quadrangle writers group through our twice monthly meetings, which allow me to participate meaningfully. This is because we present and read our writing, which we have photocopied and handed out to each member to view as the presenter reads their selection. That way, I am able to fully participate and then comment on the material in ways that we appreciate from each other. Another form of sociability that I have retained since my college freshman days is that I rarely pass a fellow resident in the corridors of the Quadrangle without at least a casual nod, or more if I sense that they are receptive.

That is because I can still speak, and lip-read their response if I am looking at them directly.

Relationship Therapy

What constitutes a relationship? I submit that any encounter is the beginning or end of a potentially ongoing relationship. Relationships, no matter what various schools of psychotherapy might tell you, are an integral part of every psychotherapy. Unintentionally and unknowingly when the people I encounter casually here at the Quadrangle pass by each other, we either feel better or worse for the experience. When I see someone dejected, impaired, and with their head hanging down, I can ignore them or maybe acknowledge their continued presence as a surviving resident with a slight nod or open smile or word, depending on how I intuitively sense their receptivity.

Let me confess that in this way, I practice a very limited form of "relationship therapy" with many of the people I encounter casually day-to-day here at the Quadrangle. It has been my experience that this has a cumulative effect. Over time, fellow residents who pass by passively have greeted me with a nod or a smile of recognition. This may not be much of a relationship to you, but it's the best that I can do and it certainly does no harm. I firmly believe that it does some good for both my fellow residents and myself.

And what should I say, if anything, to my elderly fellow residents as we pass by each other? At the very least, I can say, "Good morning," or "Have a good day," or "That's a good-looking shirt." Why do I do this? None of us is so bland or unimportant as to have no effect on each other. I believe that every encounter between us is either therapeutic or anti-therapeutic. We are aged survivors and siblings, who ought to act kindly toward each other.

Round Ten, 2009: Skin Cancers and Mohs Surgery

Among my rounds with Mother Nature, I include my three episodes of skin cancer, beginning in 2009, because each successive skin lesion was malignant, required surgery, and caused me substantial concern and anxiety. Skin cancers are very common among people my age. Mine were removed by Mohs surgery, a technique which was developed around 1938 by a general surgeon named Dr. Frederic E. Mohs. It is usually performed now by specially trained dermatologists, who remove thin slices of the tumor or skin lesion, and immediately examine them under the microscope, continuing this process until no more evidence of malignant cells are seen. The procedure is relatively easy and has a greater than ninety percent chance of cure. So, on three occasions, Mohs surgery has resulted in curing skin cancers for me.

Part Two
Some Things I Ponder and Believe

Chapter 25
Looking Back at My Choice Between Surgery and Psychiatry

I NEVER PLANNED to be a psychiatrist, let alone a forensic one. At medical school, psychiatry was often poorly taught in the 1940s and was generally regarded in low and unflattering terms. I loved everything else, from anatomy to parasitology, and pathology to obstetrics. Looking back on my thinking then and subsequently about my eventual choice, I have at a few nostalgic times as a practicing psychiatrist missed the honest, hands-on arts and crafts of surgery—not the basic cutting and stitching skills, but its increasingly impressive instrumentation and technology.

Other physicians, including psychiatrists, charge by time spent. With an insurance system like we have in this country, which reimburses more for procedures performed rather than time spent with patients, surgeons often do better financially than other physicians whose work depends in large part on fostering trust and communicating effectively with patients.

On the other hand, had I remained in surgery I would surely have missed the chance, the challenge, and professional privilege of studying the aberrant thoughts, feelings, and behaviors of persons whom psychiatrists and much of society regard as "mentally ill." Today's psychiatrists have learned much of clinical and theoretical interest, as well as some anatomic, physiological, and molecular facts about where and how our nerve cells transmit impulses and communicate with each other. However, the overall, essential, and seemingly eternal mysteries of the human mind remain as abstract, intangible, elusive, and unsolved as before.

Meanwhile, surgical procedures have advanced by leaps and bounds during my sixty years of laboring in the public and private sectors of psychiatry. Progress in surgery had enabled hearts, knees, hips, livers, and lungs to be accessed, repaired, and even transplanted by increasingly experienced, interdisciplinary teams of experts. We have no such interdisciplinary teams working regularly as clinicians together in psychiatry. This would be difficult to conceptualize in most psychotherapeutic practices. Psychotherapy patients seek an intimate, absolutely confidential, trusting, and soul-searching relationship with an experienced mental health professional, who is trained to provide clinical observations about the patient's mental processes, patterns of behavior and interpersonal relationships.

What My Body and I Owe to Surgery

What I learned in surgery is a great respect for detail, precision, accuracy, and accountability in dealing with patients. Looking back on my own career choice, I have retained the greatest respect, admiration and personal gratitude for surgery. I would not be alive today without its many advances. In the past sixty or more years since I've been a doctor, our medical knowledge and technology have changed substantially. Regrettably, as I've aged over the same time period, so has my body changed. For me as for many others, as our bodies have broken down over time, surgery has come to the rescue—excising tumors and repairing hernias and replacing hips, knees, kidneys, livers, lung, heart valves, and more.

Consider that I have had two cancers, a carcinoma of the lung and a sarcoma of the stomach, either of which would have likely been fatal had they not been surgically removed. Had I not died of either of those two cancers, I would most certainly have died of an age-related, aortic valve constriction, if that valve had not been replaced with a well-functioning artificial valve during cardiac bypass, open-heart surgery. The new valve is designed to serve me well for another dozen to fifteen years, assuming nothing else goes wrong. And if things should go wrong, many of us die with a variety of still viable organs and healthy tissues that we cannot take with us, but can bequeath to others. So, at least in that sense, all is not lost to those who are charitable—with thanks to transplant surgery. In any case, benefits of surgery have extended my life and brought me gratefully to my present circumstances and whereabouts.

Surgery is dramatic, remunerative, and stressful. Good or bad surgical results and those in between are there for all to see. From the viewpoint of other physicians, and our surgeons themselves, however, surgery is a wonderfully positioned specialty. If a condition cannot be cured or alleviated by surgical means, it is dismissed by definition as a "non-surgical illness" for the present, and turned over to an internist or another medical specialist for further treatment or supportive care. This way, surgeons are able to get high marks by calling their shots, so to speak. Along with their higher income and macho-heroic image, this tends to give surgeons a leg up on most other medical practitioners, who labor in less bloody and dramatic trenches, but equally different and important fields of health care.

Surgeons charge not by the hour but by the job, doing "piece work," as it is called in other needle and cutting trades, such as garment work or barbering. Psychiatrists charge by the fifty-minute hour, but medical insurance companies and their "managed care" experts allow for fifteen or twenty minute sessions, or enough time to check on medications and write a new prescription. All that is fine with the drug companies, which have their own bottom line problems in developing new drugs and bringing them to the market after expensive, government-mandated clinical trials to make sure that patients are properly dosed and not poisoned by insufficiently tested drugs. Many psychiatrists who minimize psychotherapy enjoy the study and practice of clinical psychopharmacology, at which they are expert.

But other physicians, like family doctors, internists, and pediatricians, miss out because a large part of medical practice requires the informative and supportive trust of the doctor-patient relationship, in which the doctor explains in terms that the patient can understand the treatment plan and the risk/benefits ratio of the available treatment options. This takes time, which is often not covered by Medicare or "managed care" medical insurance companies. Consequently, doctors feel rushed while their patients feel cheated by our enormously expensive, wasteful, and mismanaged medical care system, unless one can afford the luxury of a private contract with a "concierge" medical service.

What Surgery Cannot Cure

Our species is unlikely to get wiped off the face of the Earth by cancer, malaria, AIDS, or heart disease. The good news is that we are making steady progress in controlling or eradicating those afflictions. The bad news is that we may blow each other off the face of the Earth or pollute our planet beyond repair. There has never been a single generation in the annals of ancient or modern history when the Earth was free of mankind's habit of destructive warfare. With our newly acquired and spreading biological and nuclear warfare technologies, and our propensity for human error, is our exit from the Earth's stage only a matter of time? For now, however, the individual life spans of persons in technically advanced, hygienic countries have increased markedly, more than doubling since the ancient days of Rome, it seems. One would have hoped that as our human life spans increased, we would have become wiser in our behaviors as a species.

What do we know? What do we believe? Why do we believe? "You Gotta Believe" in something if not all that you hear in a church, mosque, or synagogue. Back in the 1950s, Edward R. Murrow, a highly regarded commentator on CBS, had a program called *This I Believe*. Audience members were invited to send in brief essays on their core beliefs. A number of these were so good that Murrow published a book or two of these collected essays with the same titled *This I Believe*. I enjoyed reading these during my surgical residency training, and it might have been one of the things that made me wonder if I might be interested in taking a year in psychiatry before continuing with my surgical specialty training.

Chapter 26
Seeking Answers. What Was It All About?

I'M NINETY-THREE AND old enough to ask what it was all about. Over the years, a doctors learns many things while listening, looking, and working with patients—things that are not always in our textbooks. I think that one of the most important things I learned is that we differ from our patients, as we do from each other, mostly by degree, quantitatively that is, and often not by that much. Some of us have a little less or more of one thing or another, of this and that, perhaps a small aberration or mutation, an over-expression of one gene or another that can have such elaborate consequences. And so, we often observe and study microscopic and other small differences in the art and science of medicine. What accounts for our differences?

Some neuroscientists regard our human emotions, attitudes, and behaviors as being hard-wired in our genes and neuroendocrine systems, rather than by how we have been subsequently shaped and programmed by our environmental perceptions and experiences in response to life's events and challenges. Although interested as a physician in all of the developments and leads that our medical science has to offer, I have personally tended to listen to my patients more from the perspective of a "therapeutic programmer," as a psychoanalyst and psychotherapist. In actual practice, as an obligatory psycho-pharmacologist, however, I have maintained a broad clinical interest, rather than any particular expertise, in neurophysiology, neurology, and the psychology of learning theory and cognitive science.

Seeking Scientific Answers to Life's Mysteries

My basic science major in college was biology, the study of living things. While earning my Bachelor's degree, I took all the biology courses that I could find, and I earned enough credits toward a Master's degree. The only requirement I didn't complete was the thesis, which I subsequently wrote in my senior medical school year which enabled me to received both my MD and MS when I graduated from medical school.

Along the way, I also studied some physics and electronics, as well as history and literature in our liberal arts college. Following this, I had many post-doctoral years leading to a relative abundance of experience, qualifications, and credentials as a psychiatrist. I still have much to learn about my recurrently frustrating and beleaguered, but fascinating specialty in which I have been entrusted, rewarded, and privileged indeed, to listen to the everyday worries and most intimate secrets of persons who often seem quite like you and me. The more I learned, the more I discovered how much more there was to learn, and how much more I needed to know no matter where or what I studied.

Neither biology, neurology, biochemistry, physics nor psychoanalysis, however, shed any further light on what I am most interested in learning—the ultimate mystery of the meaning or purpose of sentient human life. Biology did reveal for us the roles of genetics and chance mutation in the competitive adaptation to our earthly environments, and the evolution of life's species, which favor survival of the fittest.

Recent advances in the subspecialties of genetics, cytology, and molecular physiology have opened up a vast, new, miniature world that is regulated by the arrangement of proteins in each species' genome, whereby cells signal each other via special receptors on their surface membranes. These wonderful discoveries were made during the era of my own lifetime which also brought forth Einstein's theory of relativity, as well as Freud's psychoanalytic concepts and methods for exploring the Unconscious. And physicists postulate a super-explosive Big Bang theory to explain the origin of our still expanding universe. But what about the meaning or purpose of sentient human life? What science cannot yet perceive poets have long sought to provide us with as nutritious food for thought in verse. What good can it do for our species to have developed our awesome technology when we have yet to learn how to get along with each other? What, if anything, can the poets and playwrights tell us?

Consulting with Shakespeare: Is All the World a Stage?

Some scholars consider Shakespeare to have been the greatest English language poet. Having been translated into most of the world's major tongues, his work is universally appreciated. So let us take Shakespeare as an example of what, if anything, poets can teach us about the meaning and purpose of life on our world. I am far from a Shakespeare scholar, but my high school English teacher, Fredric Haskell Dole, an unforgettable and elderly New England Yankee with a loose set of false teeth that sometimes whistled when he spoke, made us memorize and recite for our class William Shakespeare's famous lines in *As You Like It*. They began with the metaphor, "All the world's a stage, And all the men and women merely players."

These enduring lines, written around 1600, were published in Shakespeare's *First Folio* in 1623. The words have been read, spoken and heard by successive generations long before such recent psychologists as Erik Erikson set down his subsequent views of the stages of child development in clinical terms. Shakespeare's "All the world's a stage" speech survived and is treasured for what it is worth. I have remembered it all these years, but does it tell me anything about what I am still seeking to learn about the purpose of our human lives? What does Shakespeare tell us, if anything, about the purpose and meaning of our lives on this Earth? So you can judge for yourself, Shakespeare's famous lines are as follows:

"All the world's a stage,
And all the men and women merely players;
They have their exits and their entrances,
And one man in his time plays many parts,
His acts being seven ages. At first, the infant,
Mewling and puking in the nurse's arms.
Then the whining schoolboy, with his satchel
And shining morning face, creeping like snail
Unwillingly to school. And then the lover,
Sighing like furnace, with a woeful ballad
Made to his mistress' eyebrow. Then a soldier,
Full of strange oaths and bearded like the pard,
Jealous in honor, sudden and quick in quarrel,
Seeking the bubble reputation
Even in the cannon's mouth. And then the justice,
In fair round belly with good capon lined,
With eyes severe and beard of formal cut,
Full of wise saws and modern instances;
And so he plays his part. The sixth age shifts
Into the lean and slippered pantaloon,
With spectacles on nose and pouch on side;
His youthful hose, well saved, a world too wide
For his shrunk shank, and his big manly voice,
Turning again toward childish treble, pipes
And whistles in his sound. Last scene of all,
That ends this strange eventful history,
Is second childishness and mere oblivion,
Sans teeth, sans eyes, sans taste, sans everything."

Do Shakespeare's poetic observations add anything to our scientific knowledge of human life's behavioral stages as we age? Why should we elevate science to be the judge of actual facts when they are disputed? Let us look at a sad example of the resistance to scientific fact that abounded in Shakespeare's and Galileo's time. Why bring in Galileo? Did you know they were contemporaries, born in the same year, but miles apart? I didn't know it either, until I looked it up. Why did Galileo's views get him in trouble while Shakespeare's lines were applauded? Let us take a quick look at a more shameful time in Rome than could be found in all of Stratford on Avon.

A Look at Science in Shakespeare's, Galileo's and Pope Urban VIII's Time

If one traveled south in the early 1600s, from Stratford-on-Avon in Shakespeare's England to the vicinity of Rome, one might encounter the famous physicist and mathematician, Galileo, who was looking though his early telescope at the moon and stars while Shakespeare was writing his famous plays and sonnets. How different things must have been for them as they aged. Shakespeare was receiving applause while Galileo was getting into big trouble with Pope Urban VIII in at the Vatican court in Rome. What was the problem? Galileo insisted that the planet Earth rotated around the sun and was not, as the gospel truth proclaimed, the Center of the Universe.

Copernicus had been the first to get it right mathematically, but it was Galileo who nailed the case closed with his telescopic observations. Bolstered by his mathematical reckonings, Galileo boldly asserted that the Earth was a planet revolving around the Sun. This was an unacceptable and strictly forbidden heresy that troubled Pope Urban VIII sufficiently to have to have the highly-regarded scientist brought to Rome's Inquisition chambers where he was interrogated continuously for days, humiliated, and further threatened with torture and being burned to death at the stake unless he recanted on his knees and begged Pope Urban's forgiveness for asserting that the Earth revolved around the Sun.

Galileo was almost seventy years old, and much respected among scientists for his carefully calculated mathematical and telescopic observations. But humbled and no longer strong, he recanted and spent his final years in isolation, poor health, and defeat. How far our authorities and the public were, only a few centuries ago, from any understanding of our human place in the Universe. Even today we still have little knowledge of where we and our small solar system might stand in the Cosmic scheme of things.

Knowing Our Cosmic Geography and Place

Until recently, we had little ability to view our very miniscule and remote place among the stars, planets, and galaxies. By obtaining further knowledge of our relative situation and position in the lineup of other planets, we might have a chance to know whether we are winning or losing in our Earthly battles for life. Simply put, we cannot win in evolution's cruel contest for survival of the fittest if we do not know our score in life on Earth. Our human score can be obtained only by recording and tallying the collective track records of human history. Archeologists, anthropologists, historians, theologians, and scholars from our various academic disciplines are busy digging and sifting through rocks and searching through books, microscopes, telescopes, test tubes, and computerized libraries to collect the remnants, artifacts, and evidence of Mankind's past and ongoing experiences.

So far, the score seems to indicate that we humans are far ahead in winning the ongoing survival race. We are the fittest, fiercest, most troubling, and troubled species on Earth. But the game is not yet over. Living in an era of technologically advanced warfare, persistent socio-economic inequities, varying ideologies and beliefs, repressive political regimes, and ongoing armed conflicts worldwide, we must acknowledge that we still harbor aggressive instincts that might lead to our self-destruction. We pray that civilized leaders will guide our species to endure, propagate, and prosper equitably and wisely. That brings me back to my recollections of and reflections on what my life was about while I was here.

Chapter 27
Some Other Things I Now Ponder and Believe

Thoughts on Early Human Life and Our Situation on Planet Earth

BILLIONS OF LIVING things from tiny microbes and viruses to gigantic whales and redwood trees shared this planet with us. Some are airborne, some inhabit the waters, and others are immobile and planted in the ground. Of the many mobile life forms, only birds and insects had mastered the art of flight, until modern mankind joined and exceeded them in human flight to the moon and back, as well as numerous commercial and daily flights to all parts of our world. The one very special thing, however, that we still share with all the Earth's other life forms is mortal life. There are no exceptions. No living organism or creature lives forever on this planet.

Our Human Heritage of Fear and Uncertainty

We were not always kings of the hill. I believe our primitive ancestors were not the marauding wolves, but the vulnerable underdogs in fear of larger and swifter carnivores, as well as Nature's lightening storms, floods, forest fires, hurricanes, earthquakes, and other awesome events. What was life like for our earliest ancestors? Injury and death were daily, nearby, and seemingly everywhere in the lives of our earliest ancestors.

There were no police or fire departments, nor hospitals, emergency rooms, or insurance policies. There were no bakeries or supermarkets. In order to live, one had to eat. In order to eat, one had to kill or destroy a living thing—animal, fish, bird or vegetable—even if only the growing leaves, fruit, or seeds of future generations of edible plants.

The daily menu was eat or be eaten. Human life was a tenuous, short, and meaningless sentence punctuated by lingering bursts of panic and recurrent fears of being torn apart and eaten piece by piece by a lions, tigers, or hyenas with the remnants left initially for vultures and subsequently as food for the bugs, worms, and bacteria that inhabited the lower rungs of the Earth's automatic disposal and recycling systems.

I sometimes used to wonder, even as a youngster, what our distant ancestors would have needed to invent in order to live, and keep from going crazy with recurrent fears, nightmares and the almost constant stress of their lives. What great things or ideas could save them? Would it have been the ability to create fire by rapidly rubbing sticks to produce friction and heat, or eventually learning to strike flint to create a spark? Yes, that was good, but would not alone have sufficed to make primitive life endurable for humans. How about the wheel? Or bronze, steel, and rubber? No? What about the long bow or gun powder? What about steam engines, penicillin, and plastics? None of those?

It was the amazingly resourceful mind of mankind that would soon rescue our early tribes of hunters and berry pickers from their dismaying and ongoing awareness of their mortality. Our individually different but amazingly resourceful human mind needed to invent some quickly effective means of escape from sentient mankind's haunting, ongoing and dismaying awareness of their inevitable and more imminent mortality. Our earliest ancestors' personal sense of mortality was much closer when sudden death lurked in every tree or bush from which a swift and hungry predator could suddenly strike with lethal tooth and claw.

What Did Our Human Ancestors Need to Invent In Order to Survive?

So, in such a world, I ask again, "What would our primitive ancestors have needed to invent in order to survive?" What I think was essential to save the tenuous sanity of primitive mankind was not the wheel, the hammer, the saw, shovels, clay pots, tents, or ingenious igloos made only with hand-hewn blocks of ice and snow by most generous men who would willingly share their warm wife for the night to thaw out and comfort a lost and passing stranger, we are told. The tent or igloo and those early inventions all seem helpful and good, but not absolutely necessary back then. What was more desperately needed was some form of mental or psychological escape from the unrelenting anxieties and stresses of primitive human existence.

The Human Concept of Immortality to Escape the Dismay of Death

What I think as an elder psychiatrist who knows something about how people think under duress is that our human species, haunted by our visions and forebodings of death and oblivion, wished, dreamed, envisioned and invented, all on their own, the concepts of immortality and immortals. And our early ancestors called these immortal gods and prayed and made sacrifices to them for protection. It mattered little if their gods were the sun, the moon, or a seemingly special rock. What mattered is that our early human tribes and ancestors endowed their gods with names and fictitiously magical attributes called miracles. The ability to perform miracles was one of the tests of being a god. In that way our ancestors magnifed and empowered their gods and worshipped them, praying for protection from nature's inexplicable and terrifying storms, hurricanes, earthquakes, and other seemingly mysterious "forces of evil" that lurked in the darkest clouds of the sky, or in the deepest of waters, as the shadows of vengeful spirits or ghosts, no doubt, of their slain enemies.

I submit that immortal gods are one of the most colossal concepts and leaps of faith that our physically weak but uniquely sentient and needy species ever made. What we wished for ourselves, but could not achieve on Earth, we attributed to our gods and granted them immortal lives. The concept of immortality was not an objective reality like the envied flight of birds, but pure wish-fulfillment. We needed that wish to be somehow fulfilled because we were always an endangered and nervous bunch. I believe that when our earliest ancestors figured out that none of us were getting out of here alive, primitive rituals, gospels, and prayers became not only human comforts but psychological necessities for our entire species. The rituals and gospels varied from tribe to tribe and eventually between nations, regions, and subcultures in the different names and attributes we assign to the same, single, and supreme deity. The human vision and systems of gods and immortality has worked to save us for literally thousands of years. Who am I to knock it?

It's true, however, that we humans have been arguing stubbornly, defending vigorously, and warring bloodily about our various gospels, faiths, and dogmas to this very day. In our current nuclear world, that gives any rational person even greater cause to pause and pray since we are a species with a very worrisome track record of violent warfare not based on religious differences alone. But, sooner or later, religions and their gods and clergy are drawn into the act to support their endangered country's cause and warriors sacrificed on the road to victory. Thankfully, however, our early ancestors had more going for us than prayer alone, and one of their early doctor-priests (called shamans) must have preached that "God helps those that help themselves." And so it seems that some of our ancient congregations got the message and got to work, planting the seeds of our civilizations with their hands, heads, communication skills, and increasingly remarkable tools.

Belief in Higher Powers is Explored by Humans Seeking Powers for Themselves

It is understandable that our not-so-distant ancestors would seek to worship seemingly immortal power in such visible and unique objects as a powerfully blazing and light-giving Sun god, for instance, or a visibly changing but distant and tantalizing Moon god, or even some specially shaped, immovable rock or mountain. Whatever their immortal god seemed to be, prayers and sacrifices to them gave our ancient ancestors, the strength to endure against seemingly all odds as a vulnerable species. If they had not done so, with their believed magic of rituals and prayers, perhaps none of us would be here to tell the tale today. The glaring exception to their immortal gods were false gods, humans who allowed people to believe, or who actually claimed and sought to have certain godly attributes and powers. Some ancient Caesars allegedly entertained such notions of godly attributes. It seems also that more than one Pharaoh had thought himself worthy of being royally embalmed and entombed in a giant pyramids accompanied by a few of choice slaves, favorite concubines, personal chariots, and other prized possessions.

The widespread human search in vain for Earthly evidence of higher power nearby has been frequently been exploited by wide variety of moguls seeking large and still larger powers for themselves. The search for princes, princesses, and royalty among us, as well our quest for heroes and heroines to worship is among our numerous failures in learning to govern ourselves.

Until we find some final answers to the infinite mysteries of our sentient human existence, we need to believe in something far greater than our species and ourselves, or we become a cowardly and ravaging race of villains ruled by despots. You don't believe that about villains and despots? Read our ancient history, the Bible stories, and the newspapers. The struggle for human peace and freedom goes on to this day and is far from won.

Our Digits, Speech and Communication Skills Made Us a Unique Species

Long before the most talented and dexterous of our amazing species learned to master concert repertoires of violin or piano concertos, most of us learned first to count mathematically with our fingers. From these early digital origins, our advanced numerical and counting concepts rank high among our currently awesome digital achievements, not only at Boston's MIT and New York's Juilliard music conservatory, but everywhere on an abacus or on ubiquitous digital calculators and desktop computers in local banks, market places, and remote trading posts where even Walmarts and McDonalds have yet to succeed in completely encircling and occupying the farthest corners of our solitary globe. But almost everywhere else, we can find mankind counting and keeping the score.

Along with our musical and manual dexterity, our thought processes or mental dexterity comprise the highest forms of our individual and combined human capability. By subjectively conceptualizing, organizing, and communicating our personal thoughts, we have succeeded in passing them along objectively to successive and future generations of our species initially as oral histories, myths, graven images, and carvings. In more recent centuries, we have first printed and subsequently recorded and stored electronically massive historical and literary digital databases for our own use and future generations' references. It took a long time for our species to develop the foundations on which it has thus far built our impressive technologies and civilizations to date. What has truly distinguished our best civilized and intellectual human behavior from the primarily instinctual behaviors of other mammals, as well as among each other, has been our unique human ability to focus on the content, quality, and rationality of each other's thoughts and behaviors. That, I think, was our greatest strength, and how we learned to build our nests, homes, and progressive civilizations together. It was not how we started out.

The Need to Believe in at Least Something

Nature abhors a vacuum, we are told. So does the mind. When we run out of important things we really know and wonder about them, we humans seem to fill in the empty spaces with speculations, conjectures, ideas, thoughts, assumptions, and things we believe. Thus, our minds are full of things we remember and things we believe. I believe there is a reciprocal relationship between the two.

That is to say that what we remember influences what we believe and what we believe influences what we remember. Of what value are memoirs that contain no beliefs or, for that matter, human lives that are lived with no beliefs at all? Many people don't care or know what to believe. But you do, because you are reading this book. People like us, readers and thinkers, cannot postpone indefinitely an examination of what it is that we believe as we get old. Not out of fear, but to take a stand. I wonder if there comes a time, just before the end, when skeptics and agnostics can no longer put things off, and have to commit and vote: for, against, or abstain. Do I believe, or do I not believe? Abstaining does no good, since that is merely another attempt at postponing what cannot be any longer postponed before the poll is closed for good. Re-examining and re-confirming one's thoughts and beliefs can be, for many, an intriguing and worthwhile task of old age.

All of us have to believe in something about God, even if it is atheism. I have had patients who were atheists who gave more time to thinking about God and why He didn't exist than religious patients who gave far less thought to God, and took His presence for granted. So who was more preoccupied with religious thought? I wondered sometimes.

Why Truth is Stranger and Less Believable than Fiction,

Looking back now, what was my long life all about? Aside from the inevitability of death and taxes, what do I really know for sure? Not that much, especially in comparison to the many big things that I still do not know at the tail and tale end of a long and privileged life. We all have much to learn about our limited existence in this enormous universe. How can we tell the truth from the many widely disseminated fictions about our mortal lives and situations? What hints do we have?

Let me start with the familiar proverb that "the truth is often stranger than fiction." Here is another proverb that you may not have heard before, because I just made it up. It goes as follows: "Fiction often seems more believable than the truth." That is because the plain truth sometimes seems too unyielding, unfamiliar, harder to swallow, and too difficult to accept. The truth often intrudes as an unwelcome stranger that threatens our familiar, friendly, and comforting concepts about ourselves, our relationships, and our circumstances.

How do we tell actual truth from imagined things, from creative fiction or, worse yet, from intentional human lies? Why are so many lies so often believable as to enable to bear false witness, and to skillfully fabricate, cheat, fool, and betray others? We are apparently born with that ability, or soon learn to fib, even as children, and we seem to refine that ability to fib, even to ourselves as we get older.

Avoiding the truth via our unconscious use of repression and denial are almost universal and daily human indulgences. Repression and denial are among our essential and most frequently used ego defense mechanisms. They allow many of us to deny, diminish, or totally ignore the hard facts of truth and reality.

We prefer our childhood fictions with their happy outcomes, easy explanations, and the sub-cultural prophecies and promises on which we still depend as adults. We are raised on stories that are embellished, augmented, and enlivened by wish-fulfilling fictions. We live within our self-created docudramas, so to speak, rather than with the cold, hard facts. We were put to sleep with lullabies and bedtimes stories about faithful princesses and brave young princes who overcome obstacles to finally marry and live happily and royally forever after. Or if we tire of these, how about a jolly Santa Claus? We become habituated to our made-up stories, to our comforting versions of things, rather than life's real and unvarnished truths.

While as little ones we were cuddled and lulled to sleep with bedtime stories and soft teddy bears, in our later years as we grow quite old and too often when our days are done, we fight insomnia alone, un-cuddled and cold. Born and bred on fairy tales, I believe we are sustained thereafter on ancient myths, the creative fiction and manufactured storylines that need marketing, retailing and re-telling over and over again as our universal tribal lore—our familiar and comforting Gospel Truths, if you will. And if you will not, then I and most others will believe. That is because, like you and I, most of us need to believe in some sustaining something when the traveling gets hard and death seems near.

Why We Need and Seek the Gospel Truth

Our need for a Gospel truth goes back a long time. How long? Probably from the beginning of human time. When was that? We don't know for sure. It is estimated by anthropologists, archeologists and other scientific experts that our human species, Homo sapiens first developed about 200,000 years ago. Despite being pursued by huge blood-thirsty carnivores and even deadlier viruses and bacteria, the infectious microbes that continue to mutate and plague us, our species has not only survived, but multiplied and spread widely to take command, for better or worse, over all the flora, fauna, and wild beasts of this planet. It is no longer the roaring lion, but our electronic and computer-equipped species that now is king of the beasts. How we will ultimately make out against the Earth's insects, bacteria, and viruses that far outnumber us, remains to be seen, but recently we have been holding our own against both predators and plagues—if not each against each other among our technologically advanced, constantly warring, and dangerously divided species.

Would You Really Like to Live Forever?

We are wisely warned to be careful of what we wish for. How sad, foolish, boring, and meaningless our lives would eventually become if we lived forever. It is actually our dreaded mortality that adds value to our transient lives, just as it enhances the precious and passing beauty of the flowering rose, as well as the fairest maiden in full bloom. By limiting our days without specifying their exact number, our mortality or death makes each of our transient lives innately precious, albeit in ways that too few of our species fully appreciate. But now, think with me. If we each knew the number of our remaining days, and had really open choices about how to spend them, and the means to do so, what would we do about that? A good question which might make a great plot or storyline for a best-selling, futuristic, and philosophical book about how people might really spend their remaining days if given free and independent choice when they are young and healthy. Try exploring and spelling it out for yourself.

What good might it do for us and our world to realize each day and perhaps especially on Sabbath, that our time on Earth is limited. If we knew we would live for centuries, if not forever, would we ever get around to digging in, working hard, and doing something really worthwhile? What great things did the Biblical Methuselah accomplish in his many years? If we knew we would live forever, would we get around to our best creative efforts at our leisure in the next century or a future millennium? It is our mortality that presses us to move forward, if only to hopefully to see the results of our children's and their next generation's creative efforts and prospects for a better future before we pass on. We are just beginning to know about our universe. It is only in the last few centuries that substantial numbers of humans have widely appreciated and accepted the basic scientific facts. The biological truth, still widely and stubbornly resisted, is that we are but a remarkable species of mammalian life astride a rotating sphere that orbits the sun along with other planets, and that our world is merely a distant speck in the vast and still expanding cosmos which likely resulted from some kind of gigantic explosion or accidental "Big Bang" rather than from The Creator's seven days of planned labor that included a single Sabbath for well-earned rest and contemplation. I wonder why it has taken us so long to recognize these truths.

Truth is much stranger, harder, and often more frightening than fiction. And so we prefer to believe fiction—creation theory vs. Big Bang. Theoretical situation and fantasies aside, I believe that Henry Wadsworth Longfellow wrote wisely about the reality and mystery of our mortal situation in his poem, *A Psalm of Life*, which I cited in Book One of these memoirs. For those who have not read that initial volume I quote it again in part as follows:

"…Art is long, and Time is fleeting,
And our hearts, though stout and brave,
Still, like muffled drums, are beating
Funeral marches to the grave."

Longfellow went on to add that:

"Lives of great men all remind us
We can make our lives sublime,
And, departing, leave behind us
Footprints on the sands of time;

Footprints, that perhaps another,
Sailing o'er life's solemn main,

A forlorn and shipwrecked brother,
Seeing, shall take heart again.

Let us, then, be up and doing,
With a heart for any fate;
Still achieving, still pursuing,
Learn to labor and to wait."

I believed, both as a wondering youngster and now as a reflective elder, that Longfellow wrote some very good stuff, and created a beautiful psalm. If we really looked for footprints in the sands of time, what kinds might we find? How about those of Buddha, Moses, or Jesus Christ ? Or the more recent footprints of Abraham Lincoln, Mahatma Gandhi, Dr. Martin Luther King Jr., or Mother Theresa? You can create your own list of prints to map out and follow. But at the very least, while looking for answers, listen to Longfellow and "Learn to labor and to wait."

Chapter 28
Our Psychosomatic Relationships

EVEN IF WE have no close family or no family at all, nor any "special other," we are not entirely alone. In our journey through mortal life, we each have a very close, intimate, and much-involved companion, for better or worse. No, not your spouse, but an even closer, lifetime traveling companion from whom there is no possibility of separation, divorce, or annulment so long as you live. Okay, you guessed it. How long has it been that you've thought about your body, except to complain about it? Let's think about how we might get to be in better touch with our bodies and perhaps something about our psychosomatic relationships.

What kind of a relationship have you had with your body? Is it a good marriage, so to speak? Because it indeed is a most intimate and unbreakable marriage, pre-arranged at birth. Or did you think it was just an affair you are having with your body, or an engagement that could be broken? We and our bodies are committed and zipped together like conjoined twins that cannot be separated. We share via our minds, emotions, and neuroendocrine systems the same vital equipment throughout our lives. Did you pay it little or no attention at all, or think that your body, mind, and soul were one and the same, always pulling in the same direction? I have no theological nor philosophical expertise, but I do know something psychologically about how we each think about ourselves as a person.

When we try to understand how we picture ourselves, I believe it is important to listen closely to our words and language. Thus, when we refer to our inner, subjective sense of identity or Self, we tend to do so in the first person: I or Me. But when talking of the body it is usually in the third person. "It" as in "It is bothering Me," and not something like, "that part of me which is my body," is bothering me. It is not myself that is bothering, hurting, or failing me, but an estranged "it," referred to in the third person. When did you separate, or were you never conscious of your mind, limbs, and fingers working together with you like those of an accomplished gymnast or soulfully gifted concert pianist?

A Brief Note on Body Language and Denial

Now there are exceptions in which our tendencies to distinguish between our mind and our body seem to be blurred, such as, "I am tired or sleepy," rather than my "My body is tired or sleepy." I believe that our conscious sense of self assumes the right to censor and deny, even to ourselves as well as others, the existence of our bodily sensations and urges that we prefer not to report or experience. And we can keep up this pretense and denial for quite some time. Sooner or later, despite vows of asceticism or abstinence, the body speaks up for itself and sends signals that persons have long recognized as the reliable and revealing messages that psychologists and others have come to recognize and study as "body language." For now, I want merely to suggest that most of us think, and often try to act, as though our bodies and ourselves were closely related, but somehow, independent entities.

Moreover, for numerous people, even in widely varying cultures, there has been a deep need for a sense of spiritual separateness. Toward that end, the powerful human intuitions of prayer and poetry have each held that, "Dust thou art, to dust returnest, was not spoken of the soul," as Longfellow describes in *A Psalm of Life*. Most people believe and behave as though body and self are somehow separable, despite being involved in a lifelong commitment that was biologically consummated without the least element of our prior consent. We take what we get, as we do in most earthly marriages in which we rarely know as much as we think we do about what we are getting.

My Body, My Bodyguard, My Buddy

My body is my buddy and my bodyguard. And I am his bodyguard, too. Political correctness aside, I say "his" because he is definitely a guy with everything flat or sticking out where it should. We guard each other, my body and I, usually pretty well. He regulates and takes care of my heartbeat, my blood sugar, my kidneys, my digestion, blood pressure, liver, and metabolism. Just by itself, metabolism has been a very big job of constantly feeding and running the "furnace" by which we generate and use glucose and other products of our digested foods to provide us with essential energy and nutrients that our sometimes noisy body propels along our digestive tract and finally dumps outside. Our body, our buddy, usually signals us when they are ready to do so, and you'd better not ignore that signal too often or too long.

Some people ignore many, if not almost all, of their bodily signals until the signals become manifest symptoms or signs of bodily distress or disorder. Persons who neglect their bodies must think their body is not only deaf and dumb, but stupid too. You can usually spot such people, who sit there with no idea that their body, their buddy, is at work non-stop 24/7 while they add abusive quantities of alcohol, tobacco, and other recreational substances to their ultimately shared problems. We and our bodies share the same space. We cannot get away from each other 'til death do us part.

Body Talk and Ongoing Conversations

Our aging bodies can't talk, but perhaps they can sense our emotional circumstances and send us signals through signs of bodily discomfort such as pains, itches, stomach rumbles, and reflex sneezes or coughs to which we should pay at least a modicum of attention. Actually, I've been giving some serious thought to my body lately, as old folks should. I don't want to ignore my body and have it suddenly conk out on me. I can't talk to my body. People will think I am talking to myself and getting senile. But some old people do talk to themselves. Why not? It often appears that no one but ourselves seems to be listening to us. And yet, throughout our lives, our bodies pay careful attention to us, and usually express themselves quite clearly by sending us feelings about our sense of well-being or discomfort. When you feel fine, who do you think sends you that message? Some stranger? No, it's your naked buddy inside, telling you that all is well. When you are feeling fatigued, exhausted, and about to get sick, who do you think is making you feel that way and warning that you are about to throw up on the living room carpet? Not your wife or your friendly bartender, but your upset body, your beleaguered buddy. And if you don't respond to those signals, your body will send you physical symptoms and signs that are diagnostic of deeper disorders.

An aging psychiatrist like myself is perhaps entitled to a few hard-earned eccentricities. Most old folks are. I believe that our bodies send out certain signals in response to our various feelings and situations. You find that hard to believe? Does your body not get red in the face when you are ready to burst with anger? Or maybe just signal with a pink blush when you are merely embarrassed? And does your face not blanche and become pale when you are suddenly shocked and frightened? There are many more such responses with our inner neuroendocrine systems at work. How can you let your body know you really care after all these years of being together? If you can't talk to your body, maybe you could write a letter. Things may soon be over between you two, but there may yet be time to let him or her know how you feel about your relationship. I tried a couple of years ago. Maybe it worked because my body, my buddy, is still hanging in with me. So, let me begin with an easier approach to getting to know oneself better. How about a letter to one's body? Straight from the heart and from the mind, that is. And in doing so, one might even find a bit of one's soul or inner spirit. If you'd like an idea for a letter of your own, here is what I wrote.

A Letter to my Body, 2012

Dear Body:

How shall I start this? We've been together now, you and I, for some ninety years, and I've never written to you before, as I recall. Nor, for that matter, intimate as we've been, we've never spoken much to each other. Perhaps I didn't listen enough. I suspect a body needs some listening to. But we've tended far too long to take each other for granted, especially considering how important we've been to each other all these years. I've written to lots of people. Maybe, if it is not too late to come to some understanding about this life of ours that we've shared so long, if that is possible while there might yet be time. So, here goes.

What shall I call you, old buddy, my body? How about Soma? That's close to my middle name, Sam, which I've never used much. So you can call me Sam, and I'll call you Soma, if that's OK. I think it's important that we address each other this way so that neither us feel that we are talking to ourselves. Because we've done that also, too much talking to ourselves when we felt there was no one around, and we still needed someone to talk to. But you were always around, and maybe talking with my living but aging Body and dear Buddy would have been better than talking to an empty room, or to a stone wall.

Maybe I should have tried it sooner. But now that we're getting old, and you and I are so often alone together, and know each other as well as we do, it's better to talk than to pretend we are complete strangers. Let's the two of us try to talk and understand each other, Body and Mind. And just maybe we might even tempt that other special part of us to join in. You know, our so-called immortal Soul that we'd like to hear from, and maybe get to know as part of ourselves that may really be, God willing, immortal. Look, dear Soma, old Body old Buddy, if I can't talk to you this way, whom can I talk to for a look inside?

So we better get started. I've meant to write for some time, Soma, I'll miss you if we're not still around much longer, because we won't be hanging in with each other forever as much as I'd like to. Frankly, it can't be much longer the way you are. With all your faults, and mine too, I still like you and wish we could be together forever. If that sounds like love, or a proposition, don't get nervous. But together forever, you and I, dear Soma, the way you are, I now really know that cannot be. So maybe it's time to see where we've been together, where we're at now, and how with luck we might spend what time that may yet be left for us to be together. You know, I've been very loyal to you—much more than I've been to anyone else. We've never gone anywhere without each other, and I don't want to leave you. But I know that, sooner or later, you are going to leave me. I often think about that these days, and what I might do to keep you around as long as possible, for better or worse, as they say. Despite all my complaints about your appearance and limitations, I've gotten used to you.

So, I'm sorry you're going to leave me, or me leave you, or however that works when we come to separating. Because I sure don't want to rot in the ground with you, if I can get away. I feel sorry about that, and I hope you can understand how awful I would feel if I ended up like you. I wish I had taken better care of you and taken you less for granted. You helped me to do everything I accomplished. But, you're not getting any younger, and neither am I.

I don't want to worry you, but I think you know that I now listen very carefully to you each morning when I get up, and each night as I fall asleep to check and see how it's going with you. I admit, I'm more concerned, and a bit worried about you once in awhile. Sometimes you even scare me—that you might suddenly quit on me, or maybe worse, that we'd be crippled and helplessly stuck together. Even though I'm still a pretty good medical doctor, you're not always so easy to read, Dear Soma, old Buddy. And I know I probably gave you a harder time than I should have, and I am sorry for that. I wish I could apologize for ringing your alarm bell, and forcing your immune system to cope with my own nagging anxieties, gastronomic and oral indiscretions, bursts of anger and periods of high stress, infrequent as they were. But I'm trying to do most of the right things now to give us the best chance of hanging in together.

Maybe if we could communicate a bit more often it might help you to deal with some of my discomforting emotions and behaviors with which you have had to cope. And I suppose I must confess some resentment that I am feeling older in you, my body, than I am in spirit. Don't take that wrong. It's unfair to criticize you. I'm sure you're doing your best for us. But let me ask, even though we're together for better or worse, how would you feel if I swapped a part of you, like a kidney or liver transplant, if that were ever necessary? I suppose if it kept the rest of you and me together you wouldn't mind. But, if it were the other way around, I sure would not like to swap my thinking brain for someone else's. There I go, putting you down after all your hard work I've too often taken for granted.

I do not know if old age brings much wisdom to the elderly. Many of us do learn some things from experience. And even though I have learned many things—enough perhaps to write a book or two—I still have more to learn than time to spend learning that many more facts in this information-technology era. It isn't more facts and information that I think I need, but wisdom. I am talking about the kind of wisdom that is supposed to accrue with the experience of living to a ripe old age—and not so many more of the medical, physical, historic, and other important facts I have picked up in my reading, studies, and conversations with others. Wisdom and judgment are not guaranteed by experience and age alone.

Humility helps, but only if we really know our stuff, including the protoplasmic and cellular signaling wisdom of the body. We are just beginning to learn, toward the end of my long life, the initial molecular details of the body's puzzling cell-signaling wisdom in its innate as well as acquired immune systems. We may be just starting to learn how to make the best use of our body's genomic potential with its inter-connected neuroendocrine and cerebral cellular abilities to set new records in the expanding history of human accomplishment. I would not bet against that, because, although fearful of our human capacity for destruction, I am ever more impressed by our human instinct to explore, create, and make the best of what may yet come our way.

Well, I've gone on too long. I know you are still there, busy because I can feel my stomach rumble. So I'll stop for now, but I'll get back to you.

A Second Letter to My Body, My Buddy

Hi Soma, I'm back. What I've learned about you, I've learned by paying attention to the numerous stimuli I initially gleaned through your keen sensitivities and perceptions, bodily gifts for which I have been most grateful, of course.

How are you doing? Neither of us are what we used to be, but with several pairs of glasses, a hearing aid, a walking stick, an occasional laxative, and a few other props, we're still functioning, thanks to you. So, my Body, old Buddy, I'm listening to you and looking to you too for some wisdom these days. I should have done this sooner because I increasingly sense that our bodies, Dear Soma, have far more wisdom and knowledge of life's grand design to impart to us than we suspect. Especially in these days of mapping our own genomes, as well as those of the other creatures large or microscopic, we should look for wisdom in sciences of microscopic anatomy and molecular physiology. We are far from having all or even sufficient facts about the hardworking bodies of life forms.

So, let us listen to each other, dear Soma, while there is yet time. What have I learned from my good seat in life's theater that I can share with you, even if only to sooth and calm us both down a bit? And what might we share with others while we still have the energy to pursue these matters together? Our old fingers which used to be so dexterous are now numb from peripheral neuropathy. But I need your formerly fine fingers since I can't type with my toes or my nose, as you know. Speaking of noses, maybe I can try to stimulate your interest and grab your attention by talking with you about sex. Yes, sex, intercourse, love-making. You were always interested in sex and ready to make love, as I recall. As a matter of fact, for too many years, as I think back, you seemed to take the lead in sex, and it was sometimes a hard job to keep you from taking over and distracting me completely from other important things back then. So you can understand that I sometimes had to take you firmly in hand, so to speak—just to keep things from getting too hot and heavy, and so completely out of hand as to get us into deep trouble, if you follow me. I hope I didn't beat on you too much or do us any real harm, although I always felt very guilty and ashamed about all that. We were so dumb, young, and well-endowed back then.

Well, Dear Soma, we're still functioning, even though not so well in that department lately. And to tell you the truth, I don't know if it's mostly your fault, or my fault. I suspect a good part of the problem is mine. Yes, it's mostly mine, because human arousal is a strange flower that blooms not only in response to touch but to erotic thoughts of the mind. Human arousal is psychological, and not merely a generalized or genital itch that needs scratching. That's the way things are with you, me, and whoever she may be. So, dear Buddy, I have heavily burdened our sex life, such as it was, with value judgments and further reflections as we have grown older, while you, I suspect, would like to go at it as we used to, less troubled by conscience and consequences. We need to talk more about these things in future letters, maybe about my sexual fantasies and our sexual functioning as a senior-citizen partnership. My wife and I needed to learn these things by ourselves as we grew older. Nobody told us these things when we were younger, and if they had, we probably wouldn't have listened.

Well, maybe that's enough for this letter. I'll get back to you, and meanwhile, I hope and pray that I'll keep hearing steady heartbeats and other reassuring sounds from you, dear Soma. You know, your usual body sounds, even breathing and the things I seem to take for granted, really comfort me. So, I really don't take you for granted and I marvel at the varied rate of your pulse in response to exercise or repose. I am also grateful for the quiet and efficient way you go about digesting, if not always easily eliminating these days. Between the two of us, I now enjoy all your intimate functioning.

We humans, so imperfect as individuals, are a miracle as a formidable and developing species. And to dwell on the fact that you and I started with the chance coming together of a unique sperm and egg, dear Soma, and all that has happened to that good fertilized egg since then is mind-boggling. Just think of that in the face of how you'll end up—"dust thou art, to dust returnest." But what about the rest of us, our minds and souls? Dear body, my buddy, we have been bound together as fellow prisoners of each other on this Earth from which none of us escapes alive. We have been cell-mates in every sense of the word. Until one of us lets the other go, I think we need to stay more closely in touch, while trying to maintain our hold on the precious protoplasmic cell we now share as wrinkled but still grateful old pals.

Faithfully, 'til death do us part,

Your Mind, Soul, and Fellow Prisoner

Is Not the World a Wondrous Prison?

Do jails have to be ugly? Does the planet Earth present too much risk of escape to be a prison? How can any of us escape from here? None of us are getting out of here alive. Just try it. The security is superb, designed by clever experts, if not a genius in prison design. Our Warden or Keeper seems to be absent, and we do not even recognize His or Her clever technology in keeping us bound down without locks, chains, and bars. Gravity under foot and firmly in place has kept us close to the ground until our present lifetimes when small numbers of brave, adventurous, and carefully selected astronauts made it to the moon and back. But for any who are contemplating getting out of here on their own, know that our Keeper binds each of us very closely and securely here by the cleverest, strongest, and lightest tether of all. It is practically weightless as a narrow tube or twig of air in our nose, throat, and trachea through which we breathe. If that thin tube is pinched off, we are deprived of oxygen, suffocate, and die.

It is even more certain than the criminal justice system's electric chair, and much less pompous and ceremonial. So understand your position as a prisoner of nature from birth on, man and beast alike are tethered to this Earth by their thin personal tubes of oxygen. The only medical advice I can give you about that is don't smoke or abuse your airway. When we get very old, we try to make the best of it while we can. OK, I've had my fun, and you get my point about our earthly home being a sometimes lovely but secure prison which none of us leave alive. Now, let's look at a real prison made by man.

Chapter 29
My Experiences and Thoughts About Prison Work

The Search for Equal Justice in an Unequal World

IN FORMER CHAPTERS, I have described many of my experiences while working in the courts and prisons of the criminal justice system. After spending a major portion of my academic and clinical career in forensic psychiatry during some fifty years of active professional life, what can I now say about it? And what must I say as a psychiatrist and physician about justice and our justice system at this point? Despite what we preach, people are not born equal, nor do we develop equally with equal opportunities and luck thereafter. What can our justice systems do about that, and the profound consequences of haphazard genetic mutations that appear seemingly willy-nilly in human and other life forms? Our ponderous American justice system tried to achieve a more equal justice, but it still has far to go.

During past years, our Courts have come down with a number of landmark decisions concerning the U.S. Constitution's far-sighted provisions for civil rights, due process, and equal protection under the law, as well as the infliction of "cruel and unusual punishment." Despite these efforts and hard-won gains, even in the best of contemporary democratic governments, humans have suffered far more injustices under oppressive governments than equal opportunities and benefits from the best ones.

The human search for scientific knowledge and truth is likely the most hopeful endeavor of modern mankind, but the human quest for justice is perhaps the loftiest and most noble goal of all.

The cry for justice and fair play is inbred in our unique species. Only the human child at play with another protests, "What you are doing is not fair. I won't play with you." A basic sense of fair play and justice then is essential in wholesome relationships and human relationships from early childhood on. This innate need for justice in human affairs is reinforced in our American schools where even young children are taught, to pledge allegiance to "the flag and the republic for which it stands—with liberty and justice for all."

Nature Favors the Fittest to Survive and Propagate on Planet Earth

Unfortunately the human goal of "liberty and justice for all" has never been fully realized as the defining feature of any of our major nations to date. There is a powerful and ugly reason for this. It appears that justice is not natural. Where are examples of justice to be found in Nature where big fish eat little fish, where powerful and wily predators hunt down and devour their weaker prey in a system which favors the survival of the fittest? The fittest for what? For survival, at all costs, no matter what? What individuals and species are eventually the fittest to survive in the botanical and horticultural prison we call Earth? I do not know, but I have spent some lengthy time working in prisons.

My Impressions of Prison Work

My impressions of prison work began in 1951 and continued part-time over the next thirty years in my academic duties at Temple's Unit in Law and Psychiatry pursuant to the University's ongoing contracts to supply professional services to our local courts and prisons. These contracted services also provided supervised clinical-teaching facilities in our forensic psychiatry fellowship program. As for prisons, I think that one of the main problems is that they were not originally set up or designed to keep people for very long times. Prisons are derived from dungeons, where people were kept at the king's pleasure until the ruler decided one's further disposition. Many crimes that receive prison terms of two to five years today were capital crimes punishable by death not very long ago. And so, a major problem is that prisons are a somewhat recent alternative to execution and exile. Our attempts to cope with incarcerated prison inmates appears to be one of our relatively newer follies.

Most of us are quite ambivalent about prisoners, and I think every one of us with any prison experience has doubts and disagreements about what the goals and functions of prison incarceration ought to be. There are those who are very certain that the functions of a prison must include punishment and deterrence, and the more spectacular the punishment, the greater the deterrence, some say. There are others who regard this as inhumane. They say that the only purpose of a prison, if there is any at all, should be rehabilitation, and that prisons should be a secure and safe place in which people can find alternatives to their previous ways of problem solving. In my experience, about the only honest function that a prison serves is that of detention. Prisons are a place where you can hold people securely, and if you hold them under inhumane conditions, they are apt to come out less human than when they went in. So much for some basics.

Encouraging Psychiatrists to Consider Part-Time Work in Courts and Prisons

WHY WOULD A DOCTOR WANT TO WORK IN PRISONS?

I cannot resist an additional bit of geriatric preaching as I type these pages at an elder age. Please bear with me, if you will as I recall and begin with my efforts of long ago to recruit physicians to work part-time in penitentiaries and prisons. I asked myself why a doctor would want to work in a prison? What might motivate a physician to do this?

There are many possible reasons, including an altruistic instinct to serve as a medical missionary. Medical missionaries have long been up to two things. They provided free medical services, but they were also pushing a product. They were selling something with what they gave away. They were selling a belief, a religion. Thus, the function of the medical missionary was not only to serve and enlighten the prisoner's so-called primitive population, but to serve the prisoner's soul up to the missionary's Almighty God. This was really the basic mission. So, I would say that persons who go into prison work with missionary zeal as their first motive ought to ask themselves, "What am I selling and why?"

Another motive for providing medical services in prison is, "Well, I can't do anything better and I need the money." A third motive might be curiosity—"I'd like to find out what's going on in there." A fourth motive is to try to improve existing conditions. The rest of the motives, five, six and seven, are probably neurotic, pertaining to combinations of narcissism, masochism, and maybe a few other things. And I have probably been guilty of each and every one of them to some extent. That is how I know them so well. Let us then say that for a number of reasons, conscious and otherwise, an individual physician who is well-trained and qualified decides to spend some time in a prison.

Full-Time or Part-Time?

If such doctors go into a prison work full-time, they may rapidly become dependent upon the institution unless they are persons of independent means. If they make their money from the system and have loved-ones who are dependent on them, and the warden or some other person tells them that they must do such and such, they begin to think twice before they might cut loose from the economic and emotional benefits of going along with the system. That's the way the system works. Doctors must be healers. To be a healer in prison, I learned that we needed to be reliable and respectful insiders or team players, but we also needed to present an outsider's mature, independent, and responsible viewpoint for the good of the prisoners, the staff, and the prison itself.

Prospects for Equal Justice in an Unfair World

There is no shortage of violence and mayhem in Nature, including frequently brutal competition and mandatory combat even for basic propagation or breeding rights. And if this were not as cruel and criminal as staged cockfights between bloody roosters, consider the widespread incidence of theft in nature. This includes the not infrequent theft of eggs from unprotected nests, for starters. And then consider the daily assaults and devouring of the weak or impaired, and otherwise vulnerable inhabitants of the forests, plains, and teeming waters of this fertile planet, isolated in a still expanding cosmos in which stars explode and meteors streak by with the destructive power of nuclear-armed missiles. There is massive violence in Nature's cosmos, but there is no crime in Nature, no honor, and certainly no justice. All such concepts of crime, honor, and justice are products of Mankind.

It took our unique human species to dream and yearn for justice and seek peace on this Earth. Civilizations, nations, peoples, and communities may be understood and appreciated historically by what they regarded and defined as criminal behavior, and how they dealt with it. Labeling another as an offender or transgressor is a community affair, grounded in the values of their society, and it is encoded in laws and regulations.

What is a Crime and Who Says So? Early Legal Codes

The ancient Babylonian laws of Mesopotamia date back to Hammurabi's Code, close to 2000 BC. Equally ancient, and perhaps the oldest and most succinct of legal codes are the biblical

Ten Commandments, as recorded and transmitted to us by Moses. Their subsequent interpretations, as part of the Judeo-Christian legacy of our Western civilizations, eventually evolved into more secular justice systems with detailed attention to civil rights and the freedoms of individuals.

Sad to say, as I look back at age ninety-three on my lengthy experiences as a forensic psychiatrist in courts and prisons, most things have not improved that much, and many have become worse. Particularly troubling has been the rapid expansion of our prison populations. The United States appears to have the highest incarceration rates in the world. Our incarceration rates have led to a serious epidemic of overcrowding in prisons, which seriously endangers both prisoners and staff.

Ethnic, Racial and Political Factors in Our Crowded Prisons

In our American prisons, overcrowding problems have been substantially aggravated by covert political, ethnic, and racial factors, the latter of which has manifested itself both openly and violently. Way back in 1951, in my new job as a prison psychiatrist at the U.S. Penitentiary in Terre Haute, I was puzzled and fascinated when I encountered my first and outspoken Black Muslim inmate. He was an openly proud and very angry man in his mid-forties, who had grown up in a dysfunctional family in Chicago, where he had been a delinquent and high school drop-out. However, as a very intelligent youngster and avid reader, he continued his education on his own by perusing numerous articles and books that reinforced his growing convictions that many great people of the past, including Christopher Columbus, were descendants of black Africans of Moorish and ancient Egyptian origin. He had strongly rejected his grandmother's African-American Baptist church affiliation, claiming that it was a religion forcibly imposed on black slave by their white masters.

He had a quick answer for every question, and there was no arguing with him. He had been referred to me for psychiatric evaluation by the Associate Warden, whose report read, "Please see for agitated behavior causing disturbances on the cell block." As for mental illness, I felt that he had some grandiose and paranoid tendencies, but did not regard him as grossly delusional or psychotic. Unfortunately, just as he was beginning to trust me and open up a little bit more, he was administratively transferred elsewhere "for custodial reasons," and I saw him only a few times.

Since then, I have seen an increasing number of prisoners who have chose to embrace the Islamic faiths. Others, of Hispanic or white racial background, have sought collective strength and identity by clustering together in ethnic solidarity and white supremacy groups. This form of inmate-initiated segregation, based on racial, ethnic, and ideological grounds, placed further obstacles in the way of practical prospects for individual treatment, prosocial learning, and societal rehabilitation. As for prison work, and prison inmates themselves, it has led to numerous assaults by prison gangs who secretly compete with and undermine the custodial staff's efforts for control of racially troubled cell blocks. There seems more anger and despair in cell blocks. What has happed to inner feelings of shame and guilt?

Court Verdicts of Guilt vs. Inner Feelings of Shame

Although our criminal justice systems are encountering many assaultive and violent individuals with antisocial personality disorders, the custodial staff and its correctional officers are being called upon increasingly to deal with prisoners who openly regard themselves, not as guilty convicts, but as politically mistreated underdogs who are victims of an "oppressive capitalistic society" that has long stacked the odds against them. This finding brought me to consider the psychological differences in a defendant's state of mind when confronted with an externally imposed finding of guilt by a judge or jury in contrast to the subjective feelings of dismay when one regards one's self as inwardly and actually guilty. The punishments for such self-condemnation are recurrent and sustained feelings of shame and guilt,. With no one to be angry at except one's self, such unremitting forms of self-condemnation can become very cruel forms of punishment, against which there are no constitutional protections, quick remedies, nor guaranteed long-term treatment. So where is the justice in all that?

The Search for Equal Justice in Sentencing

During my full-time and busy years at Terre Haute's federal penitentiary, and my ongoing clinical experiences as a forensic psychiatrist working part-time in courts and prisons, I have had ample opportunity to witness the effects of lengthy imprisonment on numerous offenders and defendants. The results of their imprisonment were not what the public had expected and paid for. Two-thirds of our released prisoners returned as repeat offenders or recidivists. Our justice system's attempts to achieve justice through punishment alone have long been one of our ongoing human follies. The simple and sad fact was that prisons kept releasing more repeat offenders than rehabilitated ones, until our prison populations and costs were swollen far beyond their planned bed capacities and budgets.

There are now more persons serving prison time in the United States than in any other country in the world. As previously noted, prisons derive not only from hidden dungeons, but from sadistic places of public entertainment called Colosseums where Rome's highly placed leaders and ordinary citizens made bloody sport and bets on prisoners who were trained to kill each other. Other, more gentle ones, were simply kept alive to be devoured by lions and tigers for the entertainment of their captors.

Even today, as a technologically advanced people, but far from a completely civilized and peaceful one, we still do not know what to do about our prisons and prisoners. We seem to be in a longstanding state of emotional ambivalence, caught up somewhere between alternating compassion, confusion, cruelty, and despair regarding our prisoners, their crimes, and punishments. Few governments, if any, are scientifically pursuing the possibilities for prevention of antisocial and criminal behavior, if not cure. As for deterrence rather than prevention, there was never any credible evidence that punishment deters violent crimes, especially crimes of passion rather than premeditated, cold-blooded killings.

On the other hand, there is considerable evidence that our justice system's current practices allow for lengthy delays and numerous costly appeals. The result is that instead of carefully delivering a clear and prompt reply to each crime, our judicial system all too often wields the dull and hesitant blade of justice delayed, which is also called "justice denied." Death penalty cases, however, rightly engender nagging fears of wrongfully executing even one more innocent person in the irreversible and haunting miscarriage of justice in our admittedly unequal justice systems, which still do not offer fair treatment and equal defense counsel to all. As in most market places, one purchases what one can afford. That generally holds true, as well, for our different neighborhoods and communities seeking equal treatment and protection from crime and criminals.

Community Security Needs: Do Good Fences Hide Bad Neighbors?

What about the basic security needs of children and vulnerable others unable to protect themselves from the risks of abusers and criminal predators in their own neighborhoods, or in their very own homes, as incest victims? Many such humiliated, betrayed, and bitter victims eventually end up in jail. Prisons are surrounded by stone walls or fences. What good do they do when we cannot and should not keep a prisoner forever? So, what about our prison walls and fences?

The famous poet, Robert Frost, wrote, "Good fences make good neighbors." That rang true in rural New England, but behind our private fences and closed doors that we value so highly among America's hard-earned freedoms, there occur painful and permanently damaging crimes, like the repeated rapes of incest inflicted on vulnerable family members within the enabling secrecy of our neighbors' own homes. We all know what Robert Frost meant when writing that good fences make good neighbors, but maybe good neighbors are better than good fences. Perhaps vulnerable kin today may be better protected by their cell phones than fenced yards these days.

I mention incest and domestic violence not to shock you, but to emphasize that our justice system, social services, and forensic psychiatry studies are no less challenging, important, or simple public health problems to solve than finding cures or preventions for cancer. During my many years as a medical doctor, I have never felt we were in imminent danger of being wiped off this Earth by infectious diseases, plagues, cancer, or heart disease. Our most threatening adversaries are ourselves, as we recurrently update our capability for all-out combat with weapons of mass destruction. That makes me wonder if our human history of almost constant wars being waged somewhere on this planet makes it likely that we may blow.

Chapter 30
Other Worries of an Elderly Forensic Psychiatrist

I BELIEVE THAT the most important and urgent question for medicine, law, and our sciences is not how we can prevent cancer, but how can we prevent all-out warfare with our nuclear and biological weapons of mass destruction. Forewarned of that, as we have been since Hiroshima, and with fanatical religious and ideological suicide bombers potentially among us, or with armed missiles already standing and aimed in our direction, where, when, and how can we live with all that and raise the next generation of our children? Instead of practicing Denial with a capital D, or Prayer with a capital P, and Voting with a capital V, what can we do about all that?

It all seems a little crazy, so maybe it does sounds like a job for a psychiatrist, but we don't have any quick-acting pills for that. And besides, no one has asked us. To the best of my knowledge, neither American, Chinese, or Russian psychiatrists have submitted requests for National Institute of Health (NIH) funding for a credible, peer-reviewed study of our atomic chessboards, which would allow for open inspections prior to the safe and reciprocal removal of our opposing pieces from the board before the whole game blows up in our faces.

In my view, avoiding all-out nuclear warfare and Armageddon requires much more than psychiatric worry. It requires sane and sincerely cooperative military planning. Absent divine intervention, our currently stockpiled weapons of mass destruction call for all of our human resources to find ways to end human warfare between major, nuclear-armed powers, which have stockpiled enough of such weapons to destroy life off this planet.

Why do I worry about such an evil and tragic outcome in the history of mankind? We have already seen the face of evil in our species. Many times the face of human evil has reared its ugly head under different names. One of the last times it checked into our history books, it was called the Holocaust. It continues its dirty deeds today under such ironic and cynical synonyms as "ethnic cleansing."

Mental Illness versus Human Misbehavior

Ethnic cleansing has a long and ancient history, both Biblical and pre-Biblical, with traces in the archeology and genetics of human evolution. Many early civilizations and peoples have disappeared through conquest by other groups that converted, enslaved, absorbed, or destroyed their populations through warfare or disease. It is possible that modern humans wiped out the Neanderthals through warfare, as well as absorbing them through interbreeding. The Holocaust was more than inter-species or inter-tribal warfare, however. It was planned and executed with the German people's genius for organization and strong habit of obedience to orders from an authority, be it a royal Kaiser, a dictatorial Fuhrer, or simply the shouting Sergeant, Captain, or Major above them. A number of very brave exceptions in the officers' ranks were quickly caught and shot, or more slowly and painfully executed.

Were the rapes of Nanking, the mass executions of the Holocaust, and the nuclear massacre of civilians at Hiroshima the work of normal persons in their normal states of mind? How do we know? We have few if any physically reliable or hard and objective signs of mental illness. We rely on grossly deviant and inexplicable behavior, alleged thoughts, and apparent mood disorders to delineate mental illnesses. In light of our violent human history, can these events even be considered aberrant? This is a question for scientists and moral philosophers, as well as scholars in any field concerned with human behavior. As a psychiatrist, I have thought a great deal about these questions, and tried to address them, in part, in a letter to my granddaughter several years ago.

Denial and Holocaust Denial, Letter to my Granddaughter, 2010:

Dear Granddaughter,

As for your school assignment regarding the Holocaust, I had no direct contact with its survivors. But I remember my mother and father's grief and horror when they realized that their own brothers and sisters, nephews and nieces, who remained in my mother's Poland and my father's Lithuania, had been slaughtered for the simple "crime" that they were Jews. I was young, your age, when Hitler came to power. I loved life, and shuddered to realize what would have been my parents' fate had they not come to America, but had remained in Europe along with their doomed siblings. I don't think I ever fully overcame the feeling of vulnerability and endangerment for having been born of Jewish parents. I've tried to fight it and rationalize it, but it is still there. And so, perhaps in that limited but still traumatized sense, I, too, am in a way a kind of victim of the Holocaust. And to the extent that we are compassionate humans, and able to empathize with less fortunate persons, we are perhaps all actual or potential perpetrators or victims of Holocausts, and we could not live with the enormity of it all, but for the mechanism of denial.

Almost all of us, man, woman and child, practice denial. We practice denial daily. How else but for denial could you and I live such relatively privileged and fortunate lives in this beautiful country we took from its natives after killing many of them and driving their remnants into segregated areas we call reservations? How can we live with that? Simple—we didn't do it. We didn't know about it. We weren't there. We weren't even born then. Get it? That's how a generation of Germans live with it, just as you and

I try to go about our daily lives while knowing that genocide goes on in Africa, the Middle East, and elsewhere.

So, what's so special about the Jewish Holocaust in twentieth century Europe? Aside from the carefully planned and brutally executed attempt to wipe out all Jews of Europe by the mass murder of men, women, and children, the Holocaust was the biggest, most successful, and best organized armed robbery and first degree homicide of the Century. The Jews were held up, relieved of all their wealth, clothing, shoes, furnishings, and even their gold teeth pulled from their corpses. In the annals of crime in allegedly civilized countries, it was the most successful, carefully organized armed robbery and pre-planned murder ever pulled off. And most of the ones who participated in the killings were never prosecuted or even brought to trial. Dead bodies without transplantable organs are not worth much, but the Nazis' haul in cash, clothing, property, furnishings, even human hair and teeth is what armed robbers might call the biggest heist of all time, except perhaps when we allegedly stole Manhattan Island for a bunch of glass beads. No bank ever held so much loot.

How do we live with this murderous record and its further potential among people who were biblically created "in the image of God"? I think we can only do so if we realize that, as much as we are god-like, we are also ape-like. We are enormously talented and partially ape-like creatures that can fly to the moon and back but have not yet learned to get along with each other. Your life is sweet and full of potential. So was Anne Frank's. That's the horror of the Holocaust as we think especially of the young ones robbed of their parents and so often of their lives as well.

Some day perhaps I'll tell you more, but now I must get on with other correspondence. Maybe, if you feel like it, tell me what you make of what I have written to you this evening. You are a very good student at school, so I have written to you as I would to any bright youngster approaching adulthood.

Much love, Grandpa Mel

My Further Thoughts on the Sins of the Holocaust

Could the Holocaust be attributed to mental illness on the part of its perpetrators? We have no scientific nor clinically reliable, objective signs of mental illness except for seemingly inexplicable behavior and bizarre thoughts of certain people who commit crimes. As for mental illness, various personality as well as behavior, mood, and anxiety disorders are described in the American Psychiatric Association's Diagnostic and Statistical Manual (DSM), which mainly is used to provide a uniform list of mental illnesses for medical insurance coverage purposes.

Sins are still with us. They have largely been renamed in the DSM by psychiatrists struggling to create a rational and orderly diagnostic system out of a disordered jumble of prior terms for the same disorder or illness. It is, I think, a bit ironic and revealing that our best colleagues, who have labored long to produce this diagnostic framework and its numerous revisions, have chosen to call their entities mental "disorders" rather than diseases or illnesses. This was perhaps a convenient way of avoiding the need to describe and scientifically define what constitutes, if not causes, the absurdly wide variety of specific mental disorders listed in the DSM.

As for sins, if a rose is a rose no matter what you call it, the widespread moral and behavioral transgressions of sins are still with us by any other name. In Chapter 8: Crime, Exculpatory Insanity, and the M'Naghten Rules, I have described some of the legal attempts to distinguish blameworthy crimes from conditions of mental illness referred to as "exculpatory insanity" in criminal courts, and which are argued about by legal scholars. Insanity is not a psychiatric term and does not appear in the APA's list of mental disorders.

Chapter 31
Faith in Life Somewhere

SEVENTY OR MORE years ago, William Saroyan in his 1934 short story, "Daring Young Man on the Flying Trapeze," reminded readers that as much as death is inevitable, so too is life inevitable. Scientists today tends to agree. Science tell us that there are billions of galaxies out there in the expanding universe, many with suns and planets of their own. Given the many potentially life-supporting habitats out there, the sheer mathematical probability is that, although we may be unique, we are not alone. And so serious efforts are being made to send signals out into the furthest reaches of the universe. These signals travel in terms of light years. Each light year represents the enormous distance light travels in a year, at the rate of 186,000 miles per second. We are talking of many hundreds and thousands of light years before our signals reach even the closest galaxies that might hold life out there, and reply. That is, if they understand our signals, if we are on the same wavelength, as they say. Then, an equal amount of time would be required for their answer to reach our planet.

A very, complex, major, and serious scientific effort is being made to communicate with whatever might be out there. Many scientists are convinced that it is mathematically likely, if not certain, that we are not alone. Now some of our parents, grandparents, and great-grandparents would probably smile at all this effort to prove what they already knew to be true in their hearts. They had been sending special signals each day and especially on their Sabbaths or Sundays. They called their signals "prayers," and in many cases, were convinced that they actually had received answers. These new scientific endeavors and old human habits are worth pondering, especially as we get older, and closer to our own mortal destination on the long train ride we have shared with our cohort in each of our lifetimes. If old age is not to be lived in fear, then each of us must find inner peace for ourselves.

Consider also mankind's "brave-new-world" efforts within our current lifetime to travel to the moon and back, and to live in scientific space stations gathering data for months on end as other scientists pursue their mathematical faith in the "statistical certainty" that there is intelligent life somewhere out there in the cosmos. Although based on a persistent faith in prayer, the old-world's quest to communicate with whatever Lord, life creator, holy force, or heavenly spirit, however named, was out there. The quest to communicate from our lonely planet was the same. The methods and faiths are markedly different, but perhaps equally brave and essential. If once told that our future world scientists had accomplished actual communication, the ancients might have regarded that as little more than the rediscovery of their own familiar prayer-wheels through which they communicated with the spirits or inhabitants of their own distant heavens. According to the gospel truth of biblical accounts, human communications with God were two-way. Abraham, Moses and others received actual replies which are labeled as miracles. So much for our new radio-astronomy, our ancestors might think. Are there no more miracles? Or is life itself an ongoing miracle recreated daily?

How and When Did Cellular Life Begin on Planet Earth?

We do not know how or when the "miracle" of cellular life on Earth first occurred. There are various scientific hypotheses, including the possibility that cellular life may have landed here on a comet or other vehicle from outer space. All we know now is that all cells come from cells. A recent fascinating theory, however, is that the first cells might have emerged from a primordial ooze or soup, according to the work of Dr. Jeremy England, a physicist at the Massachusetts Institute of Technology (MIT). Dr. England has proposed the provocative idea that the laws of thermodynamics support the concept that matter acquired life-like physical properties in a primordial soup of the Earth's chemicals when sufficiently warmed by the heat of the sun—if I understand Dr. England's theory. Now, actuarially close to the end of my lifetime, there is still so much more to be learned about the basic details of individual cellular function, not to mention the mind-boggling mystery, meaning, or ultimate purpose of our sentient human lives.

The Miracle of Mortal Life: My Creation Theory

What do we know, if anything, about the meaning and mysteries of mortal life? I specify mortal life because that is the only kind of life we find on Earth. Every living thing born here, from tiny bacteria and blades of grass to the largest species of whales and giant redwoods, eventually dies here. Mortal life is the only life that a sane person can encounter and study scientifically on this planet where all living things die in their season or time, if not sooner—and even rocks crumble. I have maintained in prior pages that the concept of immortality is a human invention and a prime example of our capacity for wishful thinking. I believe that the idea and wish for immortality is but another product of the fertile and imaginative minds of our unique species, which has accomplished such amazing technological achievements within our recent lifetimes.

What could be the purpose of such mortal life where each of us comes and goes in our time, and when creatures experience such different lives and fates? What, for example, did Galileo's scientific struggle for justice and truth have to do with poets like Shakespeare, Longfellow, and others who engrave mighty truths with their pens?

Our Purpose is to Create

In the 1910 operetta *Naughty Marietta*, Victor Herbert and Rida Johnson Young featured the song "Ah, Sweet Mystery of Life." This song was one of my mother's favorites when I was a little boy. When I was four or five, she was always singing and humming it. The lyrics by Rida Johnson Young went, "Ah, sweet mystery of life, at last I found thee…for 'tis love and love alone the world is seeking."

I'm all for love, but I think that love is not enough. Both Shakespeare and Galileo taught me that in addition to the biologic purpose of procreation, the meaning and purpose of mortal human life is to create through the sentient arts and sciences of our species. I believe that the purpose of life is to create because our species is uniquely endowed with the most creative ability of any that we know on this Earth. Loving one's fellow worker (man or womankind) is creative too, if only by enhancing and supporting the honest efforts of others. Hating, harming, or humiliating one's fellow man is the destructive opposite of human creativity.

I truly believe that, driven by the human awareness of our mortality, that life's purpose is to create and wait. That's all we can do, and it might just be what our developing species was put on this Earth to do.

Postscript
The Train Ride

WHAT'S LIFE ALL about? I don't know, but it seems to me like we have been on a long, long train ride. Among all the other biological life forms and species that are traveling along with us, we humans are probably the only ones who sense that we may be, and have been from time immemorial, on an endless trip that none of us began, and that none of us will complete. Almost all the passengers are in enclosed cars or sections without windows. Their entire universe is what they see. Some spend their entire ride unknowing that there is more outside their limited view than those with better seats and opportunities. No matter how unenlightened, illiterate, economically or culturally impoverished these human passengers are, each is capable of a uniquely human viewpoint on life, because of our species' capacity to dwell on the stimuli, thoughts, and experiences that stir the mind of even the most deprived person. You have not lived a dog's life, nor a dolphin's, but a human one. It is mainly the most fortunate humans who travel in cars with windows and have a chance to view the larger world going by.

Humans who never get beyond their little village or neighborhood, and all the rest of life's species, have little or no idea of what lies beyond the confines of their own train car, large as it might seem to them. Perhaps some species of migratory birds, soaring far and high, or even some fish, turtles, or other aquatic forms whose destiny takes them over huge distances to spawn, might share to some extent the human appreciation of the world outside our train. A romantic thought, but an unlikely one.

What is uniquely human on life's enormously long train ride is the realization that passengers are always getting off, and new ones are getting on. As much as we like not to think about it individually, it is only the human species that is aware and in awe of its mortality. That, too, is an increasing preoccupation of old age. It is only a matter of time before we get to our station. We know it cannot be much further, and is likely to be coming up soon. We usually do not know exactly how or when we will be getting off, except for some of us with a terminal illness of weeks or months, for whom their local conductor who usually is wearing a white coat, announces our own stop as the next on. You can try to fight it, and probably should, because, as they say, while there still is life, there may yet be hope. If it is really your stop, it is time to leave your baggage, say goodbye to friends and loved ones, and calmly prepare to step off lightly, and maybe see if there is anything, after all, at that last stop.

Regarding the Knocks and Boosts of Death

But hold on. While the train is still moving and we are still breathing, what about our last big knock and its potential boosts? How do you feel about stepping off the train? Are there any "boosts" or good things to be said about the feared knock of death?

I've talked about death in prior pages and expressed my feeling that it is death itself that places a great value on each day of our lives. In the face of our mortality, our individual days are limited, and therefore, as valuable as rare gems, if not much more. That concept should stimulate an attitude of gratitude, rather than sadness, anger, disappointment, or regret at the prospect of dying. Do you think you've lived a dog's life? What do you really know of a dog's life? You've lived a human life, and no matter how short or long you have been on this Earth, you've experienced the blessings of life like no dog, or any other lifeform but ours can. No other life compares with the unique sample of human existence that you've experienced. That realization can be a major boost to appreciating the gifts of life you have received.

Death presents us with yet another boost. It is the gift of Nature's justice, which at the end, makes us all equal no matter how much power or importance or wealth a person may have gained in life. At the end, kings and their subjects, conquerors and the conquered, murderers and victims, all share the same fate. In our recent time, Hitler himself, having tasted power in his Third Reich like few before him had experienced, gnashed his teeth in defeat, blamed his people for lack of motivation and bravery, and shot himself. That was because Hitler himself, having lost the war, lacked the classic warrior's essential courage to face the humiliation of a trial and death sentence. That Hitler's suicide rendered him as dead as his millions of victims seems like an injustice in his case. By way of contrast, the far loftier and royal pharaohs did not commit suicide. They made and carried out far more grandiose plans in their golden and biblical age of slavery only a few thousand years ago.

Nature merely shrugged as their looted and emptied pyramids turned into tourist traps, and their grotesquely preserved bodies were openly displayed, dishonored, and dissected as curious museum pieces and delayed autopsy objects. Death was always the great leveler of all mortals, no matter what they believed. Is that equal treatment in the face of life's inevitable injustices an undeniable boost?

The final boost of death, I think, is that it offers an end to our frustrations, pains, and fears, as well as the possibility, no matter how remote, of some kind of "afterlife." Regardless of what form our longings and hopes may take in the spiritual realm, at the very least, we may look forward to being recycled as a few chemicals of this precious Earth to which we were born.

With best wishes, good luck, and blessings to us all,

Mel Heller, MD

Haverford, PA

mheller1@comcast.net

A Family Album of Boosts
Following Numerous Knocks

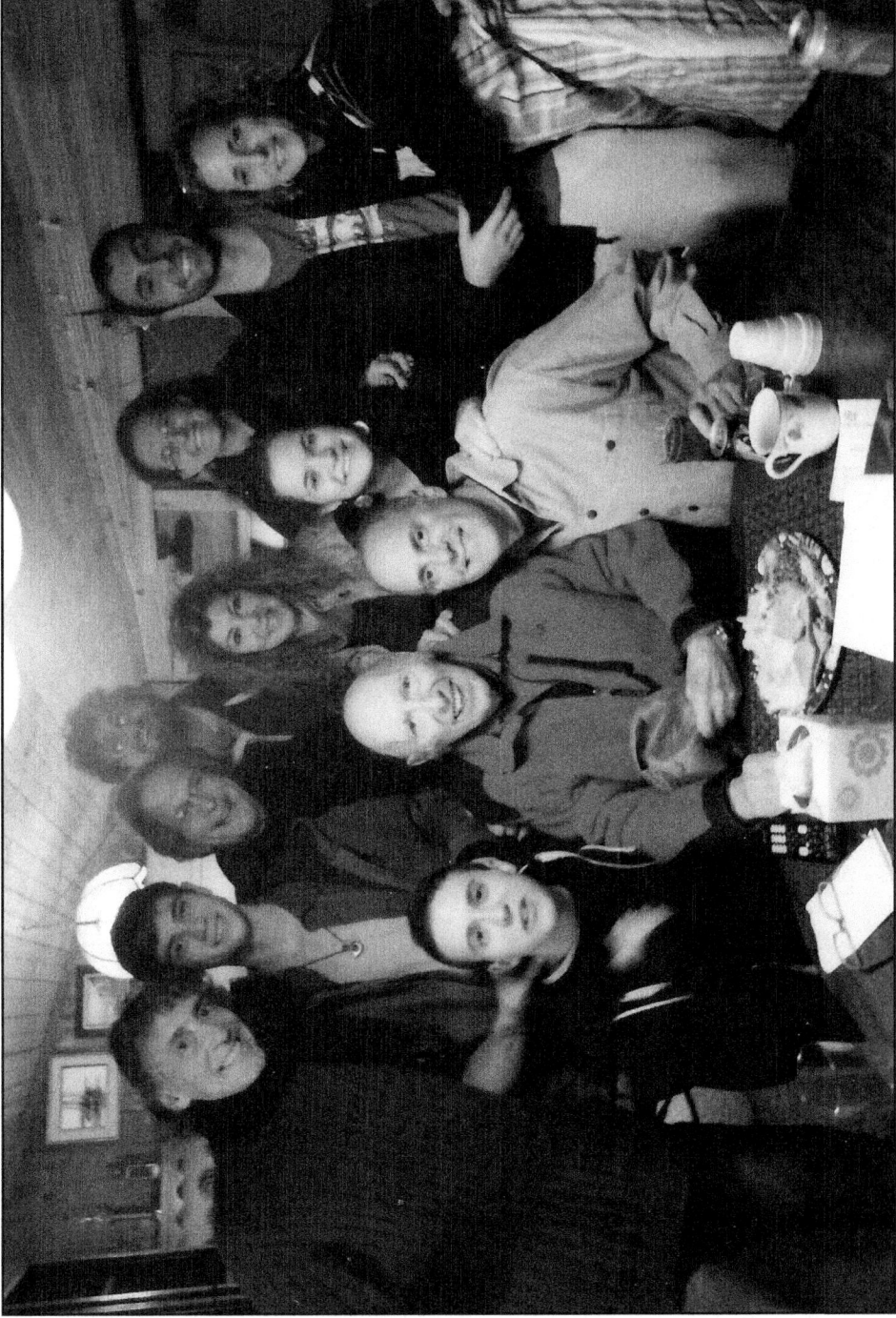

Happy Author and his grown children, their spouses, and his grandchildren assembled at Elk River home (2014).

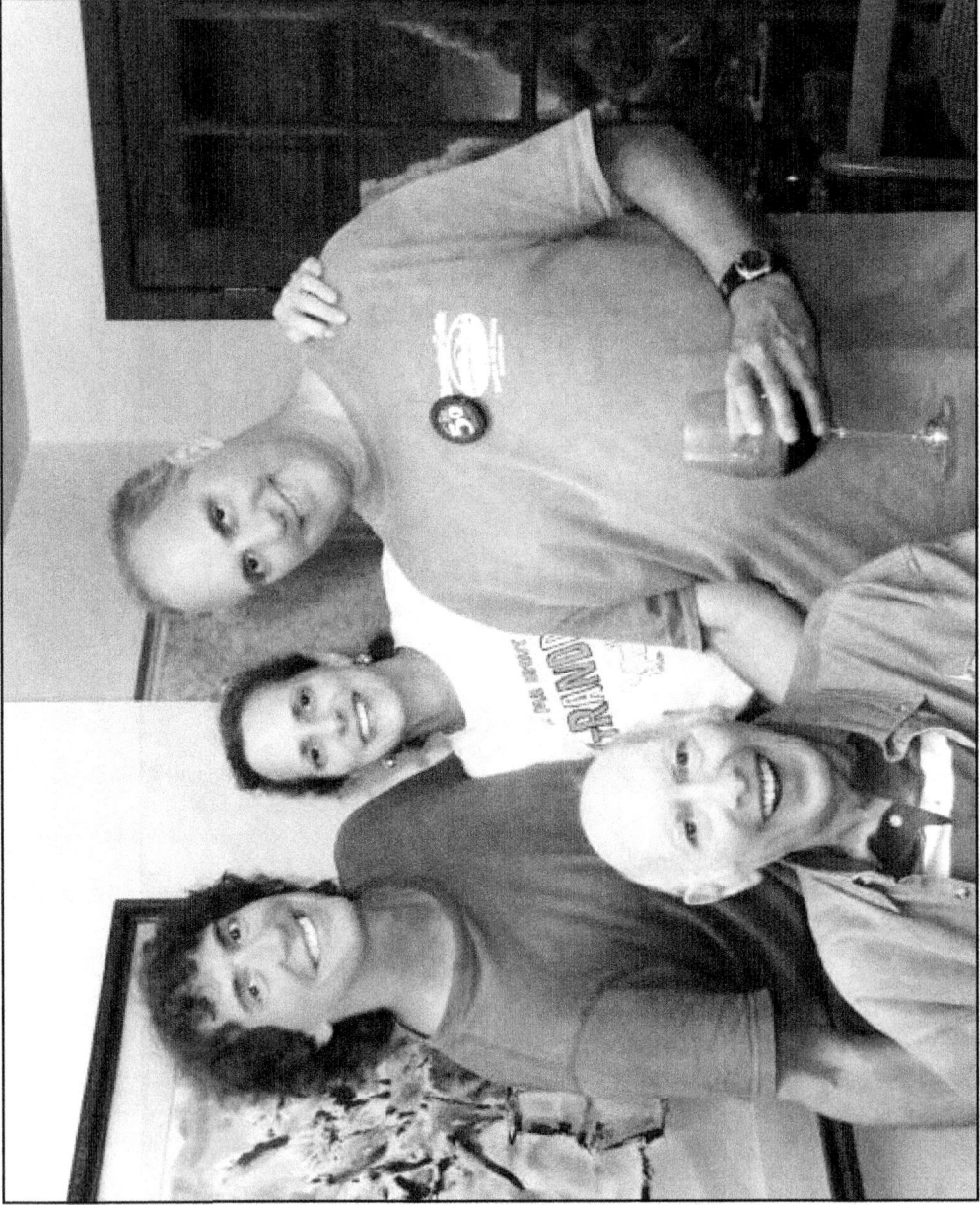

Author's first dividends, David, Joan, and Paul.

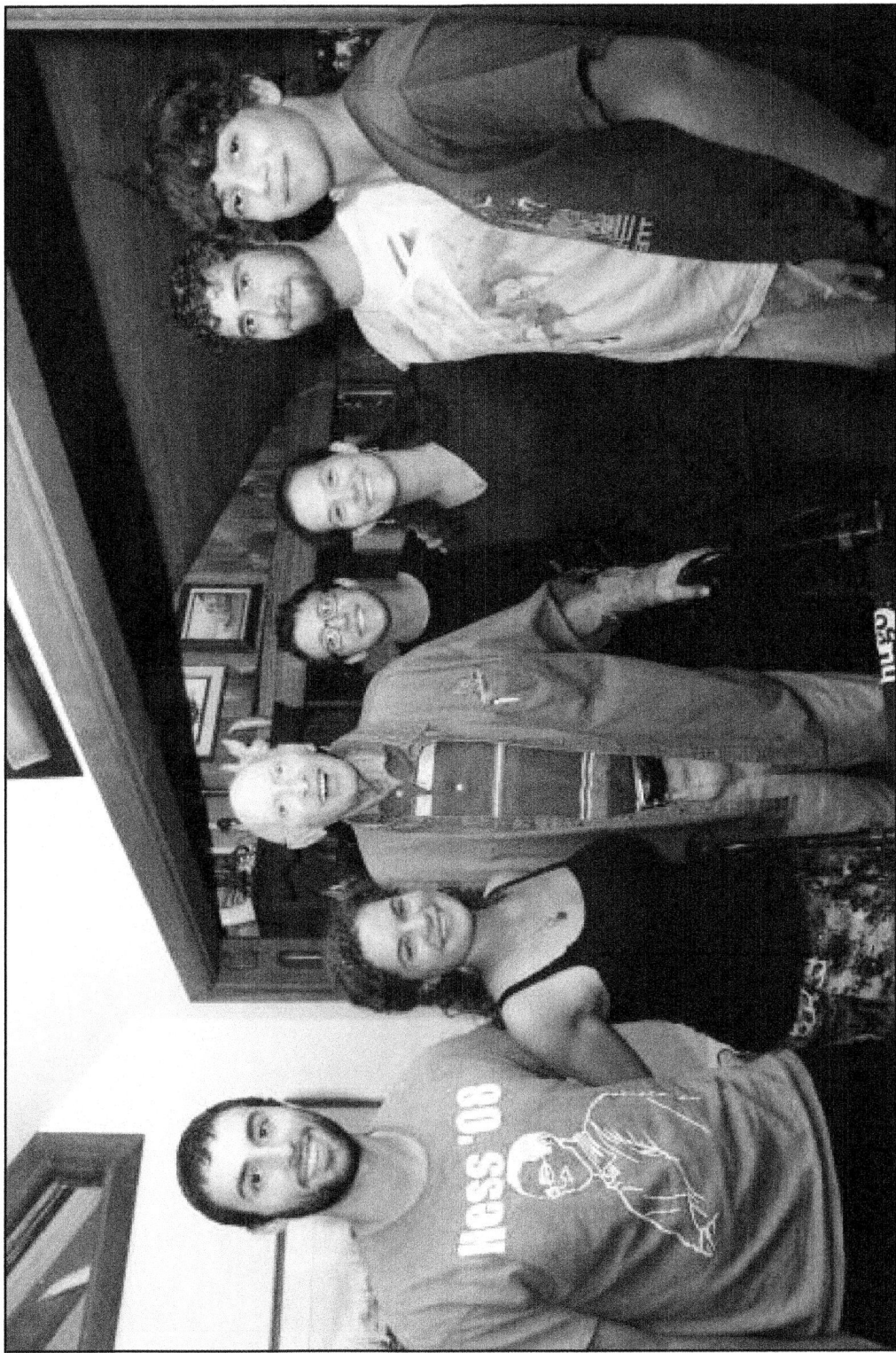

Author's secondary dividends, his prized grandchildren.

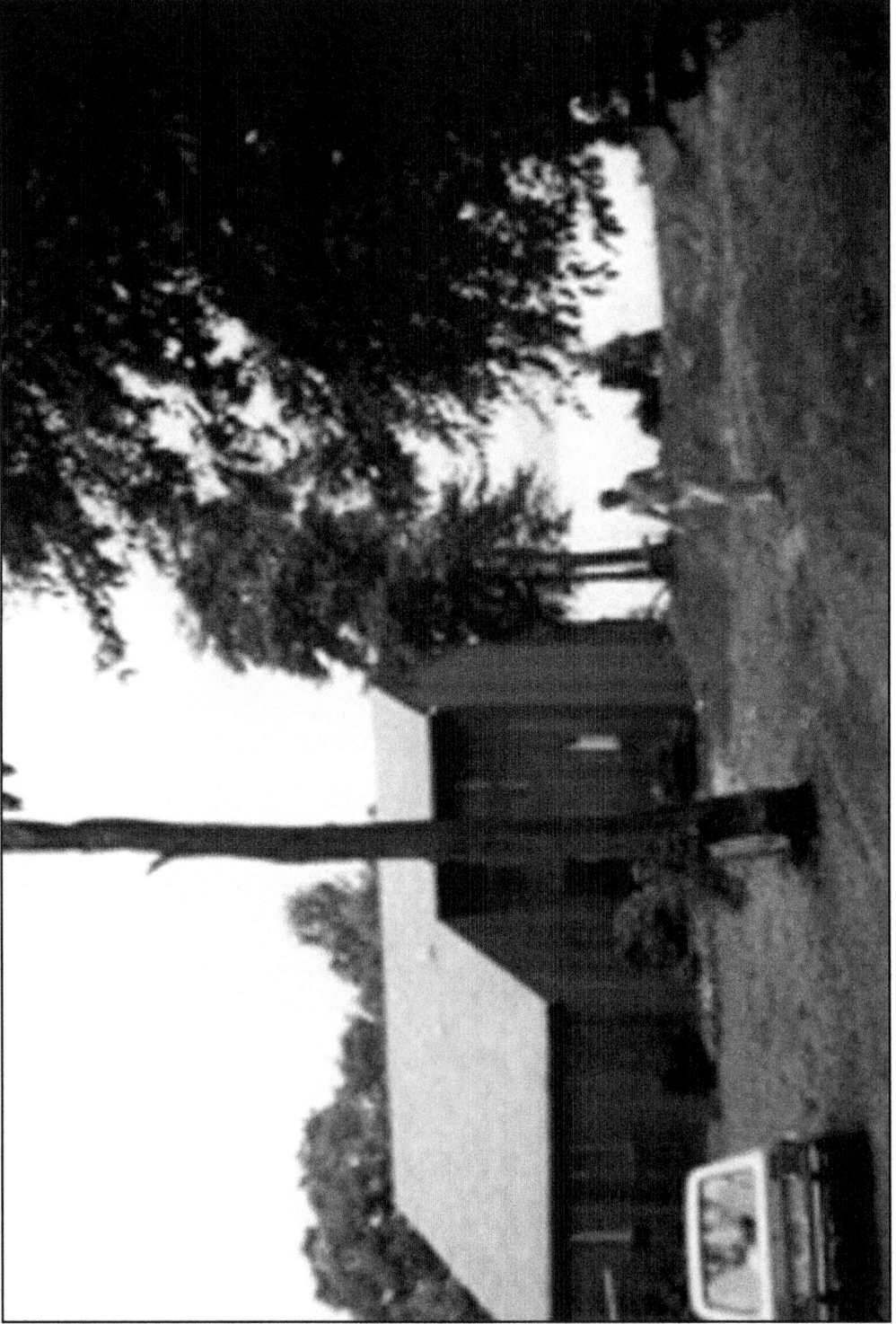

Author's Chesapeake Shore home purchased as a modest A-frame house in 1975.

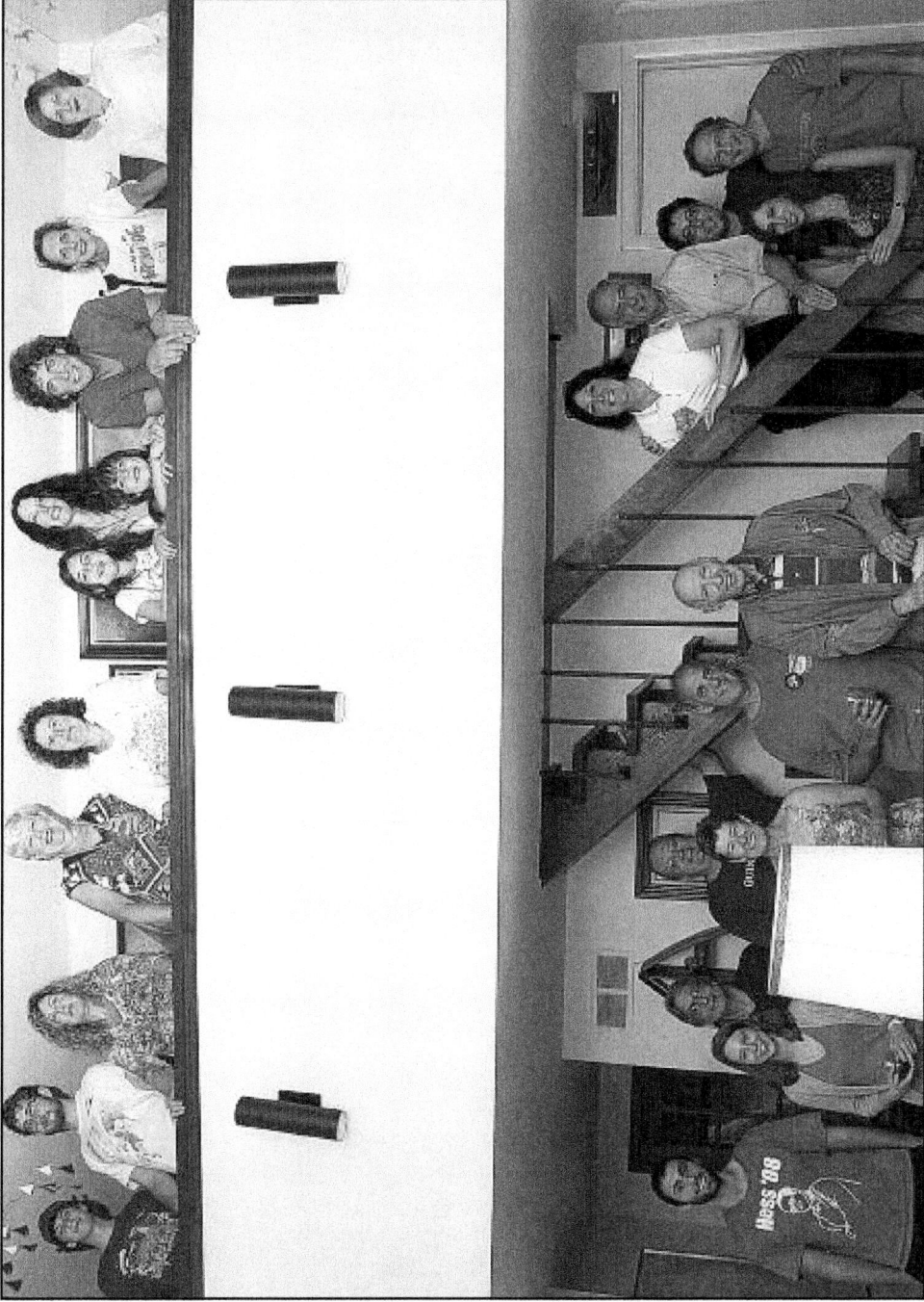

The Elk River home was originally an A-frame with a huge two story living room. We retained that and its balcony to accommodate a multitude of family and friends to celebrate our August birthdays.

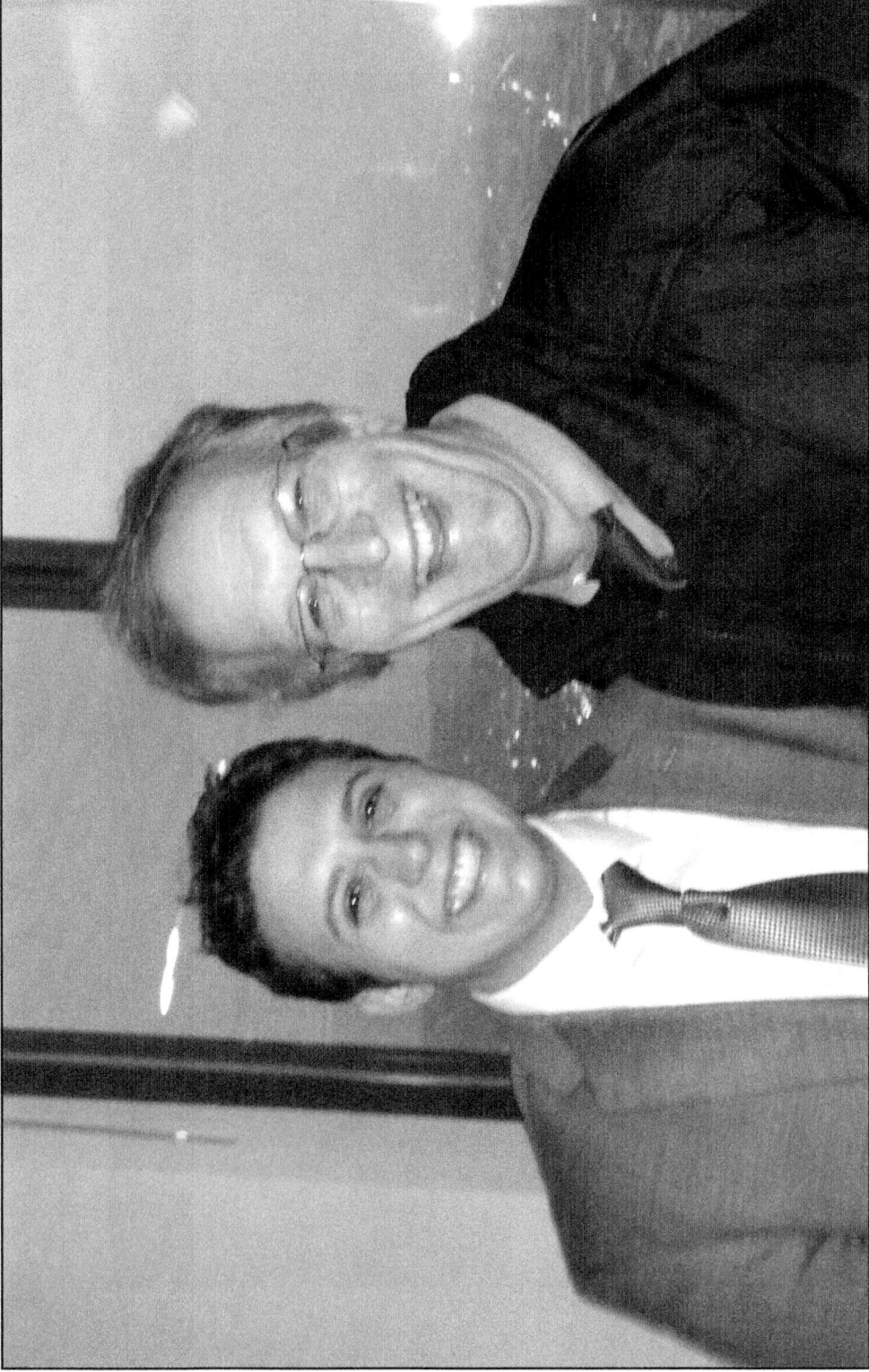

Jeremy and his dad, Dr. Ken Miller, on receiving news of Jeremy's admission to John Hopkins Medical School.

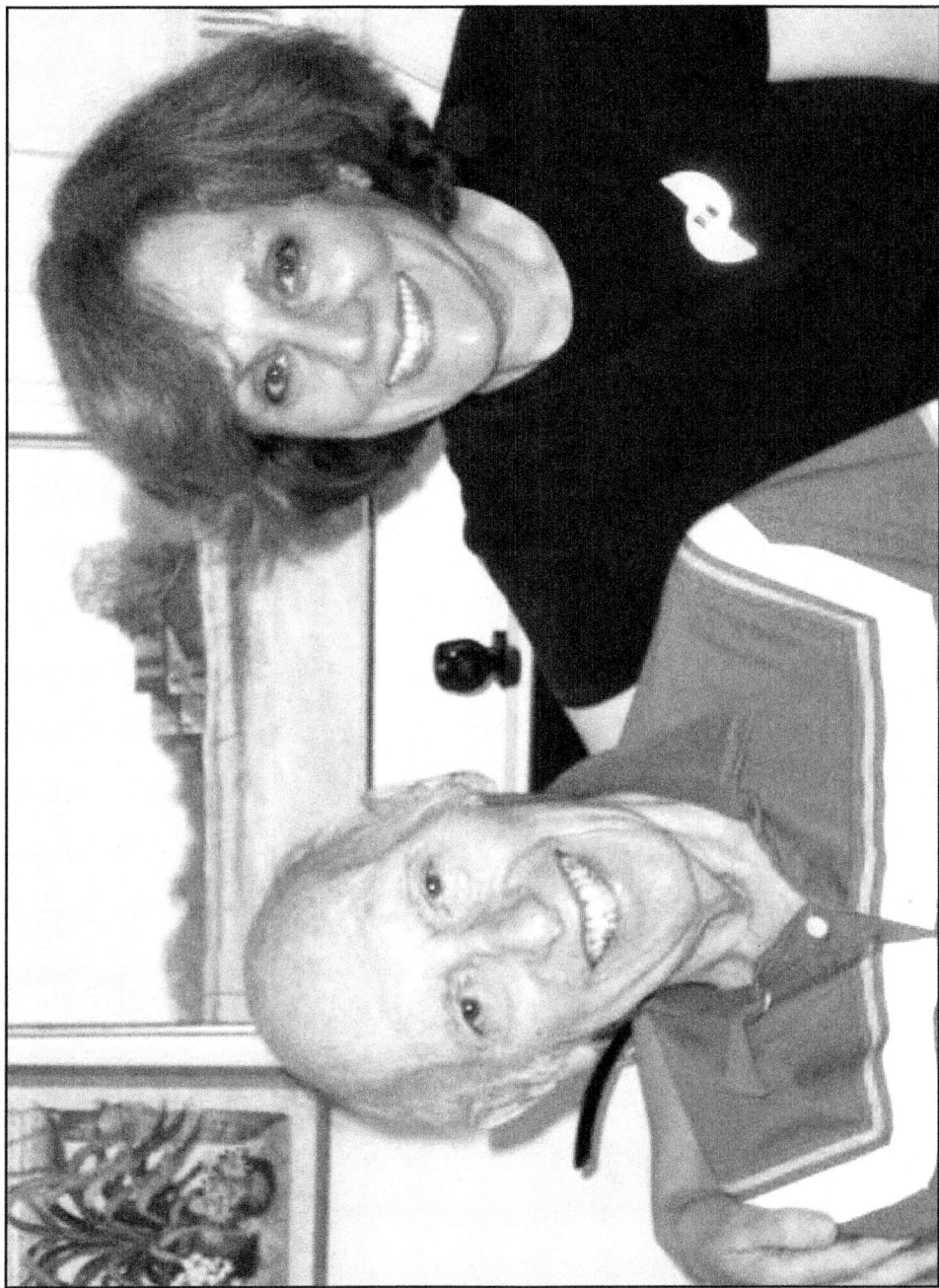

Author and brother Saul's daughter, Karen Heller PhD, who wrote the preface for *Book One of Every Knock is a Boost: The Developmental Years.*

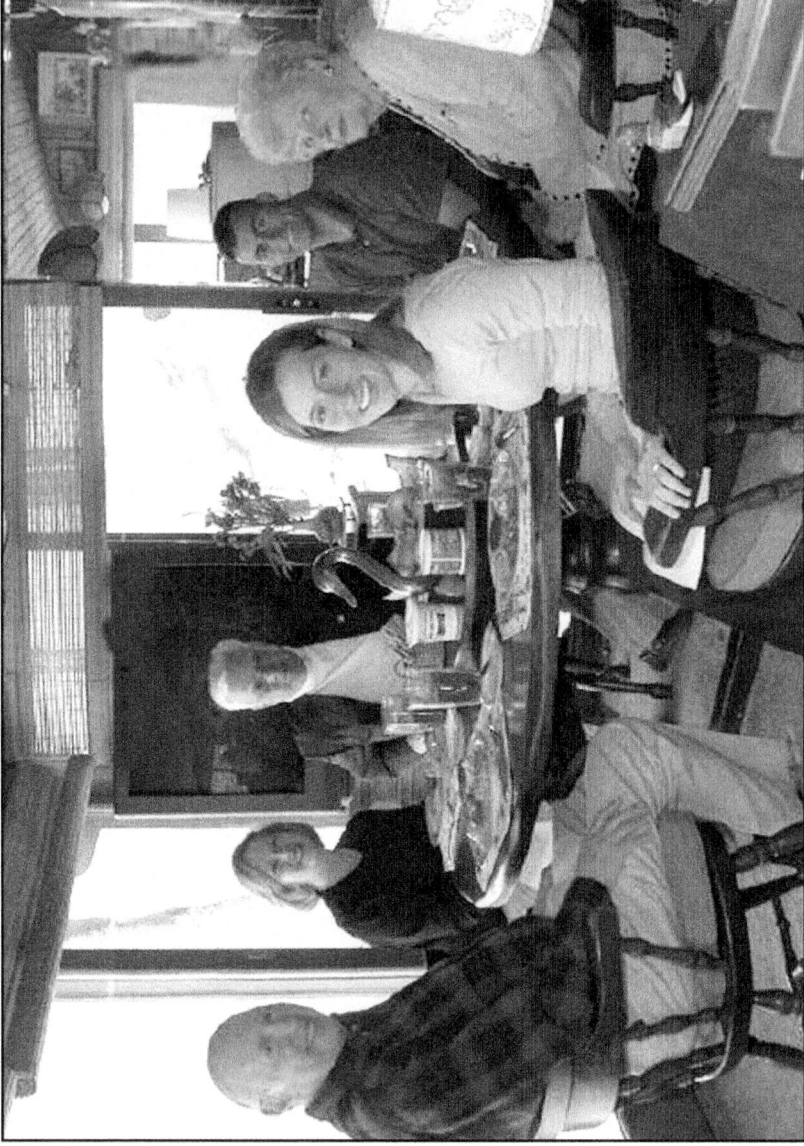

The Author and Irmgard so enjoyed melding each other's children, grandchildren, and best friends. From left to right: Author, Karen Murray PhD, US Department of Agriculture, Chief Learning Officer, Tom R. Murray, USN (Ret.), USNA '61 nuclear submarine commanding officer, Major Anthony Giardino, USMC, Irmgard, and Elizabeth Rees Giardino, in our river room overlooking the Elk River (2005).

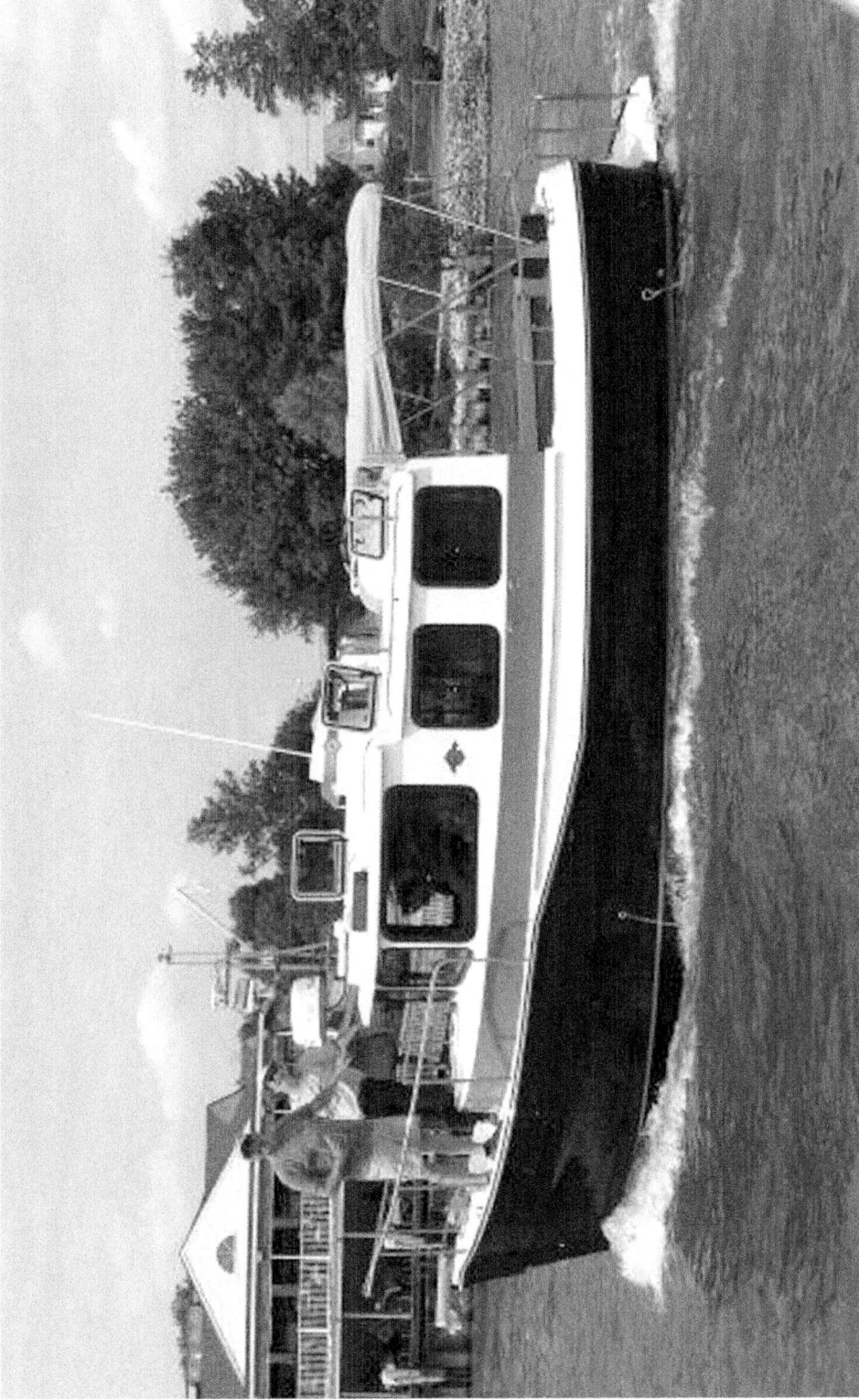

Grateful for all our dividends and Paul's 54th birthday present to himself, a brand new trawler which he named **Grateful.**

Appendix
Selected Publications

SOME STUDIES WE published some seventy-five years ago are still pertinent and valid. Here are a few from our early Temple studies in Forensic Psychiatry and Dr. Sam Polsky's and my consultation work with ABC-TV.

Forensic Psychiatry

Heller, M. S. and Polsky S. "Insanity Procedures Under Federal Law." [Report of Study of Insanity Procedures Under Federal Law", NIMH, Research Grant #OM366, 1958. (report completed 1963).Temple University Research Studies in Law and Medicine, 1965. Temple University Law School Library, Philadelphia.

Heller, M.S., and Sadoff, R.L., "Experiences with a University Affiliated Psychiatric Service in a Correctional Institution", Corrective Psychiatry and the Journal of Social Therapy, Oct.1965

Heller, M.S., Sadoff, R.L. & Polsky, S., "The Forensic Psychiatry Clinic: Model for a New Approach", American Journal of Psychiatry, 123,11:1402-1407: May, 1967.

Heller, M.S., Sadoff, R.L. & Polsky, S., "Developing Clinical Facilities in Forensic Psychiatry," American Journal of Psychiatry, 124,11:1562-1568: May, 1968 (Read at 123rd Annual Meeting of the American Psychiatric Assoc., Detroit, Mich., May 8-12, 1967.

Heller, M.S., Guy, E.B. & Polsky, S., "Disposition of the Mentally Ill Offender", The Prison Journal, 49,1:24-33: Spring-Summer, 1969.

Heller, M.S., "Prospects for the Psychiatric Prediction of Dangerousness" Presented at the Annual Meeting of the American Academy of Psychiatry and Law, Oct. 25-28, 1979.

Heller, M.S., Traylor, W.H., Ehrlich, S.M. & Lester, D. "Intelligence, Psychosis and Competency to Stand Trial". Bulletin of the American Academy of Psychiatry and Law, Vol. 9,4: 1981.

Heller, M.S. & Ehrlich, S.M., "Actuarial Variables in 9,600 Violent and Non-Violent Offenders Referred to a Court Psychiatric Clinic". Paper presented at American Psychiatric Assoc. Annual Meeting, May 1983. American Journal of Social Psychology, 4,3:Summer, 1984.

Heller, M.S., Traylor, W.H., Ehrlich, S.M. & Lester, D. "A Clinical Evaluation of Maximum Security Hospital Patients by Staff and Independent Psychiatric Consultants", Bulletin of American Academy of Psychiatry and Law 121,1:1984.

Heller, M.S., Ehrlich, S.M. & Lester, D., "Suicidal History of Defendants and Offenders", Journal of General Psychology 112,2:221-223:1985.

Heller, M.S., Ehrlich, S.M. & Lester, D. "A Consultant's Survey of Patients at a Maximum Security Hospital." Journal of Forensic Sciences, 31,4:1429-1434: Oct. 1986.

Long Ago Selected Publications: TV Broadcast Standards

Heller, M.S. & Polsky, S., "Television Violence" Archives of General Psychiatry", 24. 27-286: March, 1971.

Heller, M.S. & Polsky, S., "Studies in Violence and Television", American Broadcasting Company Report, New York, 1972.

Heller, M.S. & Polsky, S., "Children's Responses in Television Viewing, American Broadcasting Company Report", New York, 1974.

Heller, M.S. & Polsky S., "Behavioral Aggression and Television Viewing in Children: Psychological, Developmental and Clinical Factors", American Broadcasting Company, New York, 1975.

Heller, M.S., *Broadcast Standards Editing*, American Broadcasting Company, New York, 1978.

Heller, M.S., "Television, Sexuality and Broadcast Standards," Monograph: American Broadcasting Co. Inc, New York, 1978.

Contemporary Publications

Every Knock Is a Boost: Book One, The Developmental Years – Memoirs of a 20th Century Psychoanalyst. Outskirts Press. Denver, Colorado. 2015.

CPSIA information can be obtained at www.ICGtesting.com
Printed in the USA
BVOW11s0441160116

432920BV00001B/1/P